Dark C Gather

Katy Sara Culling

Katy Sara Culling

Published by:
Chipmunkapublishing Ltd
PO Box 6872

Essex
CM13 1ZT
United Kingdom

COVER PHOTOGRAPH REPRODUCED COURTESY OF ERIC

SMESTAD.

For Clare, Maggie, Lisa, Carol, Neil and Alan.

And my heart: for all those I have loved and lost to
these terrible afflictions.

Katy Sara Culling

Foreword.

If five years ago someone had told me I would be writing a foreword to a book by Katy Sara Culling I would not have believed it. From the moment I met her on the first day of a new post as a consultant psychiatrist in Oxford and for the next two years as one of my patients she was a constant and major source of concern and stress.

Being responsible for her care as a patient in the inpatient unit in Oxford was highly challenging for the whole team looking after her as she struggled with severe and life-threatening bipolar disorder, coming literally to the point of death on several occasions. I would say that in 20 years in psychiatry she is one of the five individuals who has most challenged me as a clinician, whose management most stressed and divided the clinical team looking after her. Things were not made any easier by her problems with anorexia nervosa.

Five years later, her enduring recovery is a story of hope for all those in the midst of mental illness, a lesson to those who care for them about not giving into despair, retaining hope, and having persistence in treating bipolar disorder even in its most challenging and extreme manifestations.

Getting from near death to publication of this book is a story worth telling and a story worth reading.

Dr. Alan Ogilvie
Medical Director, Equilibrium - The Bipolar Foundation, Honorary Consultant Psychiatrist, Oxford, UK.

Katy Sara Culling

Prologue: Letter to a friend…
Derby, 6th August 2004.

Dearest Clare,

I was thinking about what you said yesterday: "Thanks for being so positive Katy." As is usual for me, sometimes I pick up on things and think about them. Twiddling my toes and stretching in bed this morning, not really wanting to get up and face the world, I got to thinking about it for no particular reason. I tried to decide if I was an optimist or pessimist, now 29 with a lot of experience, and in my past with over 20 years of illness.

I think the answer is neither.

Without any optimism whatsoever, I used to be so excitable, blinded, magnanimous and *idealistic*. Pre age 26, even when depressed, suicide was romantic, anorexia beautiful, and becoming a doctor my panacea.

Now I am *pragmatic*. But without being particularly realistic, and at no time fulfilling the definition of being "level-headed." I am a pensive, reasoned sceptic. It can be perfectly pragmatic to expect the worst when that is what keeps happening to you. Transferring between idealism and pragmatism happened by effectively dying for four years when living in the wonderful city of Oxford: sinking to unfathomable depths, (and reaching heights) beyond those I had already reached.

In the depths of mixed psychotic manic depression, something kept me alive, and I can only assume it was *hope*: buried deep in my unconscious mind. Hidden optimism, apparent pessimism at an obviously dreadful situation. Such horrific mixed depression, the pain of which would make anyone want to dive freely into the abyss. *Sadness, fear and ANGER were (are) the emotions that filled my life.*

Now there is no equivocation, no bullshit, with all the risks, memories, illnesses, possibilities and consequences. Death has always seemed rational and appealing; far too often, it still does. Nothing about how I weigh up life and its gifts or blows has changed. I'm a nihilistic existentialist who appears unbreakable, but who (in contradiction) cares for people and is actually very sensitive. I will always be a manic depressive. All possibilities are considered (or more precisely, over-considered). The best possibilities are hoped for, the worst prepared for, but that is all. My life is merely an exercise in damage limitation, trying to be worthwhile & leaving a legacy. *Avoiding the emptiness that, in all honesty, is still with me every second.*

Am I to tread water all my life, occasionally going under… eventually going down too soon?

I am *so* scared of becoming ill again, but that is my expectation. And this is my sort of thinking on a "good" day. I am still *holding on.* I hope that if I hold on long enough, I will find some peace, a life: for a while at least. People prefer to think I am "fine now," than contemplate that my struggles continue. True: I am much better. Forgive me, I needed a friend's ear, and I return to yours yet again, as you understand in the way only someone who has been there can do.

Katy Sara x

JUST AN ORDINARY GIRL, WITH AN EXTRAORDINARY TRUE STORY.

"You ever-gentle gods, take my breath
from me;
Let not my worser spirit tempt me again
To die before you please."

❧ William Shakespeare. (1564-1616).
King Lear (Gloucester, Act IV, scene vi)

Katy Sara Culling

Introduction - In the beginning: *I do not hang my head in shame.*

> "The body is a house of many windows:
> there we all sit,
> showing ourselves and crying to passers-
> by to come and love us."

> ❧ Robert Louis Stevenson, Scotsman,
> writer, (1850-1894).

So how is it that a "nobody" who is only in the twilight of her twenties decides to write her autobiography? Should she copy Tarantino in a Kill Bill-esque style and call it Volume 1? She is just a girl who was born to a humble family in Liverpool, England and brought up in rural Derbyshire. An inquisitive and humanistic child who was always fascinated by other human beings; a girl who aspired to study medicine to help others, and made it in to the eminent University of Oxford in the City of Dreaming Spires to do just that. An unpretentious girl, somehow surviving all along with undiagnosed manic depression. Yes, she had a very dark side.

Maybe these events were actually far from easy or smooth, and she feels, (knowing she is in no way alone), that she has already had more than her lifetime's worth of pain. Maybe she can't shake the feeling that she better write this now because she fears that her life may still be cut short by her own hand. No Volume 2!

Is she driven by a powerful desire to help? Has she had enough of societal stigmatisation as a result of misunderstanding and fear? Maybe she has beaten all the odds and survived almost appalling depths of illness, and wants to inspire, teach, warn and advise people, and prove to them that they can survive, and even better than that, flourish too.

I wrote this predominantly because it is the book I needed to read when I was ill, and I know there are many similarly struggling people. It's a *brutally* honest real-life story – no frilly edges, with facts that cannot be ignored, however much we would like to.

This book is a conversation, or rather a soliloquy directed to you as my friend. I feel I need to warn people in advance that I am a direct person. I am blunt. Unequivocal. Some parts of this book might cover topics highly sensitive to you, especially those of you who have lost someone you love. I try to be sensitive; indeed I am very sensitive in my heart. However, experience has enabled me to talk too freely about issues such as suicide, particularly my own suicide attempts and self-harm, whilst anyone else's suffering pierces me to the core, time and time again.

If you recognise that you need to help yourself, or someone close to you is suffering, personally or professionally, you will find great help in educating yourself. Such edification and possibly inspiration, without false claims, I aim to give here. A lot can be learnt by simply *not* doing as I did! I aim to teach you to spot the warning signs, learn ways you might help, and learn ways you will not help, either yourself or someone else. Being honest, my book cannot provide the "easy," textbook, correct answers that you would like, or miraculously cure the ill, because every person is individual and there are no easy answers.

When considering the amount of explicit content, I sought advice, which came back very mixed. Thus, *I chose to write the book I would have liked to read when*

I was ill – blood and guts included. I censor little – just the small fact here and there that could do harm, especially where that information might be directly harmful to the general public (but watch out if you are a doctor/ nurse/ vet/ pharmacist/ or drug user). I have included some dangerous information that is already well known: but you will find many candid warnings. I am concerned about the bulimic looking for tips about purging, anorectics looking for tips about not eating, and the suicidal person looking for tips on how to exit this world. I must caution you that you may find the subject matter "triggering." There are no pictures that might trigger. This book is explicit and at times disturbing, but it is never gratuitous; rather it is the whole <u>truth</u> of my experiences, *<u>which are horrific</u>*.

It is my hope that this book will not be used for self-destructive purposes – I realise that some people will want to use it for just that. It would have been easy to provide more details in some inane attempt to prove to you how dedicatedly I sought death: instead I choose restraint. If you look elsewhere, (please don't), there are ways to find step-by-step instructions on how to kill yourself, and websites (please avoid) encouraging and teaching anorexic and bulimic behaviour. There are many helpful pro-recovery books, organisations and websites given at the back of this book.

There are many distressing psychiatric conditions. I will be focusing mainly on what I know best, which is depression (of several types, obviously including bipolar disorder), various addictions complicating other illnesses, eating disorders (mainly anorexia and bulimia), suicide, attempted suicide, and self-harm: though not entirely these topics exclusively. I will share real life stories from people whom all suffer, suffered or recovered in different ways: all of whom agree that sharing is the good and right thing to do. Some things that worked for them did not work for me, but they may help you.

According to the World Health Organization, 450 million people worldwide suffer with serious mental health, neurological or behavioural problems. These people suffer just as much as any other physical illness can cause them too, plus they feel additional guilt, shame and worthlessness. The severity varies from person to person of course, but any suffering requires attention and, if possible, a remedy. Understanding and reassurance is required, and in my experience there are health professionals and organisations you must approach, who are ready and want to help.

One in four people are suffering from a diagnosable mental illness in a given year. The joke goes: "Look at your three closest friends, and if they seem OK, it must be *you*." Obviously there is a spectrum of cases from extremely serious to less serious, but all these individuals suffer and take on undeserved shame. Stigma is invariably attached.

At least 1 in 10 (10%) and maybe as many as 1 in 5 (20% of) people experience a form of depression within their lifetime, and up to 15% of these commit suicide. The prevalence of bipolar disorder (manic depressive illness) is now estimated to be as high as 5%. Bipolar disorder probably affects up to 2.4 million people in the UK, 12 million in the US and 254 million worldwide.[1] The World Health Organization has identified bipolar disorder as one of the top causes of lost years of life

---

[1] Equilibrium – The Bipolar Foundation; http://www.bipolar-foundation.org/

and health in 15-44 year olds, ranking above war, violence and schizophrenia.

It's not just about appearing really sad or strangely happy: Mood disorders can manifest themselves biologically and/or emotionally, and/or intellectually and/or behaviourally, in an infinite combination of symptoms and complex presentations. For those unfortunate enough to experience any form of depression, it is most certainly true that its terrors are unique, just as every single human being is inimitable. For some it is an illness that passes; for many it is always a part of their lives. Depression, manic depression and their horrors have consumed my life and are my own personal nemeses. For some people life is about love, family and/or work. But I walk a darker, more unbalanced path than you could possibly imagine: and still, I smile.

How it actually feels: [Removing all symptoms that were eating disorder related, whilst free of drugs and alcohol, not even caffeine, many of these as young as age 5]. I would feel very low in mood; think of death, suicide, hate myself, feel worthless, feel hopeless, be unable to sleep, feel like I had wasted my life, see no future, enjoy nothing, feel really tired, self-harm brutally, seriously attempt suicide... and yet at the same time have private, angry, arrogant, irritable, expansive, racing thoughts (*constantly and distressingly so*). I would consider one topic, or more usually several, and dissect each one from every angle, down to the smallest of minutiae, then start all over again. I'd find boundless energy from somewhere, feel I had to put on a brave face, and be forcibly talkative, bubbly/chatty/active/laughing/joking. At times I thought I was the only person existing, (everyone else was in my imagination). I would be <u>certain</u> that I was right and the world was wrong – *nobody* knew better than me. Other times I felt unreal; or worse, invisible. Often I felt... *too conscious*. Although not sleeping distressed me, I actually needed very little. I focussed on exams, then towards my degree, then my Ph.D., and then later, I worked hard to find ways to harm and kill myself. I could not maintain a social life; I had no personal relationships – not even many friendships. I would *severely* over-spend, be *severely* reckless, sometimes I could concentrate, but usually I had to do many things all at once to keep busy: which was my form of self-medication for an unpleasantly buzzing-brain. I was easily distracted, yet multi-tasked with great efficiency. In the later years I experienced a lot of psychosis.[2] I even went against my normally shy disposition with regards to men when I was at my most ill. It was hell!

With the exception of manic depression where 20% of sufferers kill themselves regardless of how much treatment they have, eating disorders have the highest mortality rate (2-20%, the less treatment accepted, the higher the risk, i.e. 2% of those treated still die) of any psychological illness. I suspect this is in part due to the high co-morbidity[3] with depression, hence suicide. Eating disorders affect at least 70 million people worldwide. All these illnesses carry with them a very

---

[2] Experiencing delusions and hallucinations – in my case auditory (hearing) and visual hallucinations and some delusions, particularly a pervasive feeling that the whole world truly hated me and wanted me dead.
[3] Co-morbidity refers to the concurrent diagnosis of more than one illness, e.g. depression and anorexia.

real risk of permanent injury, death, or the finality that suicide brings.

In our Western world of plenty: the constraining, tangible corsets of days-gone-by have been replaced by a new metaphorical corset of the mind. Men and women, all of whom suffer from extreme low self-esteem and lack of validation, find themselves living out each day of their life, overwhelmed with issues of food, weight, size, self-hatred, illness, anxiety, anger, guilt, control and fear. Eating disorders are a *symptom* of deep emotional distress, which entrap sufferers and create new problems of their own. Societally, dieting is rife. Value judgements based on a person's size are copious, and seemingly up for discussion without any understanding of underlying issues. Few illnesses inspire such misunderstanding, despair and frustration, for all involved, as do eating disorders. Few illnesses are awarded such warped attention in the media; or are claimed to be "lifestyle choices" by some of those afflicted.

The term "self-harm" covers any act whereby a self-inflicted deed that causes harm (i.e. it is exactly as it sounds). People cut, scratch, burn, stab, bloodlet, bang themselves, even break bones, overdose (on a variety of substances), swallow objects, insert objects, drink excessively, engage in less obvious self-harm like eating disordered behaviour, self-neglect, and/or engaging in other risky behaviours (e.g. driving dangerously) that are likely to cause harm. All of this is because they are in *deep emotional pain*, and it actually seems "better" to feel physical pain, or concentrate on a physical injury, than to cope with feelings that are overwhelming. It can feel better to see a wound (whether kept hidden, or shown to others), as such an injury can be tended to, cleansed, and looked after, or deliberately not looked after. *Emotional pain is far deeper and far more difficult to treat.*

Do not be afraid to ask for help. Do not be afraid to offer it, sometimes repeatedly. I have learned a great deal, though unfortunately I had to learn the hard way. You may also end up learning some things the hard way, because sometimes it is necessary to find these things out for yourself. Some things have to be experienced to be believed. But try to trust my words: they are true, and my sole motivation is to prevent suffering.

Mental illness is understandably frustrating for all involved. It makes no sense. Sometimes is seems that *nothing* you do can help, you cannot magically make someone recover, and you cannot necessarily make yourself recover as and when you want to. If that were possible, no one would be ill, and psychiatrists and psychotherapists would need new jobs! Recovery can sometimes take a long time. That does not mean that you should give up or not try, for then you will certainly remain ill. Remain positive for yourself or another, and *do not give up.* Any effort you make will ultimately help you, even if it seems pointless or useless at the time. I first genuinely sought help when I was only 19, but it took 10 years of what seemed like pointless, sheer hell to reach where I am today. It need not take you so long.

I am cautious of writing that you need to fight for yourself, in case this leads someone to give up all hope because they think their illness is beyond their control. If you are very ill, too tired to fight, hopeless, and out of control, take solace in the following: trying to improve, recover or fighting for your life can be unconscious, as it was for me in the worst, darkest, most unmanageable times. We all have a conscious mind, and an unconscious one. My conscious efforts were focussed indomitably on self-destruction and suicide. I remained ill and hurtled towards death, yet part of me, my unconscious self must have been fighting to keep me alive.

Many people, in fact most people, recover totally or "enough." Reading that, I know some of you will immediately think, *"Well I am the exception; I won't recover because I don't deserve to."* Some of you will not even want to recover…yet. Such thinking may make your recovery time longer, but I recovered despite such negative thinking. Treat these illnesses as *seriously dangerous*.

We owe it to ourselves, those we love, and to each other, to educate ourselves and other people, not to judge others, or allow others to unfairly judge us. Also we must not judge ourselves too harshly, a particularly common trait in eating disorders, as well as depression, and also a trait in the families who lose someone to suicide, or have a family member labelled as mentally ill. Self-deprecation is unhelpful, painful and usually extremely exaggerated; however it is a normal reaction in today's society.

My illness was <u>not</u> a conscious choice I made for my life, but illness controlling me. The fact that you are not in control of your illness can be very hard to accept, and difficult for those close to you to understand. The individuality and complexity of these problems can mean that understanding all of this will often take a long time. Many fantastically talented, intelligent, warm, honest people turn into people they are not. They lie, run away, steal, are quiet, miserable, unresponsive, behave dangerously and so on. I knew I was ill quite early on, but I felt it was my fault and something I deserved – worsening my depression. Then I was even proud to have anorexia for a few years: a common feeling, and quite deluded. Nobody really *chooses* to be so ill.

To those of you who care enough to want to understand, read this book with an open mind, and follow the journey I take you on. If you have family, friends or patients that are ill, read on, learn, and remember to get angry at the illness and not the sufferer. It is not their fault. How you act around the sufferer can greatly affect them. Listen to them, and do not give up on them, even for a moment. You need to be positive and proactive for them when they cannot be. I am pro-professionals; I know that there are conscientious people out there who make a difference to the lives of victims.

If you are ill, this book is intended for *you*. A major reason why I am writing this book so close to my recovery, whilst everything seems so painfully raw, is to better reach those people still staring into the abyss. If you are diagnosed with an eating disorder, do not let any concurrent depression be ignored or taken as anything less than very serious, and vice versa. Self-hatred is devastating, ubiquitous, undeserved, and wrong.

> "You yourself, as much as
> anybody in the entire Universe,
> deserve your love and affection."
>
> ❧ Buddha. (563-483 B.C.)

Dark Clouds Gather

Hindu Prince Gautama
Siddharta, founder of Buddhism.

Ask yourself if there are other issues. I denied my anger, and then believed the denial; but I have since realised that for me it is a huge problem. In fact, all emotions are difficult for me. Direct your anger away from yourself but do not seek to blame everyone else for what is your responsibility. Anger directed at the actual illness, such as an eating disorder, can be most useful. Adapt this to yourself; the emotion troubling you might be different, such as jealousy, sadness, and/or anxiety.

> "The thoughts written on the walls of
> madhouses by their inmates
> might be worth publicising."

> ❧ Georg Christoph Lichtenberg, critic,
> physicist, (1742 – 1799)

This is my story. At first the words did not come as I sat blankly before the computer, numb from hospitalisation and very much present major depression; then came realisations and encouragement along with some slow words; and then (in 2005) my mind buzzed and the words gushed like Niagara Falls as hypomania set in. When I first began to write in 2003, I had been out of the Warneford Hospital in Oxford a matter of months. My life-long manic depression (mixed bipolar I affective disorder with psychosis)[4] had reached the stage where my doctors feared I would take my own life.

They were absolutely right, and I did my very best to die, even though I was also desperate to recover. I was the very definition of ambivalent, torn between two poles: life and death. Despite passionately wanting to be dead, somehow, I always survived. I repeatedly defied medical science. Unimportant to this admission, was the fact that I was still an anorectic, as I had been for fourteen years.

I've been ill with depression (of various forms) since before I was five. Trying to pick the worst year or decade is impossible, but in particular, I wouldn't go through the last three years of my life again for any amount of money. I lost my voice (metaphorically speaking) to my eating disorder and manic depression. Perhaps that is why I feel such a need to speak out now. I have screamed silently from the pain of manic depression and been unable to see any future. I have turned all my pain inwards. I lost my planned career in medicine. I have lost *all* hope. I have had all my freedom and decisions taken from me. I have had my possessions searched, and been watched twenty-four hours a day to keep me alive. And I am thankful.

Some people say that if I were determined enough I would have killed myself anyway. Firstly, I *did* kill myself; secondly, they are wrong; and thirdly such a

---

[4] Mixed states consist of experiencing manic and major depressive symptoms at the same time. As my mania was not usually euphoric but was angry, it was "dysphoric mania" – sleepless, overwhelming and busy-minded. Psychosis meant I continued to see and hear (hallucinate) things that were not there and had some very strange absolute beliefs (delusions). Basically a very severe form of manic depression carrying the highest risk of suicide of any mental illness.

voiced opinion can make a person all the more determined to prove their sincerity. It really is extremely difficult, both physically and mentally to end your life. Just because a chosen suicide method has a comparatively low lethality, doesn't mean the intent to die is any less.

People are restricted to methods they find practical, "comfortable" and/or aesthetically agreeable. This is especially true if you are like me: you think too much; you may have nothing dangerous to hand; you don't want to suffer too much pain; you want it to be over quickly; you wont risk other peoples' lives; you want to avoid anything that might result in survival combined with permanent serious mental or physical injury, or leave too much of a mess to find and scrape up. Ever the perfectionist, I had such very definite rules about how I would and would not depart this earth. Perhaps perfectionism worked in my favour in this instance? Eventually desperation would result in abandonment of these rules.

I have thought about suicide millions of times, over many years, for different amounts of time depending how ill I was. I carved my body hundreds of times; I exposed pumping arteries, hoping to die. But beyond reason, I did not die, despite repeating this behaviour sometimes daily or twice daily, purposely giving my body no time to recover. All these I count as suicide attempts that ruined my carpet and left me gasping for breath.

Absence can have great presence; any loss can cause a hole in your heart that is forever with you. Never is loss more deep than in bereavement; and never more controversial, painful, angry, sad, and altogether devastating, than in the case of suicide. The experience of losing someone to suicide is, for some reason, more unrelenting than and un-like any other loss, in its destruction of both the victim and those left to pick up the pieces – sometimes quite literally. Emotions are stirred up: commonly anger, guilt, grief, shock, pain, puzzlement... and so on. I feel these things every day: every moment that I remember every person I have lost to suicide. Their beauty as people destroyed, leaving a void that can never be filled. I am, however, a terrible hypocrite, as I am a person who is aware of all of this, and yet I have attempted suicide hundreds of times. I wanted to disappear altogether, and would have done so without hurting anyone, if I could.

There are other times that I self-harmed in the full knowledge that I was not risking my life. Different attempts had different causes, though depression was common to all, and eating disorders were common to most. When counting my suicide attempts, I have ignored the fact that eating disorders are a form of slow suicide, even though I always hoped to die.

I overdosed on sedatives well over three hundred times that I consider to be suicide attempts. I also attempted to put myself asleep permanently with chloroform sixty times. There are other distinct attempts that I made with no ambiguity in my mind. Education made me more lethal.

As a result of illness, I have lost everything that mattered to me; some of these important things I have regained – such as a close family and friends. Some are lost to me forever: such as the ability to let people get close to me, ever having children, and my medical career. When ill, I did things I would never even consider with my faculties intact. I have attempted suicide (with full intent of dying) at least *443* times, though my memory is blurry from illness, meaning the real total will be higher. Each one was different. I was damaged and ill after most of them, and nearly succeeded several times, in fact twice I received emergency resuscitation. There were many, many times where I survived beyond medical possibility. I have actually been dead, but revived from what should have been irrevocable death, or at least severely brain damaged. How I am here cannot be explained by logic. I have no explanation.

I chose long ago to try to change my thinking, to cheer up, eat better, and stop judging myself, and instead tried to just accept myself. But for many years after making that decision I was still unable to put it into practice. The noise in my head was just too loud. I learned enough about my illnesses to deserve two PhDs, yet I was still powerless to change. So I performed seamlessly the act of being perfectly fine, and went about my academic achievements. I became too good at seeming confident, fine, happy, or more usually impassive. I even convinced myself I was emotionless: whilst burning all that time with hatred, energy, apathy, sadness, frustration, desire, and most of all, anger.

Then, after years of undiagnosed manic depressive illness and struggling with anorexia, suddenly everything went WAY off whatever is the Psychiatric equivalent of the Richter scale, spinning down in to darkness. Precarious, unwilling existence was the result, for a very long three years. Frankly I am amazed to have survived after sinking to depths I could not fathom whilst in a seemingly permanent mixed state (both fully manic and severely depressed at the same time). In my case dysphoric mania dominated, i.e.

furious anger, always turned inwards; extreme irritability; and insomnia that did not end – ever. A brain that was never quiet: hallucinations, delusions, and such *noise*. And I did it all with a calm, sweet smile on my face (when anyone was looking). My biggest problem: an overactive mind – deepening, catastrophising, and prolonging every bad experience, thought, emotion and mood. Put simply, I think too much.

"Cogito ergo doleo."[5]

Then, someone apologised to me about something I needed to hear an apology about. And one day, the right doctor (Alan, who never gave up on me) put me on the right antidepressant/mood stabiliser mixture, and saved my life. The clouding of my mind parted, and I began to gradually piece together the remains of my life.

This initial recovery was only improved upon by damn hard work by yours truly, to reach where I am today: able to write about recent, raw, and almost unspeakably painful illness, motivated by a desire to try and help others. I was finally able to use the techniques and understanding I had learned in years of therapy.

For the physical side of my illness, by which I mean the manic/psychotic/mixed depression, medication has been vital. I may hate the side effects, but I gratingly (*gritting teeth*) "welcome" them as the alternative to a life of clawing my way through existence, to barely survive in the depths of mixed manic depression. For me, antidepressants, antipsychotics and lithium are essential. Without them, all my strength, and all the

---

[5] "I think, therefore I am depressed."

help and therapy in the world would have made no difference and I would surely be dead.

I am not ashamed: there is no reason to be. Open your mind. Let me take you on a true but dark journey. I am going to share with you the deepest, most intricate secrets of my own personal struggle with manic depression, suicide, anorexia, and sometimes bulimia, self-harm, psychosis, a few addictions (like exercise), occasionally complicated with alcohol or prescription drugs...or worse. Are these dirty words? They certainly are *feared* words. They are words that carry with them many connotations that people fear being labelled with. But I do not value myself less because I have been ill, very ill. And nor should you. And nor should you allow or cause others to be. In fact, when you are strong enough, you must hold your head up high and be an ambassador for those people who cannot do the same.

I am going to open my heart's secrets to the whole world for scrutiny, to show you, to show other people, both those suffering in the same way, and society in general, that *I do not hang my head in shame*. Yes, I was utterly "mad" in the clinical, scientific sense of the word, with which I have no problem whatsoever. However, I emphatically do *not* accept, when used in the derogatory sense that they are often misused, the label of lunatic, crazy person, mad person, psycho, stupid person, nor the misnomer that the label attention-seeker has now become, nor anything else you can think of. *I was ill.*

It really is that simple. I was ill for biological and emotional reasons, but I was just ill. I am a human being and I stand proud. It is about acceptance. Do not be ashamed. Do not make other people ashamed. Accept. The idea that people should just "pull themselves together" is pervasive in today's society and I can understand why. It can be very difficult to understand why a person does not just simply stop their destructive behaviour. Psychiatric illnesses are frightening, dangerous and strange. Maybe I should forgive people's prejudices, because understanding and allowing for what a mental illness is like are difficult concepts to grasp if you've not been there yourself, or have little professional experience.

Fellow sufferers *know*. They just know what you feel like without the need to explain. Although professionals can be knowledgeable, sympathetic, and the good ones empathic, I firmly believe you cannot truly understand these illnesses unless you have suffered from them; but that is no excuse for anyone being discriminatory and opinionated about something they do not understand. I do not accept this state of prejudicial general opinion… I feel duty bound to do whatever I can to change as many people's preconceived misconceptions as possible. With understanding comes the ability to help your self and those you love, and the ability to be compassionate to your fellow human beings.

I have many scars, some visible, some not. Who wouldn't? It is not the visible scarring that still hurts. I am not proud of my scars, but nor am I ashamed. I also have a terrible, hovering fear that I will become ill again, and one day "successfully" take my own life, and this will become a posthumous book. Sometimes I still consider taking my life; sometimes suicide feels like the inevitable conclusion that awaits me: the exclamation mark at the end of a haphazard existence. I have been, and might become, prepared to subject others to *my* absence: unable to see the pain I might cause, or think it "better" for everyone if I were gone.

Knowledge that I could recover did not save me last time. I might again have faith that suicide is the answer to my pain, and a way to enable other people to at least cease fearing that I may take eventually that route. Once it is done, it is done: no more pain, and no more fear. Today I am aware that it is delusional to think people will be happier should I die. I do not always sense with such clarity.

No doubt more people will buy this book if I die, but my words would have less strength, and that is a *good* reason to live. I no longer want my legacy to be that of a completed suicide victim. I am determined to fight, live, and live well! I intend to remain healthy, but that includes preventative work, medication, support, a life, and preparation for the possible return of unbalanced depression. But we do not walk this world with the benefit of knowing what the future holds. I would be lying if I said I was not very frightened, and very much "at risk."

I have spent my whole life surrounded by death and illness. I still have many friends who are at risk, and the thought of losing them terrifies me. I have friends who, like me, feel their eventual suicide is inevitable. (I must add on a positive note, that I also have many friends who have recovered). I live daily with the frustration, anger and emptiness left behind from every time I lost a loved one or friend to suicide's bitter sting. Oh how that hurts. It doesn't get any easier each time it happens or as time passes. Philosophising about suicide and death has not gone away from my life. Maybe that will change; maybe it is something I will learn to live with, and not dwell upon.

But survive I did, meaning I must make some sense of it all. Now, somehow, I have to pick myself up, smile, and carry on living. Even when ill, I always had a sense of humour, sometimes dry, usually black, or warped to the point of being disturbed. I would always appear happy and confident: the opposite of the truth inside. I was misunderstood because my outward appearances were Euthymic[6], happy, and/or bizarre: possibly because I was in a strangely warped mixed state. I was filled with suppressed fury, and often laughed[7] about my hopelessness when self-harming, attempting suicide or when "caught out" about self-harm and suicide attempts. Something others found (not unexpectedly) impossible to comprehend or understand. The answer is painstakingly simple: it was how I coped. It's still how I cope.

> "If I had no sense of humour, I would long
> ago have committed suicide."

> ❧ Mahatma Gandhi (1869-1948), written
> in 1928.

I hope you enjoy this book. I ask of you to keep some things in mind whilst reading, particularly the autobiographical parts of the book. Some of the feelings, thoughts and interpretations that I made during my illnesses, will be described as I felt them at the time. People remember the past differently. Keep in mind that judgements I made were often clouded by manic depression, my eating disorder, or both, and therefore at times are incorrect and unfair towards the

---

[6] Euthymic = of normal mood, neither elevated or depressed.
[7] Laughing at such negative issues could be construed as disorganised speech or a thought disorder – typical of psychosis in manic depression; and very hard for other people to understand.

individual(s) or experience concerned. I will do my best not to be unfair, to tell both sides of the story and try to point to what I felt but also the different message intended by family, friends and professionals, that have now been explained to me or that I have since understood. But it is important that I explain how I truly felt back then, even if I misjudged, so that you can understand the progression of my illness.

When I look at the person I am now, I am unrecognisable from who I was a year ago. I know that I completely "lost it." As my good friend Clare put it, "You were completely potty for a while sweetheart." That is true. So I am writing from a position of deep experience, extensive knowledge, and heartfelt concern. I will never be "normal."

I do not intend to preach to you, but as you might already have guessed, I am not yet *at all* distanced from my illnesses or their lingering effects, so my words are urgent and powerful. Don't ever be complacent with your own life or someone else's. Real, live, loved people who are wonderful, creative, caring, amazing, interesting, loving, talented, generous, warm, beautiful, unique, astonishing, *and by the way ill*, can and do suffer, and some die.

Realism: You seriously doubt your own value in this world. You "know," without question, that other people think you are disgusting and worthless. But you have never stopped, even for a second, to question your apparently superhuman ability to accurately interpret *for the worst*: situations, words, gestures, or even read other people's minds in order to back up your fear that everyone despises you for existing. You *are* worthwhile. You are extraordinarily valuable. You (unfortunately) must be patient. But you must not be complacent. You must not give up. Some people die: or, you can help yourself (or another), you can fight, grit your teeth, hold on and become more well.

Ultimately I chose and then achieved the latter, as did many good friends of mine. Some were irrevocably lost along the way.

They are not forgotten.

Chapter. 1. The Complex Fragility of Childhood.

"My own brain is to me the most
unaccountable of machinery - always
buzzing, humming, soaring roaring
diving, and then buried in mud. And
why? What's this passion for?"

&Virginia Woolf (1882-1941), Letter,
December 28, 1932.

From my earliest memories, and possibly from before my earliest memories, constant questioning about life, death, and the philosophy of existentialism (the belief in freedom of choice and personal responsibility but regarding human existence in a hostile universe as unexplainable), became my quiet and *seemingly* indifferent pathway of choice. What happens in childhood, and even adolescence, can scar a person for life – for some unlucky souls this scarring is vicious, permanent, and disabling.

I have never believed in stoicism, and despite appearances to the contrary, could never be described as a stoic – unlike others in my family. Appearing stoical, or being surrounded by stoicism can be serious handicaps, as they have been for me. I often appear unemotional, falsely calm or happy, because my upbringing (strongly but wrongly) taught me that emotions are inappropriate to express; and so despite being extremely emotional, upset, depressed, manic, sensitive, muted, impatient, angry, so on and so forth, my feelings were always very tightly boxed up in my head and heart.

I became something of an expert in *not* showing my feelings, devoid of the ability to complain about anything that mattered, and, eventually, unable to understand my own feelings. Because all this left me inconsolable and unable to contemplate solace, I never learned how to cope with my emotions. Nor did I realise this was happening. I was never able to predict the behaviour of other people, particularly within my family, leaving me constantly afraid, assuming the worst, and feeling unloved. (Although of course, I was dearly loved). Then I developed manic depression too, magnifying my distress and inability to cope. Unfortunately for me, this combination resulted in an awful lot of pain contained and turned inwards, and eventually, utter self-execration.[8]

All of this started when I was very young. Obviously the complexity of these thoughts began simply and increased rapidly with age and worsening illness, but one thing I have always done, is to *think too much*. Thinking like this can be unhealthy, and is probably why so many quotes about "genius being close to madness" endure. My brain, it seemed, did not ever like to stop for rest, or allow me to rest or sleep. The only relief I ever had was keeping myself busy, or eating, both of which half-cured boredom. I needed (need) to feel in control of preventing boredom.

For me, boredom is a terrible irritation, a painful hunger that I have never been able to tolerate, and the more active and hungry your mind, the more difficult it is to satiate. Of course, depression makes any coping strategies impossible, dangerous, hopeless, and yet far more desperate and important to achieve. Time loses all

---

[8] Self-execration = concurrent self-hatred *and* self-disgust.

meaning, the metaphorical thumbscrews turn, and you have no idea how long for. This obsession with time was (is) deeply linked to a mind that was often dominated by mania at some level – and I do not mean in a pleasurable way: I mean a busy, busy active mind, clawing at your sanity.

The other enduring philosophy of mine is that of wanting to make people happy and protecting other people's quality of life, even at costs to myself. World peace and happiness for all… Well meant but impossible to achieve. So in this way I set myself up for failure, and could not share my pain because I feared it would upset another person. I could not stand up for myself because other people were more important. Again, all this meant emotions would be contained but were actually intense, uncontrolled, and twirled around in my brain for hours, months or years: wearing my self-worth down and down. I felt (feel) that I needed to master time. It is no wonder then, that issues of *control* became overly important and life threatening (classic in eating disorder sufferers).

I do not even know where all of these philosophies come from: they just "are." They feel right; much in the same way a religion must feel right to someone who believes in a god. Some of these beliefs may have served me well had mental illness not been added to the mixture; although, it is also true that my beliefs have been strengthened and modified by my illness, understanding of mental illness, and "recovery."

It is impossible to say when I first became ill, or when I started to choose my own life plan, or when I first hesitantly started on my rollercoaster ride into madness that was to last for almost three decades. All I know is that actual, definable illness started with a manic depressive illness, as young as five or six, that must have been biochemical rather than reactive. In other words I do not blame myself or anyone else. It was simply a matter of my neurochemistry.

I am suggesting that I was a 5-year old with full-blown manic depression. With the benefit of hindsight, I can see that I was already symptomatic back then, and heading in the wrong direction. I moped around, cried a lot (alone), thought of suicide; I barely slept, not ever, even as a baby. My relationship with food was complicated and unhealthy. All classical signs of depression in a child, but how many people know what to look for? My lack of sleep did not slow me down or upset me. I was anxious yet felt important – the world belonged to me. I was fervent about everything; I didn't stop to rest, my mind buzzed – with both dark and pleasant thoughts: flipping from one to the other, or feeling both at once.

My mind was always *painfully* active, my body not far behind; I talked a lot and I did it quickly, I was hyperactive and definitely "guilty" of grandiosity – signs of mania. But I was always more disturbed by depression. Events in my life would contribute to an eventual emotional collapse, and years of torment. Even as a young child, I was the kind of person that worried a lot, mostly about other people. I became uneasily "comfortable" with my life of contemplating the void. Such thoughts that I have only just realised that most people never have. I thought it was normal to think like that.

The world weighed heavily on my shoulders. Depression is like a seed of misery or darkness that grows like a parasite sucking the meaning out of life: at first insidiously, then out of control, and which utterly violates the lives of people and those around them, clouding out enjoyment of anything.

I worried a lot about death, my death, my family's death, death of people I knew and didn't know, such as children murdered in the country whose missing posters found their way to my eyes, or the deaths of starving thousands in the developing world. Where this obsession with transience came from I do not know: it just happened. I lay in bed, in tears, waiting for my death or that of someone I loved from the age of five. I read post mortem books at the age of 7; morbidly fascinated by the process of death. It has been a part of me as long as I can remember. Mum tells me that I have always had an unhealthy preoccupation with death. Back then, I hadn't heard of a condition called depression, let alone manic depression/bipolar disorder, and nor had my family. Childhood depression had not really "taken off" as a medical condition back then. Anyway, people had "nervous breakdowns" in our family, not depression. As for manic depression in children – well, that was even less well understood or expected.

Following the expectations upon me, my manic depression was never visible, and although I was pondering suicide well under the age of ten, nobody would have been able to guess. I fitted very well the description of childhood manic depression with "dissociation of affect;" in other words, my behaviour was that of a happy, content, diligent child with no cares in the world – the polar opposite of how I truly felt. I thought it was normal to spend most of bedtime lying awake with terrible black thoughts and worries racing through my mind. I do not mean a "little" problem sleeping; I mean that from the age 5, it took three hours to get to sleep, and I woke three hours too early, sandwiching a fitful, half-waking few hours of relative peace. Sometimes I longed for the time-friendly unconsciousness of sleep – filling some of those hours I was having so much trouble keeping myself occupied within. I do not know the harm that was done to myself by having so little sleep – it can't have been healthy – but again, I thought it was normal.

There was no discernable reason for me to be like this, no terrible loss, no personal problems at that time, my family loved me, it was just the way I was. My mind was always unquiet. Depression grew insidiously, until, I estimate, by the age of ten, a diagnosis of manic depression could have been made. My deterioration continued thence.

> "If you gaze for long into an abyss, the
> abyss gazes also into you."

> ‰ Friedrich Nietzsche (1844-1900).
> Existentialist Philosopher.
> *Beyond Good and Evil*, Aphorism 146.

But let us step back just a moment. I was not a 2-year old engaging in discussions of existentialism, quoting Nietzsche, pondering philosophy, stoicism, psychology and psychiatry. Reaching the above beliefs, descriptions and understandings has taken many years. All I originally brought with me were some unhelpful genetic predispositions that my nurture did not suit. I revered both my parents; their opinions became mine (at first), and above all else in my life, I had to make them proud and be perfect. But *I* set unattainable aims. It is noteworthy that feelings of sadness, rejection, failure and self-hatred that begin in childhood are inescapably carried with you into adult life. But it all began so simply, so innocently.

I don't want to bore you with tiny details, so lets stick to the really relevant events. I come from a good, strong family, having two loving, hard-working parents, both self-made, and one amazing younger sister who I would give my life for. Born in Liverpool but grown up in Derby. I share my birthday (25th January) with Virginia Woolf – which is somewhat apt.

My parents tell me I was agonisingly ingenious from a young age. As a baby I slept for one hour a night. My first clear memory is of the Queen's silver jubilee, I was two and a half. And yes, one of my first clear memories is one about food. I remember being given an ice cream cornet, eating the ice cream, nibbling the cornet to make it gooey-soft, and then sticking on my face like a Pinocchio nose. I then walked from person to person with an immovable straight face, innocent eyes and watched for the reaction. I was a curious child!

Before I even went to school I remember mum (an English teacher) teaching me to read and write on a blackboard she had in the kitchen. She also provided me with endless paint, glitter, brushes, glue and paper that would occupy me all day long. At the age of five my preoccupation with death began; innocently at first, but I remember lying awake worrying about it at night. It was my deep thinking and overactive imagination that made me frightened much of the time. Nor could my own mother reassure me. I think it is very true to say I have always been almost totally impervious to solace for no explainable reason.

My inability to cope with boredom surfaced more and more as my mind raced. In class I would finish the set work in minutes and then want more to do. I demanded the teacher's attention often. I also didn't like being told when to talk! Why shouldn't I talk? I could talk, work, finish quickly and do the best quality work all at once. I questioned authority that was not (in my little know-it-all head) earned, logical or deserved. Let's be honest: I questioned any authority in anybody. But I did love to read, or be read to, and prided myself to be reading the "big children books" way ahead of my supposed book-age. My teachers soon learned the best way to shut me up was to give me books to read.

My sister Beth has always been a happy person, hyperthymic[9] perhaps, but as might be expected coming from our family, has grown up somewhat stoical. She tells me that she just didn't think about things – whereas the many issues that would stick in my head would suck me down like I was in quicksand. She has never had a mental illness, and over time has come to understand that they aren't something people choose to have.

You know, I don't actually think my parents are particularly stoical. I've seen my dad angry, and seen my dad cry. Both of my parents got angry – explosively so, unpredictably so, and punishment followed – but that is true of every kid in every family I am sure. I have pushed my mum past her capability to endure my illnesses many times – that is not a sign of weakness in her, more a sign of how ill she has had to watch me be – and she feels responsible. I am sure most people would have abandoned me much sooner. Dad appeared

[9] Hyperthymia refers to a state of general happiness & optimism that is not detrimental to health.

(appears) unfazed, although I know he was (is) not. I know he carries with him a lot of guilt and feelings of failing me. Only mum seemed to shut down into silence and apparent oblivion: which I believe is her coping strategy. It makes perfect sense that I became the person that I am: scared of my anger, scared of my sadness.

Back to childhood: I was a tomboy; I climbed the trees that lined our secluded road to desperate heights because then nobody could reach me. The higher I got the safer I felt, there was a darker side to it. I would enjoy the danger, imagine myself fall, see my broken, bleeding body: and in that way I consciously stared my mortality in the face. Yet strangely I felt immortal and powerful.

When I was six, my dad started taking me to the football. He is a lifelong Derby County fan, and we would stand on the pop side lower at Derby's old ground, the Baseball Ground. As I was half the height of everyone else, I couldn't see anything unless I sat on my dad's shoulders. When he got tired, I'd stand for a bit, surrounded by the smell of cigarette smoke and man farts. At first it was just a bunch of men running around: I didn't really understand what was going on other than our team was in black and white, and we wanted to score goals. I absolutely loved the frenzied celebration when we did score. The crowd's behaviour fascinated me.

One day, dad told me that I would have to pick which football team I was going to support, warning me that once the decision is made, there is no going back. He said that since I was born in Liverpool I could support Liverpool or Everton, or instead I could choose from the nearby Manchester United or Manchester

City. Our house had been fairly equidistant between those two great cities. Dad also said I could support Derby since that was where I was growing up. It wasn't a hard choice: I chose Derby. Football is one thing in my life that I have never connected with food or death, just with fun and normality. C'mon you Rams!

One wonderful gift that my parents gave to us, their children, was to travel widely. I have travelled widely, my favourites places being, America, Canada, Scotland and France. We often went on holiday with the Gatley family. We usually went to "le Sud Ouest," which is the south west coast of France, south of Bordeaux, somewhere around Biarritz, where we could eat seafood and dad could sniff out good wines. I really loved the trees, their musty pine smell, which changed subtly with the weather. One day I saved Beth from drowning when our dingy was capsized. I didn't know any lifesaving; I just scrambled along the seabed holding her head up above the surface, occasionally grabbing some air for myself. I would have given my life for her. I still would.

Sundays meant we went to my grandparents – my nanny Betty, a sufferer of anorexia, bulimia and depression herself, loved to fatten up the relatives with a large spread. Alcohol flowed copiously in that house. Nan told me that her sisters all had eating disorders, and I found out later that a relative on hr side of the family was bipolar and killed himself. It seems that in our family, food and mood are issues, and have been for generations. My father, brought up by an anorexic mum was influenced detrimentally. Normality to him meant the woman cooked, semi-starving, whilst the man gorged. My father denies that there was anything abnormal regarding attitudes towards food within either in our family, his parental family, or his parent's parental families. *But there were.*

When I try to remember good times in my childhood, I am lucky to have many good memories of my youngest years. I think of playing outdoors in our garden, or the very quiet street we lived on. In the summer there is a distant hum of motor racing that can be heard from Donington Race Track. There are bad memories too, a semiconscious awareness of darker issues, most obviously a constant fear, sadness, inconsolability, insomnia, thoughts of death and suicide.

Sweets and food were a reward. Bad behaviour removed sweets or treats, or the money with which to purchase them. Nanny Doris (my mum's mum) would sneak us treats all the time, even if we weren't supposed to have them. I learned young, but without an understanding as to why, that food could be comforting when battling feeling sad.

The classification of foods as good or bad is *always* simplistic, misleading, and unhelpful. It can be very dangerous. It can also encourage unhealthy dichotomous thinking, and this quickly becomes entrenched as the truth in a young, impressionable person. Many mostly healthy women (and an increasing number of men) have warped attitudes to food that spoil their happiness although they never develop a clinical condition. However well intentioned, it is potentially very dangerous if your child might be predisposed to eating disorders. My mum and dad had no reason to know it might be something that would threaten my life. With hindsight, I am sure they would have acted differently. It worries me that other parents with good intentions might unknowingly be doing the same thing at this very moment. It is vital that parents teach their children a balanced attitude towards food. Most eating disordered people I know have some element of disturbed attitude towards food in their family.

My parents had definite opinions about some foods being bad, usually described to me as "fattening." If (for example) I put "too much" butter on my bread, dad would get so angry, shout, turn purple, his temporal arteries bulged, and he looked like he would literally explode – and he might smack me. Later he would have to apologise when he realised it was only a super-thin layer of cheese spread (one single Dairylea cheese triangle on a slice of bread), not butter at all. I know my dad only did this because he loved me.

In my mind, the hardest thing to live with was the fact I seemed able to push all his wrong buttons (mainly because I simply wouldn't listen) so that he would instantly turn from his normal, calm, stoical, loving and caring self, into, in my view: a monster. Nor were his reactions ever predictable. No wonder I feared my own emotions so much: particularly my own anger. I did not want to be like that. I didn't want to make anyone feel as badly as I felt. I was actually afraid for my safety. (This was inaccurate, but it is how I felt at the time).

At first I did not understand why food was such an important issue, although over time, my opinions came to mirror my father's opinions. In that way, his negative views about food and eating lived inside my own head. For many years it was almost as though he sat on my right shoulder whispering loudly in my ear, "that's bad," lest I forget his teaching.

I love my dad very much: he has always been there for me, and I have an understanding of why he is the person he is. He has striven to provide for his family, even if at times he unintentionally or uncontrollably caused me much misery. I revered him. I still revere him. And I was terrified of him. I wanted to be like him and not like him all at the same time – early ambivalence. I felt at the mercy of my powerful and overwhelming emotions. I was even more terrified of disappointing him. I know he would be most distressed to read these words. A wise Oxford psychotherapist once said to me, "Sometimes we feel the most anger towards people we love the most." So I rationalise my father's behaviour: well meant but screwed up, because he loves me so much, acting purely out of love and a desire to protect. He is the product of a home where the men ate like pigs and the girls ate like sparrows. I have forgiven him because I need to love him, I do love him, he loves us all, because I can see where his opinions came from, and because he has changed. These days my dad is a kitten: loving, caring, providing and protective. How can I blame him for acting out of love – however misguided?

> "If we could read the secret history of our enemies, we should find in each man's life sorrow and suffering enough to disarm all hostility."

> ❧ Henry Wadsworth Longfellow, (1807-1882).

I simply don't have any memory of food being used for its usual purpose: that is to satiate hunger. I didn't know what hunger was, and probably still don't with much accuracy. I think I started to eat more than I should because of the depression or boredom. I spent hours reading, and this converted into hours reading and picking at "bad" food. Of course, I gained some weight, and my parents were defensive about this. All I saw was their disappointment.

I don't remember when it first happened, but I was encouraged to weigh myself and then had to talk to dad about it: I cannot ever remember him being happy with the result. He would burst into my room shouting, or walk in shouting. I found myself shivering in bed, my room dark, and my dad's shadow ominous and dark, illuminated by the light from the hall. Sometimes I thought I could see his bright blue eyes bulging and frenzied. Sometimes he'd just shout. Or he would drag me to the scales, kicking, screaming, pleading and crying not to be weighed.

Unfortunately the result of all this was that my parents failed their task of educating me healthily about food. This was because of mixed messages, unpredictable anger, and the fact that I was doomed to interpret things in the worst possible way, and also, I believe, because of my genetic predisposition to have an eating disorder. They were not to know how I pondered on their words and actions, interpreting them in my own way, assuming the worse possible scenario about what they said. They had no way to know how serious and dangerous my relationship with food would become, all the time with the manic depression creeping and growing insidiously in the background. They didn't know I cried myself to sleep – if I slept.

Dad said I would not get a job or husband if I were fat. Well I've got news for you my-dad-of-the-1980s! Over two decades of severe manic depression and almost as long as an anorectic *really* puts a damper on both love and career prospects! I don't blame my dad-of-2005; he has grown as a person. A select few will know I am actually being restrained and extremely forgiving. Therapy taught me to make up my own mind, but not for 20 years...

A decision was made that sending Beth and I to a private school would be extremely beneficial. At Fairfield I made some friends, namely Emma Bell and Mia Kazi. In class 3J (8-9 years old), with an amazing Evertonian form teacher called Mr. Jones, whose favourite saying was "only fools get caught," we each had to pick a different project topic, and I wanted to do one on dogs, but Mia got permission first, so I had to come up with something else. I should have chosen football... I chose "Blades." A strange choice, I think. Surely disturbing? My project was on the use of blades, knives, weapons, and sharp tools, and how throughout history, from the Stone Age, Roman times, and in Britain up to and including the present, they have been used in horrific fashions. I illustrated all my points with drawings of mutilated victims, dead and alive.

Long before the film "Braveheart" was made, a nine-year old girl researched and drew pictures of William Wallace's execution. I drew pictures that I imagined of his emasculation and ritual disembowelment, beheading, head on a spike, and a body cut into four pieces. I also wrote with wonder about the invention of the guillotine, the axe, the knife, the razor and so on. Was this a strange outward sign of my pathology? No alarm bells rang at a nine year old choosing such a macabre subject, producing such blood soaked pages of work. I got an A+.

My sister went to a Convent school, and like me, began to fill out early. I think I succeeded in protecting her somewhat. I somehow found strength to challenge my father if he castigated her about her weight. I found myself often between him and her; strength I could not find previously to protect myself. Why was it that it is easier to fight for someone else than for my own needs? In my eyes, I was already a lost cause. Beth deserved hope, and I would shield her.

My more lightly depressed years of sadness, irritability, busy mind, insomnia and unhealthy attitude to food, ended around the age of ten. I became utterly miserable, filled the criteria for major depressive disorder, and also had periods whereby my mind was so overactive it was physically painful. I was undiagnosed. I couldn't sleep; often I didn't really need to, but at other times I was exhausted. I couldn't rest or keep still. I felt awful but didn't know there was anything strange about this, so I didn't ask for help, and continued to act happy.

It was at the age of 11 that I decided I had had my fill of living and overdosed on *** Ibuprofen tablets. I lay down, listened to Queen singing *The Show Must Go On*, and expected to die. I never told anyone I had tried to kill myself. Nothing happened.

That was first of what was to become many suicide attempts. For some people one attempt is all it takes; I could have died at eleven. A lot had happened by the time I reached the ripe old age of eleven including severe depression and the firm decision that oblivion was for me. So started the really *earnest* obsession with suicide. My fear of pain and lack of knowledge of physiology and pharmacology meant most of my research was theoretical; and when it wasn't, I survived, without a word to anyone about my actively suicidal behaviour for over fifteen years.

Unfortunately for mum, dad, my sister, …and me, I now had *mixed* manic depression, (*mixed* bipolar I affective disorder). Sometimes I had depression, sometimes I was manic, but usually only briefly: most of the time I was a horrible, confused, overwrought mixture of the two. Mood disorders and eating disorders run in my family, and so I had the genes *and* personality that clashed utterly with intended messages about food, things being *only* good or bad, and being stoical (uncomplaining, patient and emotionless). I felt as if my life was chaos but my exterior was that of someone in perfect control. In reality, I hated myself with a passionate intensity.

I was, and am (overly?) sensitive, conscientious, intelligent, determined and a perfectionist. Sounds good doesn't it? But all of the above can be powerfully damaging as well as good. The brightest people can have the most persuasive and damaging demons that tear their lives apart…

I desperately wanted to make my parents proud and happy, and even slight failure was not acceptable. I did not see all the good things in me, or good that I achieved. I saw only failure. As an active person, I grew powerfully, both tall and well built; but I didn't see it as healthy, I saw it as disappointment to my parents. My body hatred became symbolic of my low self-esteem and despair. I didn't know then that there is so much more to a person than skin, fat and bones, or that I am meant to be a large person, and that actually it is perfectly OK to be like that.

I felt like I was letting my father down, and that was wholly unacceptable, pushing myself to diet, the major risk factor for developing an eating disorder. I watched my father watching me and saw him look at my developing body all the time. I (wrongly) assumed that he looked at me with disgust. I wrote many bad poems about this… and then burned them. But I kept one poem called, "Fatness" in my diary, which I can still remember. The most heartbreaking lines (for me) were some referring to my dad, who had the most powerful influence over me, and was most important person in my life:

> *"My heart breaks as I see the*
> *disappointment in his eyes,*
> *When he looks at me in that way he*
> *does,*
> *And saddens at my size."*

> ও Katy Sara, diary, age 11,
> excerpt from poem entitled
> *Fatness.*

I took the eleven-plus exam to get into Loughborough High School for Girls. The boys in Fairfield took the same exam to get into the equivalent boy's school in Loughborough. The exam is meant to be very difficult, as Loughborough High School has high standards. I took the exam, trying to do badly. I did want to go to university to become a doctor, but had reservations about this particular school, although these reservations were kept to myself. Deep down I didn't want to go, but could not explain why. I passed the entrance exam.

At the age of twelve I had my first real kiss, with a delectable exchange student from Gasny in France, who sent me love letters for a year after he went home. That year I also attempted suicide my slitting my wrists – with full intention of dying, but not knowing how hard it would be to a. cut at all and b. cut seriously enough to die. It was an art I could not perfect until years later. Instead I made about twenty cuts, but none deep enough to cause a problem.

I had never heard of self-harm; I thought it was my private discovery and rather weird. I felt nothing rewarding from my self-injury, just a mild curiosity and ferocious anger that I could not cut deeper. I judged myself as too pathetic and cowardly to cut myself: a feeling that would come back to haunt me repeatedly in later life. I hid these early wounds that were more like scratches than cuts.

For a long time up to this point, I harboured a desire to be a (medical) doctor. Loughborough High School has an excellent reputation for getting people into university to study what they want, so I decided it would be a good place for me. Despite the fact I have always wanted to work with living patients, preferably conscious ones, and even more preferably, ones with mental illness: I continued my interest in causes and process of death and read all I could on post-mortems and forensic pathology. This, I assume, was some sort of warped mixture of my interest in medicine and obsessive thinking about death.

Loughborough High School for girls was, and is, a high quality, reputable secondary school for girls aged 11-18, a significant proportion going on to Oxbridge. I was quite pleased to be in a boy-free environment. I hated the daily forced ritual of assembly and wouldn't sing hymns. If a teacher looked at me, I'd sometimes (unmistakably) mime, or more likely I'd just look straight back until she looked away. Sometimes my subdued state and lack of personal freedom made the tiniest most ridiculous choices a battle, because they were the only times I was allowed an opinion.

My work as a student was good, so why was it then, that I used to leave school each day, quietly crying to myself at the thought I would be dead the next day? Silently saying goodbye to the friends that I loved and teachers that I respected. Internally saying an angry, "Fuck you," to the few pathetic little teachers and many malicious students who made my life hell. Of course, that intended "poetic," suicidal "fuck you," would have only harmed me and my loved ones, not those bullies that hurt me.

One day in the Summer when I was thirteen, I clearly asked my dad, "Would it be OK for me to diet by eating *nothing at all*, but taking a daily multivitamin pill to stay healthy." His reply to me was a clear and unequivocal, "Yes." That event sewed the seed in my head to try and stop eating. Today, I ask myself if perhaps he misheard what I asked him? Maybe he was saying, "Yes" to a different question. Perhaps I heard the answer I wanted to hear? It certainly makes no sense that he told me to starve myself, but that was what I heard and clung on to for the next fifteen years.

At Loughborough High school I became a seriously low of mood – there was no mania, just depression. Boys and girls on the bus from our village to Loughborough would bully me on the way to school, than again on the way back. But it did not stop there. I was bullied relentlessly at school about my weight and responded by comfort eating. I did not fit in. I had friends – Emma, Antonia, Mia, Claire, Fiona, but I was not in a popular clique. I was the lowest of the low. Picked last for netball and hockey. I wasn't thin. I liked science. I didn't hunt foxes or have a dad who owned half of Leicestershire. As a kid I didn't have the reserves to overcome this maltreatment, I didn't see that *they* were the weak and pathetic ones. Bullies are cowards.

I suffered the bitchy hell that teenage girls can inflict upon another; and quite honestly, I could not deal with it. In those days schools didn't have a bullying policy, and verbal bullying was impossible to prove anyway. Not that I would have asked for help. Worst of all, some of the teachers (three different ones), bullied me about my weight. That was *totally* indefensible.

Imagine if you will, a balance or set of scales with good memories adding to the good self-esteem side, and bullying adding to the low self-esteem side. Day after day, year after year, my self-esteem was chipped away at, and the scales became very heavy on the low self-esteem side. Much of the fellow students' cruelty is lost in the mists of time, but two major events of teacher cruelty screwed with my head for years, and I am still fuming about them.

The least bad of the two events was when the ex-PE teacher Miss 'X' started teaching Technology. The sixth-form used her room to do our "Young Enterprise" project after school. I was sitting innocently on a stool in one of her classes, and she said to me, "I'm surprised that stool can take your weight without crumbling." Initially so shocked, I just walked out and never returned. Nor did I speak to that teacher or acknowledge her ever again. So many times since I have wished I had stood up to her. I'd quite like to punch her face in, for lack of a suitably strong verbal way to express my feelings.

The worst thing that happened was when I was about fourteen, and still on the large side. In a PE lesson it was suddenly announced that they would weigh us all. I declined to take part, protesting they had no need to know my weight. They said they were weighing everyone to check for anorexia – but I was *over*weight and utterly ashamed of it. I sat at the back of the gym watching others being happily weighed, content and sure within their bodies. Some people were less keen, but still acquiesced with persuasion.

The lesson ended with the teacher Mrs 'Y' telling me I had to be weighed, and me telling her (to "fuck off" in my head) it was none of her business and I didn't *have* to do anything I didn't want to do. So she let all the other girls go, and trapped me in the gym. She told me I was not leaving until I agreed to be weighed. I protested for ages, and then, my apparent strength (which let's face it, was all a façade) crumbled and out came the Katy-who-was-too-low-to-fight. I let her weigh me. "It's a lot," she said, "but not that horrific." *"Arrrgghhhhhhhhhhhhhh!"* (I screamed silently in my head and my self-esteem plummeted). I can still remember the digital readout 20 years later – 102.8kg.

Thankfully Emma had waited for me outside of the gym, and consoled me some. Most of all I was so ANGRY with myself for giving in. I should have been stronger. Why was I so vulnerable and weak? This anger became so intense I could not contain it – action had to be taken. That communal, enforced weighing was quite critical at pushing me towards anorexia and away from life. This may or may not seem like a big deal to you, but for me it was a pivotal moment in my life; the passé "last straw." It was the event that grasped from me every last remaining shred of self-belief. It was the event that pushed me almost irrevocably towards anorexia, bulimia and suicide.

My (once again) mixed depressive and manic symptoms worsened, but not so you could tell by my behaviour. I am an expert actress. I was mentally SCREAMING, *"Fuck! Fuck! Fuck off! Away. Go. I want to die. I hate everything!"* Aimed at the whole world but without twitching a muscle. I had perfected my impassive face – I had learned well and young how to keep an exterior that does not represent what lies beneath. I think I was around fourteen when I consciously realised that eating for comfort was not the answer to my problems. I have been searching without success for another answer ever since…

I still didn't know I had manic depression/bipolar disorder, or that my sleep was abnormal, or my furious anger, or my noisy brain were anything out of the ordinary. I knew I felt sad and wired a lot of the time, but I did not know there was an illness called depression or manic depression that might be responsible for my symptoms, and that could be treated. Not only did I feel that I deserved no help, I actually believed that there was no help out there.

I was just a kid. I didn't know what was wrong, but I knew something did not add up. Added to that was a turbulent school life and a mixed up home life. I felt invisible – except at times when I really wanted to be invisible. I was a sensitive, inexperienced, impressionable, vulnerable young girl with nowhere safe to run. I think I wandered around in a dazed manner; hoping lightning would strike me down because I didn't know what else to do. I was searching for an answer: a way, something, *anything* to escape from the symptoms of my altered neurochemistry and distressing life events.

At that stage, I rarely planned in detail how I would end my life. I assumed I would find the strength to cut my wrists in some way and it would be easy. Every day I cried, always alone. Later in life I lost the ability to cry, and lost that outlet for my feelings.

I read about eating disorders, finding them first in teenage magazines. I remember clearly wishing that I could have one just for a while, just until I was thin. I remember telling my mum that I *wanted* to be an anorectic. She told me it would be a bad thing to do, but she did not seem overly alerted. I interpreted that as her dismissing me as ridiculous and that I could not "cut it" as an anorectic. I tend to rise to challenges – perceived or real. I am a goal-oriented person, and I set my goals on anorexia.

I also saw the thin models in magazines I read, and wished I was so elf-like. It was not so much that they were thin: though I admit I did yearn for thinness as a quality in its own right; but it was their exuberance that I truly envied. I thought all my problems would be solved if I were only thin. I discovered the "solution" to the external pressures on me that also happened to serve quite well to numb the manic depression: *starvation.*

Yes: I made an ill-informed but conscious decision that anorexia nervosa was what I wanted to have – only for a while. I knew it lifted my mood and I wanted it to stop the bullying from home and school about my size. I had disordered eating for a while, vomited from time to time, but didn't develop a clear clinical case of anorexia until I was fifteen, though it took me a long time to lose weight enough for people to become concerned. It was around this time that dad offered to pay me five pounds (£) in cash for every pound (lb) of weight I lost. I made quite a lot of money.

The long string of As for my GCSEs gave me some short-lived reassurance that I was, in fact, intelligent and capable of training to be a doctor. During that summer I worked in the Derby City Hospital and the Derby Royal Infirmary to get experience in various departments, the Consultants taking me under their wing so I would take up their specialty. It was great.

On returning to school: we were in smaller Sixth Form classes and I liked all my classmates, but I lost the most special and comforting friend, at what couldn't have come at a worse time. I am not assigning *any* blame to her. Emma had to go: I respect that, what she has achieved, and I love her to pieces. It's just that I lost my closest ally. Then all I had in life was medicine, anorexia, and manic depression (with some bulimia and self-harm). Such would my life be for many years.

Anorexia was, for a very short time, a conscious desire, with *no* comprehension of the pain it would cause for others and myself. I had no idea about the control battleground that is anorexia nervosa. I got what I wished for, seemingly the only controllable form of "happiness" in my life. By sixteen I was anorectic, and occasionally throwing up. Starving myself and losing over half my own body weight worked for me. I actually fitted all of the diagnostic criteria of being anorectic (except the one about being 15% below normal weight) whilst I was still overweight. By seventeen I was skeletal.

Mum tells me that the Headmistress pushed for me to get help (I didn't know this happened). My parents thought it better to "keep it in the family," that I was too clever to hurt myself, and would sort myself out in my own time. But brains give no protection against developing powerful eating disorders and other psychiatric disorders, and brains have no ability to cure them either.

My favourite teacher insisted I seek help, and I ended up seeing a community psychiatric nurse once a week – but only under pressure. I was so scared about having to waste his time seeing him for assessment, because I did not believe I had anorexia, I didn't eat at all for nine days prior to the meeting. My favourite teacher drove me to the appointment and sat with me through it. He asked many questions, then told me I had anorexia nervosa.

I felt not unlike (I imagine) having been smacked around the face with a large wet fish would feel, (like in Monty Python's *"Flying Circus"*). My denial about having anorexia ended in a second. Put simply, he was an expert, he told me I had it, and I believed him. I was told that accepting the illness was the hardest part. Oh how wrong that is! I didn't want to change. I fitted into small clothes and I could see and feel all my bones. I was in control! I never looked in the mirror and saw a fat person, I always knew exactly how thin I was, and I loved it.

He told me that in order for him to help me, I had to stick to simple rules. I had to stop vomiting, and I had to stay within a weight-band, not gaining or losing weight. This seems to me now, decidedly *stupid*: for his instructions were to *remain* at an anorexic weight, and as I was at the top end of the weight-range he gave me, I stopped eating completely until I was at the bottom end instead (loosing another 14lbs). I was then able to tell all concerned that I was perfectly within the limits that had been set by a specialist. Although my weight did drop slightly further, I lied about it, and managed to cease losing any more weight because of a direct threat of hospitalisation. I was determined never to go into a place like that, where boredom and being stuffed by food would surely suffocate me. Oh, little did I know...

However, I did stop vomiting. I drove to see him weekly for a year, but didn't want his help. I went in and said, "I don't want to come anymore." He said, "OK." And that was it. I expected more pressure, but no. So I must be fine? Or perhaps I just don't matter. The first thing I did was drive to the supermarket, buy a sandwich and a tub of ice cream, go home, eat and vomit.

The eating disorder sheltered me quite effectively from the depression. It did nothing for any manic tendencies that I had – my sleep got worse, my anger and irritability sizzled, my disorganised concentration baffled me. I was still sad, but a lot better than before. Losing weight, and being the most ill person in school, gave me a boost because it gave me some control. Eating disorders were endemic in my school, and I was easily the "best" at being ill. I remember thinking how *fabulous* it was to be called thin, too thin, skeleton, bony, anorexic: anything meaning I was not fat. It was impossible to be *too* thin. As is true today, being thin was fashionable. The lower my weight, the better the anorexia worked as an anaesthetic for me, quietening some of the black-noise powering through my mind 24-7.

One way that anorexia did not work for me, was regarding getting into University. As applications were being done, I was repeatedly warned that if I were ill, it would count against me. I can still picture the day I effectively chose anorexia over medicine. My favourite teacher called me to see her, and we discussed my future. I remember having the sense that were I to choose to really try to recover from that day, I would get the necessary reference to win my desired med school place. Unfortunately the illness won, and I was stupidly honest about it. I told her that at the moment I didn't care about anything anymore, which was true. She seemed sad to see that I had "been consumed by my illness." The anorexia made me not care about what was the most important thing in my life, and as such, I lost my dream of becoming a doctor, probably forever. Losing my only dream brought back the depression despite my low weight... Bulimia's anaesthesia loomed, starting slowly at first.

Not to leave my years at Loughborough High School behind without mentioning the people there who loved me as a friend, and helped me as their student. I don't want to name names because not everyone wants their name in a book. To all the other girls at LHS with me, you know who you are. You know if you were kind, you know if you were cruel. My physics teachers were both great, and one teacher in particular was exceptional, my geography and form teacher. Some people have the ability to see through other people's apparently smiling faces, and she was one such person. I often remember her joke about being depressed being referred to as being in a geosyncline. (Which to all non-geographers actually means a large *depression* in the earth).

And so I came of age: I had bipolar I disorder, moving between being depressed or mixed; I had anorexia nervosa, just-starting-to-be-purging type; I was physically weak, suicidal, and rapidly losing hope.

I planned to enter the big wide world starting with Nottingham University, which I got into with top grades; and I could not have been less prepared.

Chapter 2. Nottingham University: ~ "The academic" on the outside and "the mentally destitute" inside where it counts.

"Out, out, brief candle!
Life's but a walking shadow, a poor player
That struts and frets his hour upon the
stage
And then is heard no more; it is a tale
Told by an idiot, full of sound and fury,
Signifying nothing at all."

∾ Nihilism by William Shakespeare in
Macbeth, (Act 5, scene 5).

University is a time where many peoples' worlds collide, careers and characters are built, friendships and even marriages begun. All my life had been preparation for studying medicine at university. That dream was gone, I thought forever. I felt like I had no reason to live or endeavour. I attended University with absolutely no idea what I was doing, what I wanted, and no care about what I did to myself either personally or professionally. Obviously this behaviour was that of a suicidal, depressed, anorectic childlike 19-year old being swallowed into the darkness of her mind. I hated being a person with anorexia, but the illness was also my closest friend.

I still didn't know I was clinically depressed (let alone bipolar). It was a bitter existence: every morning I awoke and cried because I had not died in my sleep. I wanted to vanish mysteriously from the world, and never be found, though I lacked the clarity of thought to come up with a decent suicide plan. Instead I disappeared metaphorically. I suppose I also disappeared literally, just a little bit more each day. I wrapped my shrinking body in layers of clothing to hide my perceived weakness and to stop anyone helping me. I was afraid of help and hospitalisation. I also hid my illness because I wanted to protect those I loved from the pain of seeing me in all my sorrow. I could see the infirmity in my face and body. I knew I was thin; I saw a skeleton in the mirror. I knew I was ill, but I did not understand why.

A person's university years are supposed to be amongst the best years of their life; at least that is what I had always been brought up to believe. I never even considered the possibility of not going: it was expected of me by my family and even more strictly demanded by myself, that I would succeed academically. Only I really had any concept of how ill I was, and I still did not comprehend the depths of my problems by a long shot. The only thing I still had any confidence in was my intellectual capability. But I was supposedly studying chemistry, which I hated purely because it was not medicine.

The University of Nottingham is a top British university: absolutely first class, the main campus set in the beautiful University Parks near the city centre of Nottingham, a city most famous for the tales of Robin Hood. I already knew the University and area well, as it is only about fifteen miles from my parental home – though it might as well have been in another country – I was free to starve and self-destruct.

I originally wanted to go to university far away, but when I visited Nottingham for interview, I instinctively felt it was the right place for me. This gut feeling proved to be right in ways I could never have predicted.

When I arrived, I noticed very quickly that I was amongst highly intelligent people, who also had common sense and a wonderful down-to-earth attitude. You don't always get people blessed with common sense and intelligence together. I lack common sense!

I didn't drink alcohol at all before I went to Nottingham, but spent the first two weeks totally pissed, as is fairly standard for initiation into university studentship. I was unused to alcohol so it hit me hard, and of course, I drank on an empty stomach. In fact, I spent most of year one at least merry, if not pissed. I'd only drink vodka, which I hated, but it had the least calories in it compared to other drinks. It was the start of a slightly complicated relationship with alcohol.

I am weird. I don't like the flavour of any alcoholic drink, (except champagne!) but I soon noticed that if I had had at least a couple of vodkas, I would "sleep," or at least be unconscious with fitful, violent dreams. Alcohol was my first, (poor) remedy to the years of torturous insomnia. There was certainly the potential for drink to become yet another problem, but fortunately it didn't, mostly because I was too concerned with calories. However, it was the beginning of my powerful compulsion to avoid consciousness whenever possible, and whatever the physical, psychological, legal, and monetary costs. There are many ways to seek oblivion, with or without the intent for death: I sought them all, starting with anorexia, bulimia, drinking and abusing my position as a chemistry student.

My hall of residence was Rutland Hall. For the first week or so, going out with my floor-mates, being drunk, claiming to feel ill to get out of eating: I had a good time. I'll never forget the men trying to persuade us girls to do their ironing for them, pleading incapacity and ignorance. We mostly laughed at them. As a pragmatic feminist *I* never gave in! I remember one of the lads, a law student, probably now a top lawyer, tried to iron his trousers by putting them vertically against the wall, and ironing up and down.

Fairly soon people in my corridor realised I was ill. I claimed to be vegetarian and allergic to cheese, so that I got less calorific food, most of which I didn't eat anyway. Within the Autumn Term (i.e. under 10 weeks) I quickly dropped from 9st (128lbs, BMI [10]17.9) to 7st (98lbs, BMI 13.7), and then seemed stuck at this weight.

A large part of me wanted to die: self-starvation was a passive way to achieve this. A way my family would not have to face my suicide. Only I could choose whether to seek help or not; I was now an adult, and although the reality of the ingenuity of anorexia nervosa and its terrific powers of entrapment were finally sinking in, I was still determined to keep things on "my" terms. I suppose really it was on "my anorexia's" terms.

> *"Anorexia is just another name for 'I've nothing else left to lose.' Even the food and weight control is a mirage. In fact, anorexia controls me and forces my slow suicide. But some how it feels too*

---

[10] BMI = Body Mass Index, a ratio of weight to height that gives an idea of the right weight for a certain height. It is calculated by dividing the weight in kg with the height in m^2. A BMI within the range of 19-25 is "normal." Under 17.5 is anorexic, over 30 is obese.

genuine and comfortable to be
dangerous. And that is the
delusion."

  Katy Culling, age 19,
University of Nottingham Diary,
November, 1994.

Nottingham University has a modular theme. This means that whilst chemistry was compulsory, I could choose other classes as well, and I filled my time. Of course I chose those courses medical students needed, and so, would attend physiology and pharmacology lectures. I fairly soon stopped going to chemistry lectures, and instead buried myself in the medical school or alternatively stayed in my room, Rutland Hall K-block (with en-suite bathrooms) for days, spending the time eating and throwing up. Not much fun.

The only area the chemistry department kept a close eye on, were the practical classes every Tuesday and Friday morning for 4 hours a stretch. You *had* to attend and they took a register. I've always been really good with my hands, and practical work came naturally. Some of the academically brightest students were all fingers and thumbs; setting things on fire, spearing their hands with glass pipettes, spilling "stuff," and so on. My 1st year lab partner has a brilliant mind and has gone on to great things in the world of chemistry starting with a PhD, whereas when he was a little 1st year, I had to help him set up his work in labs! (He even set fire to his gorgeous hair).

Organic chemistry labs gave me a precarious opportunity: dangerous and potentially lethal chemicals at my disposal. I'd looked for potassium cyanide in the inorganic chemistry labs without luck, which angered me, but then had a gruesome idea. A friend of mine died as a teenager, the first time he inhaled gas trying to get high; I decided chloroform, as an anaesthetic, must be far more perilous. I knew that its use as an anaesthetic in medicine had been stopped because it had an unfortunate tendency to kill people. I stole lots; each bottle with a skull and crossbones motif warning how hazardous this chemical was.

And so, depressed, not manic, I tried to put myself to sleep – permanently. This was not an act of desperation due to insomnia: this was attempted suicide. I poured a liberal quantity of chloroform on to a cloth, and lay back on my bed, the cloth flat over my face so it would not fall off once I lost consciousness. (I lay flat because I feared that otherwise it might fall off whilst I slept and therefore *not* kill me). Needless to say, it didn't work; and thankfully I did not stop to consider whether an alternative route of administration might be more lethal – something I would think of nowadays.

I tried again, daily or twice daily, forever increasing the dose; I tried mixing the chloroform with being drunk; I tried taping the cloth to my face in a smothering fashion. I did lose consciousness every time, and survived every time: although I was as sick as a dog. I did this a minimum of sixty times; I only stopped when the smell of chloroform made me instantly vomit and I was so weak and sick I could take it no longer. I was at the lowest weight I'd ever "achieved" through anorexia, and must have looked like Death walking. Apart from losing consciousness when using chloroform to attempt suicide I did not sleep, not unless I drank first. I was a complete wreck, and it took me less than ten weeks of independence away from home to reach a stage of physical and emotional collapse. Of course, I didn't tell anyone – a lot was visible – yet nothing done. I should have learned by then that I was the only person who could help myself.

One thing that started happening around this time was the sense that I was in the presence of someone or something dangerous – not lethally dangerous, no, it felt like I was at risk of emotional and physical pain. I did not actually see anything, I did not hear voices, but I felt like there was someone following me most of the time. If I was alone in my room, I felt he/it was in there with me, sometimes breathing down the back of my neck. This was of course, very disturbing, perplexing and frightening. I did not understand what was going on, and I put it down to lack of sleep. Looking back, perhaps it was more – paranoia, or even the beginning of psychosis. (I was not using drugs).

After the Christmas break, with the depression that was psychotic, things continued on their downward trajectory. I didn't actively attempt suicide, I was too depressed by that point... but I spent all day and night thinking about it. I started cutting my arm again, was sick every other day, drank every night, and with the exception of physiology and pharmacology, stopped doing any work or going to classes.

The other students on my corridor had lost patience with me – something that unfortunately happens quite quickly to people with mental illnesses. At first some tried to be supportive, encouraging me to go see a doctor. It has been my unfortunate experience that people lose patience with eating disorders *very* fast; especially where friendships or ties are not already strong, or knowledge born of similar suffering is lacking. In the face of something so incomprehensible and seemingly stupid, where you feel powerless to help, it is an understandable, if unfortunate, response. However, *bullying* me was not an acceptable alternative.

When I left high school, I thought I had left the years of bullying behind me. My corridor of student friends all seemed perfect to me at first, and I imagined life-long friendships. Ten years on and I can't remember most of their names, nor do I want to. One day, at a student party, it dawned on me that for the first time in my life *I* was in the trendy clique who everyone wanted to know and be with.

When I introduced Henry, one of my chemistry buddies, to my "friends" they were rude and dismissive. Had I wanted an easy life, I would have allowed them to mistreat Henry just because he had long red hair – but that is not the sort of person I am. I told them their behaviour was unacceptable and why; thus starting a rift between myself, and the governing clique member, who lead all the other students like subservient pets. Never again did they knock at my door to see if I was coming to tea, or to the bar, to the sports hall, or for anything. The next night, they all went out and did not invite me. I watched from behind my curtains as they sauntered off with their self-righteous walks, all dressed up for a night out. I felt lonely and cried, but I have never regretted my decision.

"All cruelty springs from weakness."

≈ Lucius Annaeus Seneca[11] (5 BC - 65
AD).

Then began the active bullying. Calling me names
because I had anorexia; throwing away or eating my
food from our shared fridge; humiliating me in the
dining hall by sniggering, name calling or stealing food
off my plate. I took to storing my fat-free yoghurts and
milk on my windowsill because they were all I was
eating, and if I left them in the fridge I'd find them
smashed or empty in the bin. I started hiding in my
room until everyone was out, avoiding meeting any of
them in the corridor. Once I warmed some carrot soup
whilst they were all out at dinner, when they arrived
back there were deliberately loud shouts outside my
door about the disgusting smell of cooking – resulting
in my soup being discarded by myself because I was
"obviously" unworthy of it.

One night, having managed to doze off slightly, I was
awakened by a thumping sound at my third floor
window. I looked out: nothing. Then just as I was about
to look away I saw a sheet that had been knotted and
weighted at one end with a boot, swinging towards my
window. Someone (I know who) was hanging out of
my neighbour's window, and had succeeded in
smashing all my yoghurts and milk off my windowsill.

The cruelty of this act still bemuses me somewhat. I
cannot comprehend one decent human soul thinking it

---

[11] Spanish-born Roman, stoic philosopher, playwright, tutor then
statesman to Emperor Nero; who ultimately ordered him to
commit suicide. He severed veins and arteries in his arms then legs
in a bath, then drank poison (hemlock), and ultimately died from
suffocation in a steam bath. Is ordered suicide, under pain of death,
still suicide?

funny. Intelligent people would surely grasp the consequences of this cruelty. Did they lack a conscience? They knew me to have anorexia, had seen me struggle to eat daily, and they had just destroyed my whole week's food knowing it would take me a considerable 2 mile walk in the freezing cold to replenish my stock, that's *if* I dared leave my room at all. They had also unwittingly (I hope unwittingly) restored my faith in my delusion that I did not deserve to eat.

One good thing that came of this was that I was so low in mood that I did not have the necessary energy with which to attempt suicide. There was none of the energy that accompanies mania. Also, the pig-headed part of me was determined not to die at that point in my life because then those cunts would know that they had upset me. I would not let them win. I was under no illusion that my suicide might be some quixotic gesture that would "teach them a lesson" and "make them better people." Instead I went to see the campus doctor and told him about my sleep problems. He weighed me and seemed unconcerned by my emaciated presence (something else which still bemuses me). I wanted sleeping pills, but I got fluoxetine (prozac). Apparently I had depression. No shit Sherlock.

So, well over a decade after I first developed some kind of mood disorder, I received antidepressant medication and had some inkling (deep) in my mind that anorexia may just be a symptom of deeper problems. I don't remember suddenly worrying that I was depressed, rather I suddenly considered it as a rather unimportant co-disorder that came with my anorexia. I had no real frame of reference for feeling "normal" with which to help me understand my emotions.

Alarmingly, the sixty-plus recent suicide attempts didn't really register in my brain as something to be worried about or mention to my GP. I think my vague awareness of low mood became apparent because I had started to vomit more regularly, and doing so distressed me greatly. It gave me a reason (I mistakenly thought there *had* to be a good reason) for having a low mood, but I did not know I was depressed when I walked in to see the doctor. He wrote a prescription and told me to keep filling it without the need to see him again: 20mg of Fluoxetine a day. The lowest dose of what was then, the *in vogue* drug of choice. It did absolutely fuck all for the depression, didn't affect my bulimia, gave me headaches, and made my insomnia worse. (That's not to say it isn't a great medication for some people).

I have to admit, the eating disorder was more powerful than any drug I've tried (which is a few) to anaesthetize my senses – which was always my aim. Detached. Impassive. Emotionless. Frozen. Deadened. Numb. Nothingness was my endeavour and the price was high. It was a compelling mind game; clamping down hard on all my feelings; forever burying more and more memories deep in my brain logically and faithfully, just like an archivist might proficiently store historical records: for later retrieval and rumination. Nothing was missed, nothing resolved, nothing forgotten.

This meant that the most forceful emotions I felt were those I experienced each morning when I stepped on the weighing scales. The result was always one of three unsatisfactory results, which set the pace for my whole day. <u>One</u>: *"Yippee I am a good person I've lost weight;*

I must strive to remain strong; and to be safe maybe I should only eat half a cup-a-soup for lunch instead of a whole one." <u>Two</u>: *"Damn, I'm the same weight; I must try harder; I'd better not eat unless I throw up."* And <u>three</u>: *"Fuuucck! I've gone up half a pound; no food or liquid shall pass my lips until I've lost weight; and I'll be off for a run now, despite my badly recovering fractured ankle due to osteoporosis."*

I spent the rest of that academic year throwing up my student grant and hiding from all the students in my corridor. At first, I rather arrogantly thought that people who ate food and did not vomit were stupid and deserved to gain weight or be fat. I am not sure how, probably thanks to reading Henry's lecture notes and a perfect practical score, I passed the first year exams and put in for an immediate transfer to a biomedical/biological sciences course, specialising in physiology, biochemistry and nutrition.

I also moved back into my parental home, screaming in my head, and prepared to start afresh, being a good student with new friends and tried to stop the tumultuous bulimia, which raged through my life unlike anything I can describe to someone who has not "been there." The bulimia proved impossible to live with or without, tearing me between life and death on a minute-by-minute basis. It's no wonder then that my nerves were frazzled beyond repair, self-harm and suicide soon beckoned once again.

"The thought of suicide is a great
consolation: by means of it one gets
successfully through many a bad night."

Katy Sara Culling

∾ Friedrich Nietzche, *Beyond Good and Evil*

Here my life split into the lives of two separate people. On one side there was the fake me: "Kate" the good student who was always punctual (to the lectures she was interested in), coursework and exams all going very well. Energetic, bouncy, "happy," chatty... But if you really looked, you could see the sleepless expression in her eyes, she was thin, so very thin, her clothes baggy, and the parotid glands on her face were swollen from all the vomiting. If you looked closely you would notice that she was always moving about, never stopping, never at peace. She arrived on campus from an unknown place, was pleasant, funny, caring and had all the answers in lectures. She'd blabber on about football, sounding confident. Then she would disappear, sometimes in the middle of the day. Or maybe she wouldn't show up at all.

The other 23 hours of the day were taken up by my eating disorder that was very effectively masking the bipolar disorder. I had a long and nasty melancholic depressive episode that lasted for... I can't really say... a long the time... all the time? Mania bubbled in and out of my life at all times, and I never had a moment of peace or decent sleep. The confidence I wore outdoors melted like snow under a blowtorch as soon as I stepped though the front door at home, and I became a nervous wreck: anxious, grouchy, angry, sad, at times bingeing and vomiting, at times drunk, many times suicidal, but just too low to bother doing anything with those suicidal thoughts.

Coping with living me was hell for my family, (remembering that none of us are good at coping with emotions). We've since spoken about their fear and upset: I can see how they all had a taste of my hellish nightmare, but it was only that, a taste. They weren't living 24 hours a day in utter exhaustion, in anger, with such self-hatred, low-moods, and a busy mind going: "*Excuse me, hello, don't forget me, hello, you despicable excuse for a human, die, die, hello, are you still listening, coz you should, you fat cow, sleep – ha, you don't get to sleep. Boo! There did you think I'd let you rest? Do some work, cut yourself, blood, blood is good, die, food, die, food, food, fat, binge, vomit, food, no rest for the wicked, no rest for the wicked...*" It was like an evil football commentary running in my head non-stop that I could not turn it off.

If I did sleep I dreamt about food – often waking in a panic that I had eaten something "forbidden." The worst dreams were ones where I dreamed I had binged but was prevented from purging. I daydreamed about death, lived in paralysing fear of almost everything, with self-disgust, anxiety, and in such *pain* that I thought my heart would burst at any moment; and I would have welcomed that end.

I was slicing my arm with a razor blade regularly, though I cannot give you any reason as to why. I don't remember getting anything positive from cutting, I just did it, almost robotically. Sometimes there is no tenable or tangible reason behind self-harm, it just "is." In fact, my eating disorder (as a form of self-harm) became such a superb distraction from my suicidal ideation: it saved my life somewhat obstinately. If bingeing, barfing, starving, cutting, and being in constant fear can be considered to be "useful" coping mechanisms, which for me they sort-of-were: they repeatedly saved my life. Only later would my eating disorder's presence be so repulsive to me that it alone was grounds for suicide. Many days I wouldn't make it in to University because the bingeing took over. I was still very underweight, not sleeping even with a shot or few of vodka, and an emotional and physical wreck. Thank goodness for Dr. Carol M.P. McGrath.

Scared to see another doctor after the idiot I saw on campus, I dragged myself, age 20, to see my new GP in Castle Donington. I think of this as the first time I genuinely wanted help and mostly recognised the mess I was in, although I focused on eating and placed too little emphasis on the depression and didn't recognise manic symptoms. I told her the truth. I admitted the anorexia, the bulimia, the suicidal thoughts, and eventually showed her my left forearm which was red raw from self-harm.

I suppose I entered our patient-doctor relationship in a very all-or-nothing way. I had nothing left to lose except my life, and that was acceptable to me, especially if there were even the smallest sign from Dr. McGrath that I deserved to die. That did not mean she would have to say or even think anything like that; it means I would be ultra-sensitive and possibly assume it if Dr. McGrath said anything that questioned my value as a fellow human being. It meant I went in there looking for an excuse: for her to tell me nothing could be done, that I was bad, or that I needed to go because she only had 10 minutes per patient. I was looking out for any sign. An exasperated look in her eye or stern tone to her voice would have been too much for me to cope with. *Perhaps I was looking for permission to die, and holding my hand out to be helped, at one and the same time.*

As it happened, I was treated with the utmost respect, empathy, importance and without pressure. Dr. McGrath's approach was gentle and humanistic. I could find no fault, and left her room feeling *just enough* that I mattered. The fluoxetine was upped to 60mg to day, the normal dose for bulimia – though it did not help the depression, insomnia or bulimia. I was also immediately referred for eating disorder psychotherapy, and encouraged by Dr. McGrath to see her regularly and as often as I wanted. An offer I took up, seeing her at the end of surgery on Fridays. People giving me their time is something I have always seen as the most precious gift possible. The only thing I wanted but was too afraid to ask for at the time was sleeping medication.

The bulimia disgusted and exhausted me, yet I could not stop. I don't think there was a single occasion that I hovered over the toilet bowl without willing my heart to pack in and end it all. I may not have been ready to give up anorexia, but I desperately wanted to stop the binge-vomit cycle. Bulimia was the most appallingly addictive experience I have had, far outweighing cigarettes, booze, benzodiazpines or heroin. I was absolutely on the edge of suicide but back in that stage of depression where you simply do not have the energy to kill yourself. Instead, I somehow maintained my academic achievements with minimal effort (if any), and continued vomiting whilst waiting nine long months to get to the top of the *NHS* list for eating disorder therapy at Leicester.

Every time I vomited I vowed earnestly that it would be the last time. Then, as I washed out my stomach with water over and over, the desire to repeat the whole thing all over again would swoop in and take over my body, and before I knew it I would be stuffing my face. At night, as I lay there sleeplessly, I would swear that tomorrow would be different. Bingeing was always on my mind; I would fight the urge, then I would snap. For what was an impulsive act, it was controlled with inhuman strength due to my fear of being caught, and worst of all, prevented from vomiting after I had eaten. I'd never risk being in public where I could get caught. I never kept food at home to binge on.

Whenever the urge became too strong, (which was daily and usually when nobody else was home), I'd go to the supermarket, the warped excitement building within me, looking at all the food, visually feeding my desires for what I craved. Even the process of thinking about food, choosing food, and imagining eating it, fitted some twisted need to quieten my brain from other thoughts I could not handle. I'd spend money I didn't really have on enough food to binge (fully) and vomit (fully) three times. By that I mean it would take many episodes of vomiting to empty all I could from my stomach – probably 30 vomits per session – all of that done 3 separate times after 3 separate binges. Doing this I would disappear into oblivion as certainly as had an anaesthetist put me under with a general anaesthetic. It was a temporary cure for my bipolarity.

I'd physically feed my emotional craving for mental numbness by stuffing myself with soft foods that were easy to vomit; then I'd be painfully full; then bending over the toilet dreading what had to be done; then vomiting; then washing out; then washing out some more; then collapsing on the floor in a dizzy, shaking mess; often wondering if I was dying; constantly hoping I was about to die. (None of this is counted in my suicide tally). All of this over and over again:

hiding it from my family as much as possible, knowing deep down that they knew exactly what was going on. Trying to grab a few hours here and there to study. Looking back now I don't know how I fitted it all in. It was all so... so... draining, hectic and totally fucked-up. I was far beyond being out of control, I had totally lost the plot.

I loved and hated my eating disorder all at once. I think I hated it more than I loved it, but it did have some aspects that I needed with which to survive on at the time – namely holding the bipolar disorder at bay. I loved the first three bites of food from a binge. I loved being thin. I still never looked in the mirror and saw a fat person: I knew I was thin. Sometimes so thin and weak that the world often swirled away for me, I had to stop, breathe in and out, calm my thumping heart and then carry on. I would drive to Nottingham and be physically unable to walk to class. I even "liked" being weak, as it brought me closer to death – I wanted to be closer to death, life was too everlasting. I felt like nothing could harm me. When you have anorexia you can almost convince yourself that you can sustain your life like that right up until the end when you gracefully disappear without trace. Of course, it is never so dignified.

Bulimia is different. Shoving your head down the toilet and retching out your stomach contents for hours at a time is kind of hard to ignore. You can't fool yourself that it is acceptable behaviour or something that you really want to do. This insight into bulimia's entrapment is one reason why depression is so common in bulimia nervosa. Although my purging lowered my mood, it still held the deepest depression at bay because the bingeing, vomiting, planning to binge, or trying to avoid it, deadened all my feelings. It was a very potent form of oblivion for me. An expensive, time-consuming, dangerous, unpleasant, unglamorous, painful form of nothingness: but oblivion none the less. If I believed in a god then I would say bulimia is (no pun intended) a sick joke of hers. Consider the irony of people using bulimia to seek temporary oblivion: to find nothingness, usually to escape from the emptiness they feel inside. To me that's just filling one hole with an even bigger hole.

Dr. Andrew M. Salter, Andy to all his students, was for me, the link between my dark life and my life in academia. He is now a Professor of Nutritional Biochemistry and it was he who fired my interest in human metabolism, particularly lipid (fat) metabolism. He also supported me when I was quite obviously *not* OK, and understood when I needed time off. Without him I would not have stayed at University, let alone have done very well.

I also managed to get the attention of Professor Ian A. Macdonald, the Head of Biomedical Sciences, who was lecturing metabolic physiology. In the lectures he asked lots of questions to try and make the students think, but nobody answered except me (even if I waited before putting my hand up). I like to think I demonstrated my ability to apply my scientific knowledge and *some* common sense to my understanding of physiology and medical disorders because that was all that I did - I used my head.

With Andy's permission, I persuaded Prof. Macdonald to let me do my final year research project with him in the Medical School with human volunteers, the subject matter: alcohol.

It's odd what trivial food related facts eating disorders make you remember. I remember thinking it odd that Andy, a top nutrition expert ate (aghast) white bread sandwiches and (evil, fatty) salt and vinegar crisps for lunch. Obsessions with food are normal for a brain undergoing starvation, as is becoming fanatical about food, and judgemental about other people's food choices. My eyes followed food around the room, distracting me from anything else. Such frequent, intrusive thoughts may impede painful thoughts and issues, *but they block out everything good as well.*

Then I finally got to the top of the *NHS* waiting list. The first thing that happened at Leicester General Hospital was that I saw a psychiatrist who swapped me from fluoxetine to the tricyclic lofepramine to alleviate the blatant depression that I still wasn't taking seriously because I didn't appreciate its importance. I assumed lofepramine was chosen, as it is less dangerous than some other tricyclics in overdose. However, it is saf*er*, not safe.[12] I don't think it particularly helped my mood, but I stopped drinking alcohol. I'd like to claim that was a sane and healthy choice that I chose to make, but in honesty, I felt so ill if I drank whilst on lofepramine that I had no choice but to stop.

My therapist was actually a clinical nurse specialist; she was young, quite kind and soft-spoken, but I felt no connection. I was her last appointment on a Wednesday afternoon, and she was always just a bit too keen to end the session and go home, even when it should have be blatantly obvious that I needed her help (time). We always started late despite the fact I was always waiting

---

[12] Portrayed in *4:48 Psychosis* by Sarah Kane; as given to me by Zee when I lived in Oxford, although the OD didn't kill her, she actually hanged herself.

early, and with one exception we had always finished and I had been ushered out by 4.55pm. To me that signalled that I was just a job to her: unimportant, unworthy, and it lacked respect of myself as a deserving person.

Of course, my low self-esteem may have been a factor in my assumptions there, but people with anorexia are sensitive to small issues – which I expected her to know, so I assumed she didn't care. I also felt like I was not a "good" enough anorectic for her. Because I am so tall, my weight never sounded that low, even though for my height, it was desperately problematic. I hated being weighed at the beginning of every session: triggering of memories of my dad weighing me, and thoughts that I was fat and useless. Progress was decidedly absent.

At the end of my second year on my new course at Nottingham, I told Andy and Prof. Macdonald about my anorexia (I neglected to mention that it was purging-type). Andy looked surprised but the Prof. had known all along. It was then agreed with Dr. McGrath, Andy, Prof. Macdonald and my Leicester therapist that I would spend time over summer and four weeks into my third year as a day patient in the Leicester General Hospital Eating Disorders Day Unit. What fun (not).

I could go on for pages about the Day Unit but I wont. It was well set-up, if a bit claustrophobic; the staff were great, the patients wonderful. I did not respond well to the control the staff assumed, being generally angry and non-conformist, but I did as I was told and ate what was placed before me. We were not given a choice in that matter, which actually made it easier to eat. The food was bland, repetitive, and portioned out for you. Drinking two glasses of water with each meal was compulsory. The patients ate on one big table whilst being watched by at least three members of staff who just stood around and watched, which was rather off-putting, but everyone coped – mainly by the patients helping each other through.

Talking about food whilst at the table was absolutely banned, and there was rarely any discussion about difficulties with eating afterwards; the emphasis was on distraction and "just getting on with it." There was a time limit within which we had to finish everything, even our water, or it was treated as a "refusal" to eat. The place operated on a three strikes and you are out basis; three refusals of any kind resulted in being sent to see "god," (Dr. Bob Palmer, consultant psychiatrist, hairy beard and brilliant). After meals we had to sit in the room for 45 minutes to stop you throwing up (yeah, like that's long enough). I certainly threw up, and I know others did. But very importantly: this day treatment did help stop me bingeing.

I was fond of all of the patients, but one in particular, Julie Potter-Tate, became and remains a lifelong friend. I call her Julius, (OK, Julius-Woolius to be precise) and we were "the two people there who self-harmed," although mine was well hidden until I spotted hers and consequently showed her mine. She was an inpatient, at times sectioned, attempting suicide twice whilst I was there: once found by me on the toilet floor with cut wrists. We understand each other without needing to speak. Here's how she describes me now, thinking back to then:

> "I remember you came one Monday morning. My first thought when you came was 'oh no not

another twig.' I was surprised that you wanted to know me when I found out about your background. I remember you coming all that way to see me on Christmas day when I was alone in hospital, and it really meant a lot to me. I thought you were a genuine friend from then on. I loved chatting with you and I felt somehow connected to you, don't know why! I remember you wore purple a lot.

You didn't have much respect for your therapist or Dr. Palmer. I presumed because you didn't agree with their theories and methods. I thought you came there with an attitude that they weren't going to help you, but not because they couldn't if you understand me, but because you knew more than them. Also, you weren't gonna let anyone in. You were very angry with them and most people.

I liked you because you listened to me and we could talk about self-harm without prejudice. You diced your food in salt to make it taste bad; I did the same with pepper. I liked the banter we used to have about football. I remember calling you a Derby sheep-shagger and you laughing and saying something worse about Forest F.C.

You made me laugh with some of the stuff you said about that place – identifying all the bureaucratic bollocks, and the way they treated patients like children so that when they left they weren't ready for the outside world.

I think you have every right to be angry about many things you've told me happened to you - I would never have been so forgiving. But you are wrong to be angry with yourself, none of what happened is your fault."

Julie's perceptions of me are accurate. I may have eaten when told to, but generally I was resistant to help: I threw up a lot and exercised like mad before and after hospital. Another patient there, Claire, was even madder on exercise than me, and we used to talk a lot about running. She sat next to Julius at the table, across from me: we all tried to help each other get through meals. I remember she was mad on fruit, and would eat apples I brought in from our garden. She died from her anorexia just after her 30th Birthday. Next to me sat a very quiet, gentle young woman with anorexia and OCD (Obsessive Compulsive Disorder). She hid it well, it took me five weeks to realise that she was scrubbing the sink 30 times every time she went near one. I was just as fond of other patients there, but do not feel I can write about them without their permission.

I actually started to lose weight, though they never knew that because I resorted to the tricks I had read about in so many anorexia autobiographies. I'd drink lots of water, weigh myself down with heavy clothes, and have bags of coins and stones in my pockets. The experts congratulated me for doing well and looking better, (which in *anorexic-speak* means *looking fatter*). The only person to outwardly disagree was Dr. McGrath. When I told her, (taking care to *not* essentially lie), that *the hospital scales said* I had reached my target BMI of 20, she shook her head in disbelief and said "No."

All the anorectics would try to exercise when they thought nobody was watching. Towards the end of my time there Julie used to be allowed out to walk in the hospital grounds with me for about 15 minutes, and I (in theory) had to stop her running. After my fleeting ten weeks on the day programme I went back to University, but could not cope with my mood, I couldn't work or think, and I felt too far behind: so I took a year out to try and sort myself out. My therapist was furious with me for that decision, which pretty set in concrete the headstone at the burial site of our professional relationship. But I remained polite, appeared contrite, and kept seeing her because I didn't know what else to do.

Although not technically a student, I spent that year in the Medical School working on my alcohol studies with Prof. Macdonald, which I enjoyed, although I was very stressed. If I wasn't in the metabolic laboratory, I was sat downstairs in the Medical Library because I knew I had to get myself out of the house. I didn't just research alcohol, I read widely: torn between a love of physiology and psychology, which, of course, overlap in so many areas. The Prof. told me he thought I should go in to research and do a Ph.D. His confidence in my abilities gave me a very crucial boost in morale, at what could not of been a better time.

The rest of my time I spent gradually gaining some weight and vomiting less and less. I did this by creating my own secret diet (not recommended) of drinking Baileys Irish Cream. Then I gritted my teeth, and put my stubborn nature to better use, and found strength of mind, helped by Dr. McGrath. I saw my therapist less and less and was discharged despite the fact I had not actually improved anything but my bulimia. (Which was a tremendous achievement, but so much else was still wrong). It was an example of a very common misapprehension – people mistakenly assume weight gain is the only, or best, sign of recovery, when in actual fact it means very little and can be faked.

My diet was fat-free yoghurts, branflakes and Baileys Irish Cream. Assuming recovery is marked only by weight gain is a potentially fatal flaw, and unacceptable with the insights we now have about eating disorders. I felt like my therapist couldn't wait to get rid of me, which may well be true. That I was discharged whilst still so ill makes me very angry on behalf of myself and other sufferers, but it was actually the only way forward for me since I had lost all trust and respect for my therapist.

That winter I went to see Julius in hospital on Christmas day because I couldn't allow her to be alone in a psychiatric ward on Christmas day with no visitors. It didn't even enter my head that one day in my future, I'd spend Christmas in hospital on suicide watch. No visitors.

Over my year off, I stopped vomiting completely. I still desperately wanted to binge all the time, but didn't. It wasn't an overnight thing, but gradually I was able to focus more on the pain and disgust of having to vomit, than on the food and oblivion I craved. Then I just stopped. This success boosted me quite considerably for a period. I had what I wanted, no bulimia, and just enough anorexia to be thin without being overly weak and skeletal. You'd have thought that after all those years I would have learnt that there is no such thing as having anorexia and being in control of it, instead of vice versa. I suppose that was fairly arrogant of me, but it felt so real, and I hadn't actually dealt with any issues in therapy, nor helped my latent bipolar disorder.

Before I knew it was time to go back and be a full-time student again. My final year flew past. I maintained a weight of approximately 10 stone (140lbs, at 5'11'' a BMI of 19.5) technically low for my height, and under the "magical" BMI of 20 that eating disorder clinics like their clients to achieve, but the numbers seemed quite large enough to me. I preferred to be 9st 13lbs (139lbs) than 10st because it felt like such a large jump.

Physically I was quite well, existing on yoghurt, milk, bran cereal, tuna and salad. I'd cut the Bailey's to stop further weight gain. I worked hard on my alcohol project, which interested me in research and included learning medical procedures. I also worked hard-ish on all the other subjects that interested me, mainly physiology, nutrition and some areas of biochemistry, which fortunately was enough for me to do very well indeed. Perfectionism demanded a First *and* being top of the year. Despite being absent for most of the first two years of my course: I graduated proudly and successfully in the Summer of 1999.

☙

I think, on that day, I felt my parents were really proud of me.

❧

And so ended my Nottingham University years – years that I avoided becoming a suicide statistic purely by chance and lack of "helpful" research into how to kill myself efficiently. My mood disorder (bipolarity) remained unrecognised, my anorexia improved, my bulimia gone but not forgotten.

As a result of the near 2 years in the med school, an excellent degree, and two amazing references, one from Andy and one from Prof. Ian Macdonald: I was offered a Ph.D. or as they call it at Oxford and Cambridge, a D.Phil. studentship studying Clinical Medicine at the University of Oxford. This was an amazing achievement, working clinically, pushing my brain into action enough to calm it. Close enough to being a medical doctor, which was my real but suppressed ambition. I thought a D.Phil. from Oxford would look quite good on a medical school application in a few years time. I didn't know I would grow to love research itself.

Outwardly I appeared relatively normal and was obviously academically up to the challenge of Oxford. I was exceedingly proud of my achievements, as were Nanny Betty and the rest of my family. If anyone any fears about my health they were not mentioned. Dr McGrath had small tears of happiness in her eyes when I told her. Here I was a reformed anorectic/bulimic/self-harmer who was "better" and going to Oxford. She hugged me goodbye. I wasn't recovered, but I was improved, which I felt she understood. I felt the best I had in a long time, apart from the depression, which I could hold at bay if I kept busy.

I packed up and moved away from my home in the East Midlands, and headed south to Oxford University and the Department of Clinical Medicine. It's at this point that things start getting really scary.

The remains of my story takes place in OXFORD at the University of Oxford.

Chapter 3. Oxford, The Early Years.

"I wonder anybody does anything at
Oxford but dream and remember, the
place is so beautiful. One almost expects
the people to sing instead of speaking. It
is all . . . like an opera."

     ❧   Yeats (1865-1939), letter to
        Katharine Tynan in 1888.

Oxford is truly beautiful and awesome: I loved it from day one – helped along by euphoric mania. A tree-friendly city, filled with old, substantial buildings, charismatic gargoyles and grounds, all of which are beautiful and alluring. Everything seemed so solid, with history and tradition oozing from every ancient brick. The famous "City of Dreaming Spires," and *I* lived there, *I* studied there: it was like an unbelievable dream that I expected to wake up from with a sharp bump.

One of the most ethereal Oxford experiences comes from a custom dating back to the sixteenth century means that the choir sings to the crowd from the top of Magdalen Tower every May Day morning, as the sun slowly rises through the mist at dawn: forcing police to stop excitable students jumping off the Magdalen bridge into the River Cherwell – in frenzied celebration, not to harm themselves. It is an experience not to be missed.

You became used to tourists photographing you when you are paraded through town in your academic gown, such as for Matriculation: a service held in Latin at the Sheldonian theatre, which welcomed new University members. There followed a speech telling us that we were the most privileged people in the world – haughty but true. We were told to study hard and play hard: to enjoy and not waste our student years at the University of Oxford. Mortarboards with gowns and *sub fusc* (yes, more Latin, meaning sombre clothing) were expected for particular events and exams. All Oxford men take pride that they can tie "proper" bowties. There were commoner gowns for the undergraduates (which are short) and graduate gowns for the likes of me, flowing down to my ankles.

After final exams, students were subjected to a celebratory shower of flour, eggs and champagne: wandering around the City in their christened academic gowns grinning whilst heading to favourite Oxford pubs like the King's Arms and The Turf. Sombre statues heads in Broad Street were decorated by students after exams, crowned using traffic cones; which always made me grin deeply as I cycled past. Every year the students would do it, probably thinking they were the first. Some of the statue heads were very high, and I wondered how they managed to reach them. After a week or so, someone would take them down. Everywhere there were wonderful, intelligent people with whom you could conduct interesting and well-thought discussions; although I couldn't help but think common sense was less apparent than intellect (as in myself).

As a perfectionist, I felt truly satisfied that I had achieved something worthwhile by achieving a D.Phil. studentship at Oxford. Me: a country girl from Derbyshire, born in the North West, an East Midlands accent, humble beginnings, used to the countryside, with a brain that equally helped and hindered my life; surrounded by the brightest, wealthiest, vibrant, most interesting students, who would no doubt become some of the most influential people in the country... and world. A lively city, a top University: I sensed that almost anything was within my grasp, the possibilities endless. You can't really outclass getting into the most competitive department in arguably *the* most prestigious university in the world. I spent the first few weeks cycling here and there in a bubble of disbelief that they had let me in!

I spent just under five years living in Oxford: the best and worst years of my life all violently smashed together in a enigmatically complicated mess that ended in my utter mental collapse and oh so very near death.

At first things went well. I was happy for the first time in my adult life, I felt great! Because of my slightly eccentric sense of humour I chose to join Linacre College for the decidedly tenuous reason that it is pronounced the same as Lineker (li-neh-kah) as in Garry Lineker, a famous, if slightly goofy ex-England football player. Linacre College is the oldest graduate-only College, founded in 1962 and situated on St. Cross Road next to the University Parks, which are beautiful, especially on a summer's evening. One of the other reasons I chose Linacre was because of one particular photo in the prospectus: that of Linacre students (in the College's traditional black and yellow) celebrating rowing win on the river. Much like I had chosen Nottingham on instinct, I chose Linacre in the same way, and once again my intuition was proven right in ways I could never have fathomed at first.

The Linacre College motto is "No end to Learning." It is a small College by Oxford standards, which I felt made it more personal. There were usually 50 Fellows, 14 Junior Research Fellows and 270 grad students. I also liked that it was named after Thomas Linacre (1460-1524), who was a distinguished Oxford humanist, medical scientist and classicist; thus commemorating an outstanding academic and Renaissance figure. (And I am a fan of the Renaissance period, along with anyone who is both artistic and scientific). Linacre is proud of its tradition of diversity and balance; with students from all around the world – 50 different countries, an equal divide between male and female, and students reading for a vast range of higher degrees, both taught and research disciplines.

Linacre College is a distinctly coloured red-bricked building with rows of bicycles lining the entrance. It boasts the best College food in Oxford (not a reason I chose it). Formal dinners *were* fun, especially when we invited another College to join us; all in gowns, a Latin prayer read out before the meal, a gong sounded to begin the meal and end it. I got to know a few students at Keble College this way.

Within Linacre there were specific social gatherings for all the Clinical Medicine students, both medical doctors-to-be and those of us in research: really just an excuse for an evening drink and discussion! Linacre Seminars (which were less formal) and Linacre Lectures brought together the College and some very special guests, in an intellectual and stimulating atmosphere, to discuss a variety of topics from the environment to astrophysics.

The Collegiate system at Oxford works very well, once accepted, you are looked after for the duration of your Oxford career (and beyond), and supported through *any* problems. Some Linacre alumni return to get married in the College where they met and found love – as happens in all Oxford Colleges. Linacre quickly became my home: my tutor and other staff helping me though any problems with concern and without reservation or prejudice. Your College and College friends become like your family. Linacre certainly stood by me to the bitter end.

My manic depression, anorexia, and anxiety meant that my experience of Oxford was somewhat different to normal. I was well aware of the contrast between my existence, and the lives of people going on around me – and it saddened me. I was always alert, looking for people like myself, with problems. I suppose it would be fair to say, that my experience of Oxford, whilst wonderful in many ways, was always tainted by my mania depression, and anorexia.

Initially I was manic. Woo hoo! I tried joining in with College life, sipping water at the bar. I was still taking lofepramine at the maximum outpatient dose – it was not helping, but I was too scared to change anything in case things got worse. I went to juggling at St. Johns College, and joined the Oxford University First Aid Unit (OUFAU) at St. Catherine's. I joined Linacre's Women's rowing team, although work commitments made it impossible to continue, since my hospital working hours started earlier than for most people (especially students!) Rowing was fun for a while, and I will always support Oxford for the boat race.

There was a time when I arrived and started Oxford life that I was "happy." It's the only time in my life that I recall feeling such a way. I lived between happy and euphoric. I had an important job, my mind was on fire, my career was heading to the stars and beyond, I had a supervisor who was a truly accomplished brain, my eating was OK, I lived in an exciting, lively city, and for once: I felt *proud* to be me. My career, patients, research, lectures, clinics, Linacre friends, other Oxford friends, aspirations, dreams, books, writing, cycling, walking, grinning inanely, joking, talking, debating, buzzing/humming and a *mind that wouldn't ever shut up*; meant I barely slept or stopped running this way and that. My days started at 3am and finished at 1am. Then I tossed and turned in bed or listened to music. The not-sleeping and high levels of activity didn't bother me. I was truly manic.

However, it was not all good. Those levels of physical and mental activity were draining. Before I arrived at work, before I spoke to anyone, I would have been out cycling in the wee hours of the morning for miles. I had to go for walks in the day, mainly to expel some of my nervous energy (it was also partly due to the need to maintain my weight); plus I always had about 20 jobs running all at the same time, flitting from one to the other and back again.

Whilst a post-doc research assistant took a week, I'd write a perfect abstract in 10 minutes. I looked as if I wasn't busy, but actually I'd complete 3 days of lab work in a morning. I would run several experiments all at once, *and* read research papers, *and* trawl Internet for information, *and* email people, *and* research which med school to go to next, *and* plan/run my clinical days, *and* be on-call to my patients/volunteers, *and* go to lectures/presentations, *and* put on an indomitable façade of normality.

Like always, it was the masquerade that took the real energy – energy like you would not believe (unless you've been there yourself). Money was a big problem: I spent triple of what I earned whilst deliberately not looking at my bank statements – I enjoyed spending and didn't care about the consequences. If I *tried* to stop everything, my mood CRASHED. I could soar and swoop within a day – this rapid cycling of my mood becoming more persistent, whereas in the beginning, I had just been manic. Of course, in time, this all had to catch up with me; the world started to crumble into pieces right before my eyes.

My first coping strategy for the depression that hit me was withdrawal: even though I *knew* it would be deleterious to my health, and had sworn not to fall into that same trap once again. Fairly early on, I began to beg out of social events, tired of what my depression saw as the competition to prove who was the most academically brilliant according to scales I disagreed with. My insomnia left me too tired to dance that dance. I didn't get into Oxford to *feel* like I had to prove my talents over cornflakes in the morning.

And so I isolated myself from the many social pleasures of Oxford – angry with myself because I realised there were so many better, more positive options. Soon I noticed I was living the lives of two people again. There was a super-efficient, fake-happy, eager, manic Katy Sara who went to work in the Radcliffe Infirmary, forcing herself to remain hopelessly busy, committed to medical research, and endlessly-caring provider of time to all patients and volunteers. A Katy Sara who had voluntarily forgone her long summer holiday to move down to Oxford and get started on her D.Phil. early. To a large extent, that version of Katy Sara was true: just not something I could maintain 24 hours a day. All in all, I was on top of the world, independent, fit, happy with my career, and loving Oxford. There really was no immediately tangible reason for why I became so ill again, and then more ill. It just happened, as it can happen to anyone.

There was also another Katy Sara, who had manic depression and other issues she had not dealt with; who went home as soon as possible to hide; who was isolated; who cycled with increasing frequency and distance; whose eating was fucked up; and who shut herself away at night, reading papers about medicine, diabetes, metabolism, nutrition and more and more psychiatry. On Saturdays she would travel to watch Derby County play, on Sundays she would mournfully watch (wanting to join in) as the Linacre School of Defence met in the College gardens, and students took up swords to fight each other! On a good day she would make it into the city, and settle herself in a bookstore or coffee shop, enjoying the buzz of people all around. Often she'd walk around the huge University Parks, just to be around people. I guess she was lonely.

There was a presence in my room that I knew to be a hallucination. I could not see or clearly hear "he" or "it," but I knew he was there; following me, watching me, talking to me – his presence struck me straight into my subconscious mind so that I felt terrible and did not know why. I began to feel more and more like a male semi-human creature was just over my right shoulder. And whilst this felt very real, I knew it to be madness for I hold no belief in the paranormal or ethereal.

If concentration abandoned me, or sleep eluded me, (which was often), I'd open my huge fourth floor window and sit on my windowsill with my legs dangling down into the darkness, the night breeze on my face, playing music: alone with my thoughts – dark thoughts. I liked to watch the sun go down, looking towards the city, seeing the spires and turrets. I liked looking outwards in the dark, because there was always light and noise, the city was always awake, like me. So I'd play Green Day... either to sit motionlessly on my sill, mournfully, or to dance around my room, bursting with energy and shaking my head so hard it might have fallen off. Had my own brain chemistry not been providing me with enough magical fantastical visions and interest, I would probably have taken drugs.

> "O sleep, O gentle sleep, nature's soft
> nurse, how have I frightened thee, that
> thou no more wilt weigh my eye-lids
> down and steep my senses in
> forgetfulness?"

> ❧ William Shakespeare, *Henry IV Part 2*,
> (Act III, scene 1).

Now, I don't "do" being bored very well. The addition of insomnia, that often accompanies depression, means a forced endurance of even more, still-elongated hours of mind-numbing boredom. Even worse, these are dark lonely hours when the rest of the world sleeps, making you feel so very much alone and out of place. That feeling of "aloneness" is extremely wretched. It is like everyone has vanished, you are alone in the universe and going mad. And as the lonely

time drags... It feels like someone scraping their nails down a blackboard making that high-pitched, tingling squeak; except feels as if
it is physically inside my own head. Someone is scraping their long nails down the inside of eye sockets, drilling into my skull, and my head is *screaming* in the agony. High buildings, cyanide, fast trains and pills suddenly become strangely attractive.

Depending on my mood and the hour, (let's face it Green Day needs to be loud and it isn't soothing music), I'd also play Robbie Williams, Matchbox Twenty, Queen, The Beatles, U2, Radiohead, Holst, and lots of other music; whilst I watched the traffic dawdling past below. Cyclists (with and without helmets or lights on their bikes) weaved in and out of bicycle lanes; tipsy students would wander past singing loudly and laughing at all hours, obviously having fun; noisy ambulances roared past every so often, but the noise didn't annoy me, it lulled me, it brought me closer to life. Even in the quietest hours, the Oxford seemed awake. I was a country girl from "up north," feeling at home in Oxford city "down south." Although isolated and feeling low in direct contrast to my Oxford surroundings, I still felt very much a part of Oxford, in touch with the pulse and excitement of the wonderful city, Colleges and University.

Oxford is a city with absolutely everything you could want, and the wonderful thing is, everything is close together, and with a bike, the world is literally at your feet. There are all sorts of short cuts and little cobbled streets you can dart down. I could reach anywhere I needed within ten minutes on my bike. The traditional image of a student peddling away on a bike with a basket full of books, gown flowing behind in the wind, is quite fitting. Cars and buses seemed to want to murder all cyclists: I didn't care enough about that. *"Me... versus a big bus..."* Mockingly, I thought: *"Sure, why not, bring it on; I'm up for it."*

I arrived in Oxford at a "normal-ish" weight, which I maintained at first, and despite social pressures to the contrary, abstained completely from alcohol. My diet was restricted, but I made a deranged effort to get all the dietary requirements I needed... except for calories. There was food available in Oxford to suit any palate; so many shops, restaurants, take-outs, College dining rooms, pubs, hotels, and even greasy kebab vans where you get the Oxford special "Cheese 'n' Chips" at pub closing time. And no, I never tried it, but I was very much aware of all the food circling around Oxford and in my head it felt almost like the food was predatory and I was the victim. On the whole, despite depression, my thinking capacity and concentration seemed easily sufficient to cope with my work, even though I knew I was well below my full capabilities. Remember, I got my first degree whilst bulimic: anything else seemed easy in comparison.

I had a good supervisor, world expert in his field: Professor Keith Frayn – Professor of Human Metabolism and a specialist, as, I suppose was I by this point, in Metabolic Physiology – specifically Lipid (fat) Metabolism, Cardiovasular Disease, Diabetes and Hyperlipidaemia. I remember the first time I met Keith, to me he was the author on the best metabolism book I'd read and it was sort of like meeting someone famous. Keith pushed me gently in the right direction and all my work fell into place. I absolutely loved the medical techniques I learned, some of which I would put to bad use later (as you will see). I went out of my way to apply psychology to all my studies because that was what really interested me.

I spent day after day taking and then being buried in blood samples. I loved the responsibility of working with patients/volunteers and everyone trusting me to look after them. Lab work was less stimulating, but I was good at it and didn't waste time getting my results in. The research equipment at my disposal was first rate, and I soon discovered that if I needed anything, dropping the name "University of Oxford" would open doors. For example, I needed pure macadamia nut oil to feed my patients in a test meal, and was sent a gallon for free from Hawaii! Within Clinical Medicine, our department was initially called The Oxford Lipid Metabolism Group, though it changed to The Oxford Centre of Diabetes Endocrinology and Metabolism (OCDEM) whilst I was in Oxford.

Shortly after arriving in Oxford, I had to find myself a new GP. Part of the process of Colleges looking after their students was to automatically have a College doctor. Linacre College students were allocated to the practice at 19, Beaumont Street; were I met, and immediately liked Dr. Neil MacLennan who was always empathic, funny and obviously highly intelligent. The three attributes I value most highly in a person, especially a doctor. I easily forgave him for not comprehending *at all* that eating wasn't fun, for thinking my excessive cycling was fine, and even for supporting Manchester United.

The letters after his name were most impressive, but not as impressive or important as his approach that made me feel valued as a person. He was patient, soothing, understanding and would pre-empt my dangerous thoughts and behaviour. Every visit he would sensitively check my arm and comment on how well the old scars had healed: an action that made me hold out against cutting it (for a considerable time). I needed to feel respected, which I usually did: an achievement of his that is not to be underestimated, as I was ultra-sensitive and always looking for "proof" that he (indeed anyone) hated me. My suffering, intelligence, and over-active suicidal brain needed to be recognised as dangerous by my doctor if by no one else. And that is how our doctor-patient relationship continued and worked. Dr. MacLennan became my confidant: the only person in Oxford, indeed the *only person in my life* who knew all was not well.

For my first autumn term at Oxford University, known as Michaelmas Term, all seemed well. There were many guest lectures (e.g. by Michael Jackson, who I did not go and see) at the Oxford Union, and in the Clinical Medicine Department by top professionals all around the world, another benefit of being at Oxford University. I had been so keen to stick needles into people at every opportunity, that Keith gave me a tourniquet for Christmas! (Please note: I don't mean I liked to hurt people, rather I liked to be good at taking blood and *not* hurting people). When not in the lab and learning procedures, I attended clinics to observe Oxford's Consultants at their work. Within a month of my arrival, my former desire to study medicine and practice as a medical doctor was revisited and magnified. This brought back all the feelings of loss I experienced when I was eighteen and was turned down for Med School. The strength of this sense of loss was (is) overwhelming.

Just before the 1999-2000 break for Christmas and Millennium celebrations, a post-doctoral physiology researcher in our department effectively put a gun to my head and pulled the trigger. I do not believe it was intentional, but she should have been more sensitive. I had been totally honest in my application to Oxford about my history of anorexia; in return the University had been completely understanding, supportive and unprejudiced. (I hadn't mentioned the manic depression because I still didn't realise that was actually the major problem). I had wondered if my colleague was anorectic or eating-disorder-not-otherwise-specified because she was skinny and didn't seem to eat anything except Pot Noodles.

She made comments about my behaviour that I knew only a "fellow" sufferer would pick up on. A spiteful comment about my going for walks in the day, "to burn off all the calories in that water." Then she said she *had* had anorexia. I took this to mean that she understood, like I assume all people to have shared anorexia - to *understand*. Eating disorder sufferers, in my experience, are terrific, thoughtful people, who share a horrific illness and want the best for everyone, even at their own expense. She asked me what treatment I had received, so I told her about Leicester. Her vitriolic reply was, *"Yes, you let them make you too fat at Leicester."*

This was below the belt. This was something cruel to say to anybody, let alone someone trying to cope with a recovering anorexic state – and also inaccurate, as I was a normal weight. But for me, the thing that made this situation deplorable was the fact that she should have known better. I have never met a "fellow" sufferer with more vindictive, atrocious behaviour, personally aimed (intentionally or not) at another's well being.

I should have been strong. I should not have let her words effect me because by doing so, I was letting her win. I had too much to lose. But I was not strong enough. I had not yet learned how to contradict those anorexic thoughts in my head. I am not claiming this was all her fault: no, *much* else was wrong in my life, none of it anything to do with being at Oxford. But just like being forcibly weighed at school, one event can tip the balance. All I required was this one last push over the edge: *and this time it nearly killed me.*

To celebrate the Millennium, I went not to Sydney, Paris, New York, Edinburgh or London, but fantastic Sheffield (yeah!) with my sister and some friends from all over the country. The night seemed so intangible and unreal. I was still at that point refusing all alcohol, even though people kept trying to slip it into my orange juice. My sister drank all of my surreptitiously spiked vodka and oranges that night, as well as her own drinks! I danced around Sheffield in a slinky black evening dress and my beloved and lucky Derby County scarf. (Only I could have come up with that outfit and dared sing songs about my team very loudly in a rival city). I hugged my sister and some sexy stranger kissed me at midnight, whilst Semisonic played *Secret Smile* in the room.

It was a good night, though already the dark seeds of illness were blossoming and I knew it without a doubt. More as a symptom of increasing melancholy than anorexia nervosa, I began to lose weight yet again. Losing weight did not afford me any pleasure. I felt ill, I felt sick, I felt stupid, I was risking a fantastic, once-in-a-lifetime opportunity, *and* I knew it, *and* I couldn't stop. The insomnia was paralysing yet I forced my body to carry on at superhuman speeds. To this day, I don't know how I did that.

After the New Year, I asked Dr. MacLennan to put me on the waiting list for eating disorder therapy even though I was at that point, only a few pounds lighter. He did so, based on my previous eating disorder history. It was unusual for the eating disorders Unit to accept GP referrals, but they accepted mine. Oxford, it seemed, was a good place to be ill.

I struggled constantly with mixed manic depression; *surely*, I thought, *my mood problems are only a side issue, caused by the anorexia, due to malnutrition.* I didn't recognise the mixed episode for what it was, and still did not ask about changing or augmenting the ineffective lofepramine. Nor did I push for any further help with this strange buzzing depression that overwhelmed me. I did, to an extent, self-treat it by thoroughly indulging in any sort of eating disordered behaviour or self-harm. It is possible (not-infrequently in people with bipolar I affective disorder) to experience a mixed state for varying periods of time. It can be very confusing to yourself and others trying to judge one's mood (however experienced), even when obviously depressed *and* manic. Black-fire rips through your body and mind; there is no solace to be found. Mixed states (using current DSM-IV criteria of full-blown mania plus concurrent major depression) occur in an average of 40% of bipolar disorder patients over their lifetime.[13]

---

[13] Akiskal HS., Bourgeois ML., Angst J., Post R., Mo¨ller H-J., Hirschfeld R., (2000) Review article: Re-evaluating the prevalence of and diagnostic composition within the broad clinical spectrum of bipolar disorders. Journal of Affective disorders 59 (2000) S5–S30 www.elsevier.com/locate/jad

It is depressive pathology that leads most people with all forms of depression to suicide. Mixed episodes are particularly dangerous as the person has both the inclination to die and the energy to go about the killing. Patients who are psychotic and have severe depressive symptoms concurrent with mania (i.e. are mixed) are most at risk of harm to self or others, including suicide.[14] I fitted the bill perfectly, although the only person who was at risk was myself.

The presence in my room had taken form, although it was still a hollow form that was less powerful than it would become later. This male creature looked like a deformed man of sorts. His spine was twisted, his skin was burnt black, not like the milk or dark chocolate colour of dark skin, but absolute black, jet-black, *charcoal* black - and it was cracking to show blood red and white skin beneath it. It was almost as if he had been roasted on a barbeque spit, and as soon as I had that thought, that was what I could smell too. He wore a hat like Freddy Kruger (in *Nightmare on Elm Street*), and his clothes were all rags, black rags, all torn, all swirls, and covering him from neck to the floor which he floated just above. He was big, twice the size of a man – the size a normal man might seem to a child. He moved when I moved, going wherever I looked, or alternatively he hid at the corner of my right eye – always bothering me. Only his eyes and mouth looked human. His mouth was pink, too pink next to all that black, and his eyes were bright blue – piercing me. Again I feared for myself and so needed distraction from this "thing" and what it probably represented in

[14] Strakowski SM, McElroy SL, Keck PE, West SA. (1996) *Suicidality among patients with mixed and manic bipolar disorder.* Am J Psychiatry;153:67 p 4-6.

my subconscious. At least he faded away most of the time – at first.

This necessitated self-harm to cope. A glossy magazine article in Cosmopolitan, (yes really), that I'd read several years earlier, gave me the idea to try bloodletting. For my clinical work I'd been trained to take blood with needles and to insert venflons.[15] It became an alternative to cutting that I preferred, as I felt like I was successfully punishing myself, without the pain. I was never a big fan of pain; my self-harm was driven by other motives. Losing blood soothed me, made me ill (which I liked because I "deserved" punishing), it made the Dark Man quiet, made me feel less angry, made me sleepy, and I got a weird kick out of playing with medical equipment (which was probably yet more suppressed anger at my perceived career failures – despite actual success). Most of all, it calmed the noise in my head that was agonisingly uncomfortable.

Bloodletting enabled me to avoid cutting, which would have immediately alerted Dr. MacLennan. An interesting question, to which I don't know the answer is: *why* did I bother to hide it from him? I started with equipment I "borrowed" from the hospital or bought on from shops in town. (It's amazing what you can buy). If Dr. MacLennan spotted the neat puncture wound(s) into my cephalic vein at my anticubital fossa (inside bend of the elbow) he didn't say anything. I'd insert a large needle or venflon, and let my blood trickle out into a measuring cup. If you are familiar with venflons, you

---

[15] The trade name for cannulae, a needle and plastic tube assembly to allow continuous infusion or multiple blood samples to be taken without repeated needle-sticking, known as catheters in North America.

imagine putting one into a your own arm using only one hand; it takes real "skill." I set myself an _unsafe_ "safety limit" of 250ml.[16] But if I did that several times a week (or within a day) it soon added up, leaving me feeling very weak. However I forcibly soldiered on, cycling and running about at work, my heart pounding like it would burst.

Dr. MacLennan thought I looked anaemic: and fancy that, the blood test agreed. He knew I wasn't cutting my arm because he checked the relatively small number of scars I had back then. He asked me if I'd cut elsewhere, to which I truthfully (at that time) answered I had not. He asked me directly if I was losing blood in any other way, so to avoid lying I diverted his question and asked him, "How else could I be losing it?" He said, "Heavy periods or bloody stools," to which I could honestly reply, "No." He put me on iron tablets, assuming my poor diet explained the low iron levels in by bloodstream and I did not correct him. I knew it was depression related bloodletting and I wish I had been honest, but somehow I was unable to make the connection in my brain that my depression and my "clinical" pursuits were serious problems.

Some time around this point I realised I had lost the ability to cry – however melancholic, my tear ducts were barren.

"I'll not weep.
I have no full cause of weeping; but this
heart
Shall break into a hundred thousand flaws

---

[16] Note I am **not** suggesting or recommending that 250ml of blood loss is safe, either alone or repeatedly: that was merely my deluded thinking at the time.

Or ere I'll weep. O fool, I shall go mad."

જ William Shakespeare, *King Lear* (Act
IV, Scene 1)

Oblivious as I was to the real severity of my own situation, my eyes sought out familiars. Because I saw the world through depression-tinted goggles, I was acutely aware of people with eating disorders and mood disorders. My mind was never free of thoughts about illness, and whether or not my judgement about seeing ill people all around me was strictly accurate is debatable. I did my best to ignore the fact that I saw more severely anorectic students/young people wandering Oxford than I thought had ever encountered in another area of the country. On my dark morning cycles I would pass a student from New College always out running, his parotid glands were so swollen from vomiting that they made his face diamond shaped, and his legs so skinny they looked like they would snap. Now and then our eyes met in a knowing appreciation of our common circumstances. As I came towards the end of my pre-dawn cycling, many women would be out jogging: some far too thin (at least in my opinion).

Now and then I'd see girls walking to lectures so emaciated the wind would practically blow them away. Some would try to hide their thinness; some would flaunt it. I found all of this extremely painful to watch, turning away quickly as if acid had been thrown into my eyes. That is how painful it was to see. Yet despite my insight, I could not help myself, or these other sufferers, and that thought suffocated me in its inescapability. Perfectionism and intelligence breeds both top class students and people with eating disorders, indeed eating disorders are more common amongst university students everywhere. I knew that all those people who actually appeared ill were just the tip of the iceberg of eating disorders in Oxford because most people with eating disorders look completely normal.

One day a young, six-foot male student from Hertford College (a beautiful Oxford College with the famous Bridge of Sighs, and where I had some friends, all content with their studies, only one with "mild" depression) fainted in the tiny Westgate Centre's Sainsbury's. I jumped to assist him whilst the staff and customers stared. Straight from work, my hospital ID badge was still clipped at my hip: everyone assumed he was in safe hands. He was thin. Not emaciated, but just too thin that an experienced eye would recognise it as definitely problematic. I asked if he had hit his head then or at anytime that day, he hadn't. He was pale, and confirmed he had given a pint of blood that day, which I had already deduced from a single new puncture mark on his arm, and a slight rash from where he had removed the dressing.

I got him to rest with his head between his knees and suggested he drink something and get some sugar. (It's far easier to tell someone else to be sensible, than convince yourself to do the same). I doubted he had eaten or drunk anything after giving blood. He refused the Sainsbury's assistant's offer of free chocolate and/or coke, but finally gave in after some persuasion from me about how "healthy" fresh fruit juice was, and, I reminded him, he had given blood, some juice would be "safe." Such talk appealed to his eating disordered thinking and enabled him to agree, although his cautious sipping was overtly (at least to me) symptomatic of an eating disorder. He reminded me much of myself in my first year at Nottingham University. I didn't push him to seek further help, but as we parted I whispered to him that I knew what was wrong. He went quiet. I've always wondered how his life went from that point.

Nor do eating disorders have the monopoly on mental health problems at Oxford University, or indeed any university. Drink and drugs were easy to find and abuse (although I didn't do so at this point). Depression (in particular) and manic depression seemed frighteningly common, although in my own way I sought out people with such problems, so my view may be biased. My floor in Linacre College held five students. In my first year, three out of five had significant mood disorders, and one of the other two girls never came out of her room. In my second year, two out of five had a Mood disorder.

My Clinical Medicine D.Phil. studentship predecessor, under Keith's supervision had attempted suicide by injecting herself with insulin in the department. A friend of mine at Teddy's (St. Edmund Hall) had depression and "successfully" committed suicide. There were also many people that I wondered about: quiet people, anxious people, angry people, and sad people – those were the people I had a tendency to notice.

There were many, many more people I knew who seemed completely "normal," and who had a terrific time at Oxford. I was only too painfully aware that in an amazing University filled with brilliants minds and all sorts of odd-bods, I was a total misfit. I felt like an oddity and sank into my music more and more. Oh, had it not been for Green Day I would be long dead by now. I played their song *Minority* over and over again.

I continued to work hard because I was committed and needed the distraction for my brain. My research was progressing nicely. I did my reading, spent several months setting my dietary work up, I saw my patients and volunteers, I wrote up as I went along, I gleaned all I could from what other research was going on in the department, I looked after the undergraduates allocated to our department, I set my dietary studies going, and was on call 24 hours a day to all my patients/subjects for the four months each was under my care. Postprandial study days (where a subject would come into the hospital, have blood samples taken, eat a special meal, and have various blood samples taken) were stressful, but I prided myself on looking after my subject. Several were so impressed that they asked to speak to my supervisor to commend me. The rest of my time was spent doing lab work: a very detailed analysis of my subjects' blood, in particular the lipid content in all its various forms (which gets quite complex), and the mechanism behind the lipid metabolism (also complicated). I must have been doing something right. My supervisor's reports to Linacre College were excellent, and I got sent to conferences, including the American Heart Association conferences in New Orleans and the International Congress on Obesity in Vienna, where I presented my research. Our research department even went punting together in the summer – a true Oxbridge pastime.

Seven months after referral to Oxford's eating disorder Service, I had my first individual therapy session with someone who turned out to be an exceptional CBT psychotherapist. By this point I was considerably underweight. Once again I thought to myself that Oxford was a good place to get ill if you were going to. Keith agreed that I could have every Tuesday afternoon off to go to therapy, totally supportive of my decision to face my problems. My initial fears were that I didn't deserve help, and that they would only be concerned with returning me to normal weight, and then politely shove me out the door. (I was wary of being dumped and hurt again like at Leicester). She calmed me.

I told Dr. MacLennan that my new psychotherapist was good, and that her name began with "L," as had been true of my therapist in Leicester, and my counsellor when I was at high school. He quickly replied, "Well, you've had one 'L' of a time." I smiled.

Looking back at the situation now, I needed help with my mixed manic depression/bipolar I affective disorder far more so than anything else. Fortunately my new therapist helped with both my mood disorder and anorexia, though the emphasis was always on the anorexia (as that was where I put it). Then over a period of months, my trust grew. We talked about many things: my dad, high school, Nottingham University, my eating disorder history, treatment at Leicester, work, being turned down from medical school because of my anorexia when I was 17, exercise, sleep, self-harm and mood. In fact, we talked more about my life than we did my being a person with anorexia – and that is how I think it should have been for me. My therapist had a great memory, and would remember facts as if she had re-read my entire file before each meeting. She was able to take in current problems, remember past ones, digest, and turn things around so that it helped me see where the problems were. Her talent for remembering names and facts made me feel that she really listened. That was truly helpful. I know that her patients were more than just a job to her.

I ate more (well I mostly drank fluids and ate runny-foods like yoghurt) enabling me to gain weight to eventually be low "normal" weight, despite a totally deranged diet. Of course, most people assumed weight gain meant I was getting better, although I note from my medical notes that I was not considered to be at a safe or normal weight. My therapist kept her promise and did not assume a gain in weight meant I was recovered or even particularly improved. In fact, I was worse because of my depression became more severe, my self-harm reappeared (secretly) and I spent three hours a day cycling. My diet consisted of *lots* of soya milk, yoghurt, soup, fruit juice, and solid fruit on "happier" days. I also ate very small amounts of tuna or salmon. Cycling many hours a day is fine *if* you enjoy it and if you eat well, but I didn't. Apart from feeling fit, I hated it; but it commanded me, not *vice versa*.

Two years into my D.Phil., after a lot of hard work and a fridge and freezer full of plasma and delipidated samples, my therapist asked me if I would like to attend the Eating Disorder Day Programme. I can still picture the session when the idea came across her mind quite evidently. I remember her appearing struck by my explanation of the depths of my depression, when for once I managed to express my despair. She told me the support I would receive might be helpful, and, it would be a chance to get me eating solid food. It is true that my mood was very low, and the suffocation of having anorexia was killing my hope, but my depression was far more dangerous and powerful than she, Dr.

MacLennan or I realised. Nor was it getting better, it was getting worse.

I spoke to Keith: asking him for time off so that I could attend the Day Programme, being completely honest about everything. My other supervisor suggested I use the time to write up what I could: and I did. I checked the University rules about having time off, and found that I could take up to two years. Keith was (at least verbally) fully supportive of my decision, although in my opinion, he did not look too happy about it – and who can blame him. I planned to have just three months off. With hindsight, I wish I had continued with weekly therapy and full-time work because I placed a great part of my self-worth on my academic success. Losing my career, even temporarily, and focussing on the eating disorder made me more depressed. I had little else to do in the day than focus on my eating problems and cycle fifty or more miles a day.

Time off was probably unavoidable, but despite the apparent practicality of my choice, it was one of the worst decisions of my life.

Chapter 4. Anyone for torture?

"How dreadful knowledge of the truth can
be
when there's no help in the truth."

❧ Sophocles.

Not wanting to alarm people: I must qualify the title. I knew what was wrong with me and what I should do: but I could not do it. For me, attending the Day Programme at the Eating Disorders Unit (EDU) was sheer torture and did not help; for many people it was extremely difficult, but helpful. Some people lasted only minutes before leaving, many lasted the maximum nine months. Some gained weight, some lost weight, some self-harmed, some were absent a lot, some vomited less, and others vomited a lot. *Everyone* struggled. Everyone there had a co-morbid mood disorder, though I was the only bipolar patient (though that was not known at the time).

Some, including myself, were deceitful out of fear, and/or anger, and/or jealousy; others were so strong in their desire to get well, it was *inspirational*. They were so fervent in their painful actions to make themselves better that in fact, I questioned if I really wanted to get better at all. I thought that I did, but then why was I different from them? I blamed myself for failing to do be "good." Why couldn't I just get on with it (eating) like the others?

I was dubious and cynical. I was the oldest anorectic there, desperate to make sure that all the "apprentice" anorectics did not fall into the same trap as me and become chronically ill. Ultimately I was the only one who ended up with a long stay in a mental institution, because my volatile, nihilistic, mixed manic depression was so severe that I could not be helped by the Oxford Eating Disorder Service: which at that time (2001), had no inpatient facility.

Before I officially started on the Day Programme, I had to have a meeting with the dietician (who I superciliously felt far better qualified than), a family therapy session, and meet the current members of the eating disorders day programme. I hated meeting the dietician because I hated talking about food; but to do her justice, having read her entries in my medical notes, I can clearly see that she knew exactly what she was doing, and had a lot of insight. I promised to follow the meal plan, and I *really* meant it at the time.

You were allowed to choose three dislikes, just like on the Day Programme at Leicester. I was more honest this time: instead of choosing foods that scared me, I chose foods I truly hated, which was the idea. Green beans, rice, and anything lemon flavoured. Other people made choices that were obviously driven by fear rather than dislike, such as choosing butter, or salad dressings. Jane, (a patient who left the Day Programme before I joined, but who I got to know), said that her three choices were "carbohydrates, proteins, and fats." I enjoyed the humour in that answer. As much as I enjoyed hearing that on a day when it was pizza for lunch, she waited until nobody was looking, and popped her pizza down behind the radiator! A sense of humour was, as always, invaluable.

The family session included just my sister and myself; seeing the family therapy specialist, with my individual therapist present. We talked about our family, our childhood, and how my illness affected the family as a whole. I learned that my parents tried to shelter Beth from my illness at first, but that once I started throwing up she realised immediately. She told me she used to sit in her bedroom and listen to me being sick in the toilet. I felt a cold shiver down my spine. I had the water running in the sink, but she still heard me. Would that knowledge have stopped my bulimia? No, I think I would have carried on regardless. Deep down I always knew people knew. However good I was at hiding it, there were always too many clues.

I also learned that she was extremely angry with me. Angry because of the mess I made in the kitchen and bathroom. Angry at how the family was strained, angry for making her the "well child," angry for upsetting her, our parents and for behaving as I did. I realise how badly I behaved, but I was living on my nerves, utterly hating myself, ashamed, and even angrier with myself than she was. It is true that when my eating disorder surfaced, as it did around my family, I was not a nice person. I was mean, snappy, manipulative and introverted. I was not myself.

Back in those times my sister seemed to think I was doing it on purpose and that I should just bloody well stop. Stopping should be so easy: all I had to do was "get a grip." During that family session, my sister showed me that she had gained awareness that just maybe it wasn't quite that simple, that I wasn't being ill just to annoy her. My need for control was so absolute that it was beyond my control. Fuelled by frustration, everyone, myself included, was so very angry with me. A mistake: we should all have been angry at the *illness*.

The final meeting before starting was to greet the current Day Programme patients. I was led into a dark room with chairs in a circle, so I sat down. My

immediate thought was: S*hit!!! I'm the fattest one here.*
I expect everyone thinks that when they join. The girl
sitting to my right smiled comfortingly, and introduced
herself. "I'm Clare, and before you ask, I'm the bulimic
one." I nodded in acceptance. Her full name is Clare
Baker; I liked her instantly. She would tell me later that
she was relieved when I joined because she was tired of
being the only bulimic. Technically I wasn't bulimic,
but as I wasn't underweight so I wasn't precisely a
person with anorexia either. I was "eating- disorder-
not-otherwise-specified (EDNOS), with a history or
both anorexia and anorexia purging-type: in other
words, an enigmatic, vulnerable, totally fucked-up
mess.

I could smell their lunch being cooked in the next
room, potatoes I think. I remember being relieved that I
wasn't going to have to eat it. Today was Friday, and I
wasn't due back until Monday: a three-day stay of
execution. The slight girl sitting next to Clare, with
funky, spiky, black hair introduced herself as Becky.
She wore short sleeves and her arms were like
matchsticks. She said she didn't know what eating
disorder she had. She ate loads apparently, and never
threw up. I didn't really know her well enough to make
this judgement, but I thought to myself, "Yeah your
idea of 'loads' is a slice of cucumber mate."

I nodded and said to the group, "I'm Katy Sara."
There was a small girl there, maybe eighteen. She said
"Hello" but left the Day Programme the following
Tuesday. Immediately to my left was a tall, wispy girl,
I (wrongly) thought might be about nineteen. She had
strawberry-blonde long hair, tied back very neatly. She
introduced herself as Rose, and then warned me that
she would not be at the Day Programme next week

because she had to have "a week out." I asked what that meant and Clare said "They'll fill you in next week in weighing group: Thursday mornings." Then she added sarcastically, with more humour in her voice than she could possibly have felt, *"It's everyone's favourite group."*

"Of all tales 'tis the saddest, and
more sad,
Because it makes us smile."

∾ Lord Byron, George Gordon Noel
Byron, (1788-1824)
Don Juan, Canto Thirteenth, st.9,
lines 65 and 66.

I asked everyone there how old they were and how long they'd been ill. Everyone looked far younger than they were. Clare was twenty-four, and had been bulimic since she was thirteen. Becky was twenty-five and had first been ill when she was fifteen, getting worse when she went to university. Rose was twenty-five and had first started to loose weight deliberately at the age of 18, but had always been naturally thin. Part of her problem was a deeply rooted belief that people had only befriended her because she was thin. I used to tell her that I liked her *despite* her being too thin, but I don't think she ever accepted those words. She first attended the Oxford Adult Eating Disorder service in 1997, and was back for another attempt. For my interest, I asked them if they had depression as a co-disorder and if so, which came first. Like me, all suffered from significant depression, and all developed depression first, except Becky who thought she got depressed at the same time as she became anorectic. I later found that with the exception of Becky, all of us had self-harmed and attempted suicide.

I was the oldest, had been ill the longest, and so I *hopelessly* assumed I was the most ill. The longer an eating disorder goes on, the more entrenched it can become, hence harder to defeat; especially once you are past the distinctive five-year barrier after which you "become" a chronic anorectic. The others there may have been thinner, but anybody who knows anything about eating disorders, will know that weight is only one indicator of poor health. I was killing myself faster than all of them, although it was a close "competition" between Clare, Rose and myself. I thought (pragmatically) that as I had been ill the longest, and as I had suffered from anorexia *and* bulimia *and* severe depression *and* serious self-harm (including attempts on my life): I was least likely to recover …or survive. As it happens, I was wrong, but only just.

The summer of 2001 was exceedingly hot, and I have never liked hot weather. I started on the Day Programme on Monday 30th July in sweltering heat. I cycled 70 miles that day before even reaching the Day Programme. That meant getting up at 3.00am. For the first and *only* time, I ate all the breakfast as prescribed. One and a half cups of cereal, 200ml semi-skimmed milk, 200ml of fruit juice, and a piece of toast with a level teaspoon of butter and teaspoon of jam. I had to ask one of the nurse specialists how to spread my toast because it frightened me so much and I couldn't quite remember how to do it – Yes really, I couldn't put butter on a flipping piece of bread. I thought I would burst. "Well done," I was told. *"Shove it up your arse,"* I thought to myself. I had a lot of anger in me, and somehow it was being directed undeservedly (and albeit silently at first) towards the very people trying to help.

Day's were planned: breakfast at 9am, a group session, snack time, a break or individual therapy, lunch (a main meal with dessert), an afternoon group, and then home at 4pm. Clare had her individual therapy on Monday, and as Rose was on a week out, so I went on a walk with Becky during our free break before lunch. We sat in the sun, her arms painfully thin, yet still on display, and we got to know each other better. She insisted she ate well, but had trouble gaining weight. I remained sceptical, but believed that she believed herself.

I don't have to check my diary or my medical notes to remember exactly how much I ate every single day on the Day Programme, and I do mean *exactly*. Some of my avoidance techniques were caught, but many were not. For lunch on my first day it was pie, my worst nightmare (at least until the next meal). A dry meat pie served with new potatoes and peas. I genuinely hate new potatoes, but I had used up my allotted three dislike foods. I tried to eat, and I did eat most of it. It sat like lead in my stomach. I couldn't eat it all, but was congratulated by the staff for trying so hard. My silent thought processes went like this: *"Bullshit, bullshit, how do you know what it's like? Don't patronise me. Ah the pain, the pain. It hurts. Fuck off. I thought you were going to help me, not hurt me and leave me. Not only do I have to eat food, I have to eat disgusting, crappy food that I wouldn't feed my dog."* Excessive I admit, but truly how I felt.

After lunch I just wanted to lie down on my left side because it hurt less that way. I did get up and join in the afternoon group, but only because it was my first day and I hadn't built up the strength to say, "Get stuffed." Snack time at 3.45pm. *"No thanks, I wont be requiring one of those, so kind of you to offer,"* my teeth grating with sarcasm, as that all played out in my mind. I believe my actual answer was a teeth grinding "No." I might have mumbled something about it being my first two weeks.

I had read the "guidelines" and knew that for the first couple of weeks on the Programme, a member may choose (without harassment) not to participate in snacks to allow for a "settling in" period. I *always* read the small print. So at the 11am snack, and the 3.45pm snack I, (of course), refused. And as it happened I never ate snacks in the morning or afternoon for the entire nine months of my time on the programme. Occasionally I appeared to eat it, for an easier life. All the usual tricks, hiding food in pockets, in tissues, putting a mouthful into my mouth, then fetching a glass of water, a subtle disposal of the said mouthful into the bin as I passed.

Other people played games too, opening a packet of crisps, sitting there for 10 minutes, and then going to throw them away as if they'd been eaten, so on and so forth. Sometimes I'd get up and look in the bin to see what people had been disposing of – let's just say that at first, everybody there played some "games." Of course, these games ultimately hurt the person playing them, not the professionals trying to help.

At home time on my first day, Clare asked me to walk back with her, as we were both students living in our Colleges, albeit at opposite ends of the city. So, the end of what had seemed like an endless day that I didn't think I'd ever be able to repeat (and I was right),

Clare and I sauntered home in the afternoon sunshine of an English summer's day in Oxford – quite beautiful. We walked from Littlemore back along the river Thames, which becomes the river Isis as you enter the City. Clare was relieved to have a person who could relate to her problems and vice versa. I was very aware (even on my first day) that if I spent time with Clare that evening, I might help her to avoid bingeing and vomiting. Apparently that plan succeeded, though most Programme days ended almost inevitably with her spending the evening being sick.

On that first day we went to The Head Of The River pub, well known to all Oxford students. I had a pint of lager, too scared to consume more, my stomach still feeling full of lead. We laughed at the way that alcohol calories seemed different to all other calories. Clare had two pints. We talked for hours: depression, bulimia, anorexia, medical treatments both pharmacological and therapeutic, and then about love, our families, and academia. Clare got a 1st from Southampton and was at Oxford reading for an M.Phil. in philosophy, a member of Queen's College.

I instinctively suspected that alcohol was a problem for her from the moment she suggested we go to a pub. I guess my own dabbling into alcohol misuse triggered alarm bells in my brain. We went our separate ways at about 8pm by which point I *knew* alcohol was a problem for her, although she had not verbally hinted at it. Two years later she would tell me she was amazed that I noticed, but it seemed obvious to me. We had the beginnings of a firm, close, understanding friendship well in place.

Recently, I asked Clare to describe herself and her health up to our meeting at the Day Programme, so that

I might include it in this book to help others. What she didn't offer is that she is a vivacious, gifted, fiercely intelligent, beautiful young woman. She would probably argue that she only appears effervescent and intelligent, a mask that is maintained for the world to hide her insecurities. I must acknowledge that there is obviously some discrepancy between how confident she appears, and what she actually feels. But her intelligence could not be faked; her loyalty and genuine compassion towards her friends are incomparable and resilient. Clare is another person to whom I owe my life. Here is what Clare described about her earlier life and illness:

> "The first time I got drunk, tried vomiting, and felt really low was when I was 13. Depression came primarily: feeling different, not fitting in, feeling isolated, and hating myself. Then the eating and drinking became a way of solving those problems (my drinking has been a factor for longer than I realised).
>
> My first memory of being aware of my weight was when I'd been feeling these lumps under my arms and made them sore, and the doctor said they were fat pads and I was devastated. I was wearing all pink at the time (a pink sweater and pink cords), and I felt like a big fat blancmange. Mum says I was only five or six at the time, but I remember it so clearly.

I had taken 4 overdoses by the time I came on the day programme. Number 1 was a suicide attempt involving "x" prescription painkillers (Tylex - paracetamol with added codeine). I freaked out when I started to feel ill, and a friend took me to get my stomach pumped, (I was eighteen).

Number 2 was the day after the first overdose! I freaked out as soon as I'd taken them and made myself sick. I think that one was quite impulsive.

Number 3 was definitely a suicide attempt, foiled by my own lack of knowledge about drugs. I took at least "x" Ibuprofen and went to be with friends so I couldn't get scared about it like the first two attempts. I woke in the middle of the night and went to hospital. I didn't know that Ibuprofen was unlikely to kill. (I was 20). I had also cut myself. Kindly, I was told by the emergency staff that I would lose all my friends if this behaviour continued.

Number 4 was when I was drunk during the summer of my graduation (2000). I had returned to Southampton to get back on antidepressant medication. I don't even remember what I took, but it included my antidepressants and other things like headache tablets. I spontaneously threw up once in the night but still had to go to hospital, as I was very ill the next day. The friends I was with called me an attention seeker, and were annoyed that I had interrupted their party (nobody called an ambulance). I was 23. This was impulsive, self-harm, under the influence of alcohol, rather than a definite suicide attempt. Still, it was rather dangerous.

I took another overdose in 2002 whilst under the influence of alcohol, and cut my arm badly under the influence of alcohol, after we had become friends and which you know all about."

(Please note: there is no such thing as a "safe" overdose. What doesn't harm one person can harm or kill another).

As you can see, Clare had a desperately troubled history, and I empathised with her. The comments she remembers from bystanders and her own friends: lacking sympathy, understanding, or even common courtesy, added to her problems. She carried extra mental wounds (*more* guilt, self-hatred and shame) as a result. A cruel word, whether educated, thought through, or not, made the suffering greater.

Clare and I shared depression, but not exactly. She knew I was terribly low in mood and getting lower by the day. She knew I was suicidal, self-harming, and cycling for 4 or more hours a day, and said, "I don't understand it, we're both depressed, but all I can do is lie in bed and sleep, you do *so much*." Reflecting on this, it made perfect sense: we both felt depressed, but only I had the concurrent mania to deal with too. In other words, I was still in a mixed episode, if the word "episode" can really be applied to something that did not change for over 4 years. It was an episode that was to go on and on, becoming more and more painful. That is how I got "so much done," most (all?) of it self-destructive.

There were many very well thought through aspects of the Oxford Eating Disorders Day Programme. The menu, as much as I hated and failed to eat much of it, was very well planned, with lots of variety. Unlike at Leicester when you ate the same thing every other week, the menu was repeated in three-monthly sections, hence far more variety. Instead of the staff standing around watching us eat lunch, two staff members would actually sit down and eat with us: much less intimidating and far more convincing to us that the food was "normal." Some meals we actually cooked together, learning how to deal with being in the kitchen and handling food – invaluable experience.

There was a time limit by which we were supposed to finish eating, but this was flexible if people were still earnestly trying to eat. There was no rule about how much water we could or couldn't drink. Food was not all dished out for us, we had to serve ourselves from dishes on the table: the understanding being we would be corrected if we took too little *or* too much. Of course, I was terrified of being told I'd taken too much and would serve up by the teaspoonful – on a *cooperative* day.

Unlike at Leicester, talking about food and the issues of eating were not banned, rather they were encouraged. We all sat around the table to discuss each meal, to raise personal issues we were struggling with, to lavish praise or raise problems we had with another patient's behaviour. A lot of people had problems with me, all of which I fully deserved. It was doubly hard for them to eat when I sat there wilfully refusing. *"Fuck off. FUCK OFF. I'm not touching that filth, I don't trust you, FUCK OFF..."* came out translated into a single-but-firm word: "NO!"

All patients kept a food diary in which we wrote about our feelings, and which we could share with the group ...or not. The staff did not guard over us after meals: we could quite freely have gone to vomit, although it would have been obvious to all the other patients. To my knowledge, nobody actually vomited at the Day Programme. Staff and patients all supported each other as much as possible. It felt like a much less clinical environment: far less prescriptive and domineering, but unfortunately still *too* controlling for me personally.

The philosophy of the Oxford Adult Eating Disorders Service was different than at Leicester (where you *had* to eat everything). Thankfully there was none of the bulk-you-up-fast then discard you attitude (although there were two big meals and two snacks crammed into just seven hours of the day). Patients are treated as adults and staff-patient relationships are kept as equal as possible. The idea at Oxford was that you chose to eat what was provided, trusting the eating disorder team that it would be "normal." At first I thought this way sounded great, more empowering for the individual: giving back the freedom to choose what to eat rather than that choice being controlled by the eating disorder. However, for me, this did not alleviate any guilt for eating. If you "have" to eat, you do. If you are told it is your choice, however strongly you are encouraged, you *can* say "No." For me, even though I trusted the people working with me, since I could say "No," a guilty conscience demanded that I did exactly that.

As I was rather angry in general I would usually imply or say, "Fuck off!" I expected (and my fears were confirmed when I later read my medical notes), that this behaviour would appear as distrust of the Oxford eating disorders team. However, I did trust them, very much so, but my mind twisted the whole "your choice" idea into making every mouthful I ate a personal failure. My anger and increasing frustration with myself did not help the situation. At first I tried to get away with the old tricks of hiding food up my sleeve, dropping it on the floor under someone else's chair, putting it in tissue on my lap, or "accidentally" spilling it on the table, and leaving food mashed on my plate as if I had finished. Some of this I got away with, some of it was challenged only for me to say, "So what?" To prove my point, I would then retaliate (hurting only myself) by eating less. An entry in my medical notes reads:

> *"Katy was discovered placing her toast into a tissue, and after this was challenged she has refused to eat toast altogether. Katy was also found to be diluting her fruit juice with water. When this was raised she stopped having any juice."*

133

That's right, I was obnoxious and difficult: ruled by fear, anger and frustration. I suddenly became very good at letting people know exactly what (my anorexia demanded) I would and would not agree to do. Perhaps this rebellion was something I needed to go through in my life. In some ways it was liberating to finally stand my ground after so many years of being walked upon. I was also rude! I was on self-destruct by this point and I didn't give a flying fuck if their advice was good for me or not. I was going to state my feelings, and not be swayed. It wasn't stupidity, it was anger: definitely against my long-term best interests, and very much a waste of my time and the time of many caring experts. However, it was the only way I could survive.

In 2001, for the whole of Oxfordshire there were eight places on the Eating Disorder Day Programme and a long waiting list. Nobody really wanted to be there. A couple of people attended for a day or two, or even for half a morning, then left. So, unusually for a service in huge demand, there were only four of us attending regularly: Clare, Becky, Rose and myself, for the first few months after I started. We all became quite close, despite resentful feelings towards each other at times.

The Day Programme ran on weekdays except Wednesdays. The food routines were rigid, and each day had different distraction/learning sessions. Monday morning was Relationship Group: meaning a discussion about any relationships within the group, at home, past and present. I gained some useful insight into the problems of Becky and Rose, but Clare and I seemed to prefer to stay silent. Monday afternoon was the Day Activity Group: for planning distractions, a social life and enjoyable things to do. At first I allowed myself to be dragged to this session but did not really make use of it. I think I avoided it because I did not want to face up to planning any life. It was a useful session: just not for someone who expects to die soon, and cannot get past that particular prospect.

Tuesdays were my "favourite" day! In the morning we had Art Therapy, which I absolutely loved and created many very expressive pieces of work. I mostly created collages of pictures that I spent all week on the Internet looking for. There would be pictures of death, suicide, pills, drugs, drink, cycling, emotional pictures and my favourite Art prints. I didn't go for the subtle approach that needed to be analysed. A photo of a bloody torso and a severed head lying on train tracks is fairly candid.

Alternatively I would just write out long quotes from favourite films. Any of you who have seen Monty Python's "*Flying Circus*" will be familiar with the huge foot the comes down from the sky to splat people or objects together with a squeezing-farting sound. That famous foot is actually taken from a Bronzino (1503-1572) painting called "An Allegory with Venus and Cupid." I had a reprint of this, and cut out the foot, took it to Art Therapy, and created a picture of the foot coming down to squash various people, mostly those who bullied me as a kid and at Nottingham. Is it bad that it felt good?

On Tuesday mornings I saw my therapist for my individual session – handy for getting out of the morning snack with little fuss. In the afternoon we had Emotional Coping Skills Group where we learned about Dialectical Behaviour Therapy (DBT) in an effort to help us develop coping skills, and learn to recognise then challenge unhelpful thoughts. We learned to be *mindful* of our behaviour and choices, and we encouraged to be acquiescent instead of *wilful*. (I am too wilful – apparently). I quickly learned to recognise unhealthy, eating-disordered thinking, instead of blindly accepting and acting on those thoughts, however *I still couldn't help myself.* Clare described the same phenomenon. Eventually what I learned helped, but back in 2001, I was just wilful and frustrated.

Thursdays were the worst day, which everyone hated because it was Weighing Group. That meant everyone had to be weighed, and then there were consequences. I had refused to be weighed, and based on my abhorrence of someone weighing me thanks to my dad, the staff agreed to let me weigh myself at home: I promised them and myself not to lie. We all had weight graphs; underweight patients had to gain weight at approximately 1lb a week minimum, until they reached a Body Mass Index (BMI) of 20. Patients at a BMI of 20, which included myself at first, and Clare, had to maintain it.

I was quite please to read in my notes that the professionals noted the fact I had a BMI of 20 did not make me "fine" because all the exercise (around 400 miles a week cycling – creating lots of muscle) would have given a falsely high BMI. Every few weeks Becky or Rose would have to have a "week out" for falling behind on their weight gain: a perceived punishment that was apparently to "give people time to think about their goals."

Everyone fought against enforced time out, and no matter how the staff dressed it up as being "for your own good" and "to make sure you really want to choose to gain weight and/or get well," it felt like punishment, and it really was that simple. Even as a fan of psychology, I thought that it was psychobabble-bullshit to turn anyone away like that. Those people needed help, not abandonment.

It doesn't take a stretch of the imagination to see why we all hated the group: if we'd been good and stayed within our weight band, we felt like fat cows. If we hadn't, the perceived threats from staff made people feel abandoned, bad and worthless; plus some group members got pissed off with others whilst emotions ran high. I found the focus on weight made me want to lose weight. Clare's face always looked like thunder as Becky and Rose complained about how hard it was to gain weight. She almost never spoke in Weighing Group, and neither did I. It was the day everybody was most likely to not attend. Thursday afternoons were for more DBT.

Fridays were strange. In the morning we had Menu Planning to discuss the following week's menu, which invariably got very complicated, and I would get caught up in the whole affair and angry. From the beginning, I often went in late to avoid this group. I felt offended at people telling me what I should eat: even though I know they were trying to help. It felt too dictatorial, too critical, reminding me of family battles about food. Being a Nelly-know-it-all who practically had a Ph.D. in Nutritional Medicine and deserved a Ph.D. in anorexia meant it felt insulting – to me.

Friday afternoons were recreational, with us playing cards or watching a DVD. Strangely, I found it very hard to play and would just sit there. It wasn't just the pain I felt from eating, if I had eaten: I was incapable of having fun.

The opinion that people receiving hospital treatment for anorexia or bulimia love their treatment because they "love food and living a life that revolves around food" is (in my humble opinion) erroneous and offensive. I agree that such hospital treatments lead to a life that is planned around each meal or snack, but that does not make it fun. Whatever I ate or did not eat, I felt like the food was piling up inside me, suffocating me. All my fellow patients consistently appeared to be in great distress: I don't believe they were all consummate actresses who kept up a 7-hour-long performance each day. I do know for *absolute* certainty that I hated every single moment of it. I have never met anyone who appeared to, or admitted to enjoying this treatment, however much they "enjoyed" their illness.

I would also dispute the common insinuation that all eating disorder patients want other patients to gain weight and eat out of any malicious or manipulative intent. I would concede that eating more than others, weighing more than others, or gaining weight when others don't *is very hard*: but that is part of the illness due to ubiquitous perfectionism and self-criticism. Some patients do get into competitions with other patients to be the "most sick," but this is only done to hurt oneself, *never* another. Some patients are aware that part of them is trying to be the "most sick," but still fight to overcome that.

Certainly gaining weight is hard for anyone, but I truly and honestly wanted my new friends to recover for their own sake; and my definition of recovery had only a very small part to do with their weight. It was easy to see "simple" ways for the others to get better, but impossible to put any of those suggestions into practice for myself. I *desperately* wanted recovery, but that heartfelt desire didn't help me. In honesty, I think I put my own recovery above anyone else's – and yet I continued to watch others improve whilst I got worse. Wanting to put myself first doesn't make me a selfish or bad person, just a desperate, distressed, tormented, ill person. Ideally I wanted us all to recover.

Recently I asked Rose to remember how she saw me as a fellow patient at the day programme. It is interesting to see how people saw me as happy. I was far too good at hiding my feelings. Rose said:

> "Memories I have of you. Well firstly you always put on a smiley happy face, even though some days were hell. I remember the influence your childhood memories had on your eating and the terror of sausages and desserts you had. So much that sometimes you couldn't even sit at the table with it in front of you. Sometimes you avoided coming in because of the terror.
>
> You had so much courage though as you fought your extreme exercise addiction. You had to cycle at least 50 miles every day before the programme whatever the weather, and it caused you great anxiety when you tried cutting it down in tiny steps.
>
> I remember your compassion and gentleness when you often cleaned and dressed my cuts from self-harm, and the kindness you wrote on a card to me, when I was very

low. You noticed everything that went on.

It is so sad that you had such a horrible controlling illness Katy. I would love you to be well and free."

September 11th 2001. What were you doing that day? My fellow eating disordered friends and I sat around the lunch table crying and moaning about having to eat a roast dinner. As we moaned, and I probably moaned the loudest, the Twin Towers fell. Lunchtime in the UK corresponded to the start of the working day on the east coast of America. In the evening, I got home and turned on the news. I sat there fixed to the TV for about 5 hours. I realised that when we had been eating, not-eating, crying, and hiding food under the table, other people were dying in the most horrific way. I can't say that September 11th "cured" me, but it started my very gradual recovery from the anorexia. It made me really see how ridiculously I was behaving, and take responsibility for my conduct.

Unfortunately, it also made me hate myself even more. (Mindful of harsh self-judgements) I decided I was a stupid, ungrateful cow who refused to let a roast potato touch my lips whilst thousands of people were crushed, or jumped from high windows when faced with the choice between falling or burning to death. What a choice?

The following Tuesday in Art Therapy, I came in prepared. Whilst the others drew, I stuck lots of large black pieces of paper together, and then plastered them with newspaper articles on September 11th. Ninety-five percent of the paper was death and mayhem, the remaining five-percent all squashed unimportantly into a bottom corner were some pictures of a roast dinner.

Despite my initial hopes that the Day Programme would help my mood and eating, it seemed it was not meant to be. Every day I excessively exercised and refused lots of food. I don't think there was a single day where I didn't feel a failure both as an anorectic and as a recovering anorectic: i.e. a *total* failure. I wanted to recover from my disordered eating, but would not allow anyone to help me: I saw it as controlling. I stood firm on my imaginary battlefield: I would not give an inch.

I did not intend to lose weight again. I wanted to be well. I did not intend to start self-harming either, mainly because I knew it really distressed my therapist who I cared about. But the depression was growing exponentially, and I started losing weight. I think, perhaps, I was making an unconscious statement. Gaining weight, therefore eating would mean I was feeling better. I quite certainly was not feeling good, better, worthwhile, human, or at all recovered.

Losing weight and self-harming showed both myself, and the others, that I felt like death. I entertained death: I "enjoyed" entertaining death.

Unwise.

Chapter 5. Sometimes things just go Awry.

"Not I - not anyone else, can travel that
road for you,
You must travel it for yourself."

☙ Walt Whitman (1819-1892).

So, things went awry. After four months at the Day
Programme, I'd had the usual three-monthly review to
see if I should stay, and for which I filled in an
achievements record: on which I politely wrote "FUCK
ALL." And on weeks 7 and 10 I'd had "extraordinary
reviews," which were called if problems were arising –
giving a feeling not unlike being called to see the
headmistress for bad behaviour. I was allowed to stay
on the Programme because my mood was so low they
knew I needed support. I was low, that part was true,
but it was a confused depression: mixed with anger,
hopelessness and unquiet desperation. I saw no way
through the obstacles of life, and I was furious at
myself.

Pathologically I fitted into nice neat boxes by this
point. I had anorexia nervosa and by this point severe
mixed bipolar I disorder[17] – which presented with
depression, psychosis, and intense anger (i.e. dysphoric
mania). Confusion was rife. To look at or talk to me,
the severity of my problems were almost invisible –
even to the trained eye. Indeed, my bipolar disorder

---

[17] Type I bipolar disorder is characterised by periods of *mania*
and/or *mixed* episodes usually together with depression of varying
severities, in my case, very severe. Type II bipolar disorder is
characterised by periods of *hypomania* and periods of depression.
The length of any episode varies from person to person.

went undiagnosed. I was suicidal: thinking all day and night about a way to kill myself. I spent hours on the Internet researching suicide and ordered various drugs (all legal to import and possess at that time) with which to either kill myself or help myself sleep. I couldn't sleep, I couldn't really eat, the whole world seemed black, and on occasion I heard, smelled and saw things that weren't there – i.e. I hallucinated.

I saw the Dark-Man-over-my-shoulder every night, though thankfully during the day I did not. Self-harming kept him at the far end of my room. Anger was my primary emotion, but I did not express it; instead my mind simmered, bubbled, and then boiled like a witches cauldron of malevolent, smelly gunk. Then it boiled over, boiled dry and burned. I turned it inwards by starving, exercising, cutting, bloodletting, searching for ways to die and generally throwing myself here, there and everywhere, as being in constant motion seemed best. Sadness was also present – it paralysed me. If I stopped moving I would be stuck, helpless, unable to defend myself or move... Anger made my mind race faster and faster, sadness made my body slow. Everything was overwhelmingly intense: a painful combination.

Whether or not I was technically delusional is debatable. I believed people hated me and wanted me to die, which partly came from my low self-esteem. I thought people wanted to give up on me, or that they already had given up on me. In my opinion, my fears of being hated went deeper than the usual eating-disordered low self-image I had been somewhat accustomed to for some years. I believe that I was delusional and I would become increasingly more so, including some distinctive paranoid delusions.

I was also suffering from what could be described as flashbacks that left me detached from reality. I was told I had PTSD (Post Traumatic Stress Disorder). Many of these were actually "small" auditory (at first) and then auditory *and* visual hallucinations that took place at the Day Programme, often at meal times. I felt like I was young (the age varied), lost, and afraid of what I can best describe as loud NOISE surrounding me from all directions, suffocating all my senses. Imagine yourself dancing at the loudest rock concert, (think Ozzy Osbourne), where you cannot hear yourself speak, let alone think; one minute you are being blinded by light, the next in absolute darkness. It was not unlike being surrounded by bullies leering or subjugated by something/someone powerful: but putting it into words is hard. I lost contact with the real world on many levels. I was mostly lucid, as if clinging to reality by spidery wisps of web, stretching, breaking, but strong enough to maybe, with a miracle, hold.

Increasingly I feared leaving the Day Programme at the end of the day because I knew the Dark-Man-over-my-shoulder awaited me. I used to hang around until the place was shutting. I knew self-harm was inevitable, however bored and tired I was of it. I also knew that my cutting was taking place with the major intent of killing myself, quietening my demons once and for all. I could often see "him" out of the corner of my right eye. He was not always there, but most often he would be there at night, threatening me.

He seemed concurrently ghostly and solid – I never touched him because my muscles would freeze if I tried. I never saw him move, he would just "be" somewhere. I never spoke to him, or him to me, but we knew what we were both thinking. It felt like he was waiting to get me alone to hurt me. He'd always stand in one particular corner when I worked on my computer late into the night. Sometimes he'd block me in my room, standing between the door and myself. I'd scream (making no sound) that he wasn't real, or self-harm to bring myself back to reality. I did not require pain to ground myself, just the absolute concentration that my surgical/medicalised self-harm demanded.

It didn't matter how unreal the Dark Man was; I was still afraid. I always "slept" right in the corner of my room, with the Dark-Man-over-my-shoulder in the corner, so that there was no room for "him" to get behind me. Lying in bed, I'd feel like he was standing in the dark corners of my room watching me. I'd close my eyes to try and sleep, but then have to quickly open them out of fear. Sometimes, in the blink of an eye, he'd have crossed my room, and when I opened my eyes, he was right in front of my face. It was a real-life horror movie. His head was on my pillow, his eyes glaring wide, our noses "touching," suffocating me, but I couldn't feel his breath.

Other hallucinations/dreams/feelings seemed less malevolent and rather like I imagine LSD (Acid) to be like. They would come and go rather than always be present. The world would seem wobbly, stationary objects would move: and this was without a drop of alcohol or any drugs. I'd stopped taking my antidepressant lofepramine; I do not recall why. I sometimes tried to write about what I saw. (I don't make much sense). Verbatim from my diary:

"I sometimes <u>hear</u> banging. Sometimes <u>feel</u> it. Have u ever seen words move around on a page? I'm sitting at the

computer – I think it is floating. Screen is all wavy. Makes no sense, like writing on a tile?? Are letters doing 360 degree rotation on the page or in my head? My words melt. A person's face, a book, a pen, a screen... the darkness. All are suspended from long, dark cords which I can see moving and I shouldn't."

I continued with my "life," and told nobody any of this. It surprises those who knew me at the time when I tell them about the activity in my mind, the things that I saw, the terrible feelings I had; all hidden away, kept to myself. I deserve an Oscar.

Becky left the Day Programme in order to study, although she was still greatly troubled by her problems. In quick succession, two new members joined the Day Programme: both so very young, both of whom I implored not to be naïve about the seriousness of their condition, and to whom I stressed the benefit of getting well sooner rather than later (unlike me).

Harriet was an effervescent first year medical student from Oxford's Worcester College, and a person with anorexia. Ayeesha was a stunning young woman: aged 19, studying history at York, but originally from Oxford. She always wore beautiful clothes and accessories: a delicate necklace, or a stunning hair clip in her strikingly beautiful, dark, shiny hair. She was so emaciated all the patients knew at a glance she was under the normal minimum weight for being a day patient, and we all wondered why she wasn't hospitalised. Maybe some of us were jealous... No, let's cut the crap, in a warped way, we *were* jealous.

Harriet's first day went by without much happening. She was obviously finding things hard, but dogmatically focussed on eating what she was told to, and joined in with all the groups. I admired her courage and her determination: both good qualities in a young doctor. I learnt that she believed if no one spoke in a group session, she felt compelled to. Unfortunately for Harriet (or Harry as we called her), Rose had lost her voice due to a psychological condition possibly linked to anxiety and stress, which lasted for many weeks. As that just left Clare and myself who spoke very little, Harry was under constant pressure to speak up.

A week later was Ayeesha's first day; and thankfully she spoke often, with honesty and competence. I saw her struggle, her pain; and thankfully, her unusual innocence regarding calories and fat in food. She also placed less importance on other numbers, such as her weight. This, to my knowledge, is rare in any person with an eating disorder. Most of us could pass as qualified nutritionists, and most are obsessed or at least markedly focused on the number on a set of scales. Straight away Ayeesha made it clear that she was worried she would learn about calories from the other patients, and thus develop more obsessions. So we all tried not to mention those things in front of her. She had a fair point: I learned a lot of unhelpful "tips" from other people with eating disorders.

I went the opposite way when it came to calories. I used to sneak into the kitchen and look at the packets of what was for lunch, add up the fat, and then tell the staff that I wasn't going to eat it (hopefully without scaring the others). Eventually the staff used to remove all the labels, or colour them in with black pen to stop me looking. So I used to look at the products, cycle to a supermarket in snack time, and find the identical items to read the labels. Clearly none of this was helpful.

Ayeesha had been an anorectic for a year. *"A year,"* I thought: *"It seems like no time at all, yet I know it would have seemed endless."* Ironically Ayeesha told me that when she met all the patients, she though I was one who had managed to do well and gain some weight, because everyone else in the room (Rose and Harry, no Clare) that day happened to be severely underweight. One thing that struck me SMACK in the face about both Harriet and Ayeesha was their obvious strong will to recover and their determination at the meal table, no matter how upset they were. There were no games; they just did as advised. Without wishing them any harm, without seeing them as weak: I was jealous.

I worried that I made things hard for other day programme members, guilty with the certainty that my not eating some or all of my food at the Programme made eating harder for them. Not only was I playing tricks on the staff about what I ate, but now with some of the patients (who were far less easy to fool). It's not huge leap to understand why they would feel resentment towards me for "getting away" with behaviours that they did not. Of course, I wanted to *scream* that the only thing I was getting away with was hurting myself.

Sometimes, especially when we sat around the lunch table to discuss the meal, some or all of the other patients verbalised their feelings about my behaviour, more usually I saw (or assumed I saw) the anger, despair, confusion, irritation and sadness in their eyes. I think that Clare found it really hard to be angry with me, despite actually feeling furious. It was very hard for her to speak out because we had become very close. (But don't worry, that didn't stop her). Somewhere in my brain a connection was not working, and my deceitful behaviour at the meal table is something I am now very regretful about.

One wonderful thing was that none of the patients took failures with food personally: we all knew the illness was at play. We were all friends, and although I know I upset people, we moved on quickly, and supported each other. Interestingly Ayeesha wrote to me:

> "The Day Programme staff and my therapist often asked me about how I felt about you. I think I just accepted your behaviour as part of a treatment programme. It was only after you left that I realised you weren't at all normal! I very clearly remember thinking that this was absurd and I was 'not going to be beaten by a bloody yoghurt.' This remained my attitude for much of the program. I didn't really think 'why should I eat if she isn't' because I became totally and selfishly focused on my own recovery."

Obviously it wasn't selfish to want to recover. I asked Ayeesha to think back and recall just one event where I pissed everyone off:

> "Ok, chips. It was the first time I had had chips since I had been on the Day Programme and they were most definitely on my list of 'danger' foods. We passed

the portions round, I was sitting next to you, and you obviously took less than you should. I took the required amount. One person taking less meant the bowl being passed around again, and everyone else had 'more.' I ate everything, you didn't. I guess it was obvious that I was fairly angry with you for what I saw as 'cheating.' Afterwards I cried. I remember saying that it just wasn't fair. I don't remember your reaction. To be perfectly honest I feel embarrassed about it all. It was a plate of chips for God's sake. This kind of memory makes me determined never to go back to the situation where I get that upset about food."

I do remember that day and my completely internalised reaction: I was *gutted*. I nearly walked out for good, and I wanted to die (as per usual). I didn't want to hurt anyone, nor did I know the chips would be circled again. I was acting out of fear and anger. Fear to put food on my plate that I knew I couldn't look at, let alone eat; and misdirected anger making me think *"why the fuck should I put food on my plate"* if I didn't want to. My argument, rightly or wrongly, was that the staff knew that I took too little, I owned up to it straight away, and the others should not have been made to pass the bowl around again. If I recall correctly, this point was discussed and learned from.

So I asked Ayeesha about how depressed and angry I seemed whilst on the Day Programme. Her insight was surprising until I thought about it, and then I realised her view was spot on:

"You had the most impassive face I think I have ever seen. It was impossible to tell what you were feeling. There was one incident when this really hit me: Clare 'had a go' at you right to your face; she was in tears, but you did not show anything at all."

And so I had to ask: did you ever think I would try to kill myself?

"Oh yes."

People struggled to understand why I was allowed to stay on the Programme whilst still cycling, or whilst actually losing weight quite quickly. But everyone had difficulties. Other people also weren't gaining weight; one person was faking weight gain for a while; others weren't eating well at or away from the Programme; I was not alone exercising in my free time; some people were bingeing and vomiting, albeit away from the hospital. Rose, Clare and myself were all self-harming. I may have been a mess, but I wasn't alone.

Despite being very pleased for Harry and Ayeesha progressing well, it also really upset me by highlighting my own failures. I was not upset or angry with them, I was upset and angry with myself. I would go home and stew about how disappointed I felt in myself. It upset me that they could do so well, with less experience of eating disorders, and about something I had been *earnestly* trying to recover from for years. I chastised myself for my self-indulgent, and above all else stupid behaviour in "choosing" to be an anorectic.

I am not claiming it to be a lifestyle choice; I hated anorexia. But I did enjoy fitting into smaller clothes, dancing around my College room at night, all night, wiggling my loose hipsters to the music to get rid of all my nervous energy. But I gave up on the possibility of recovering from anorexia, and hence I gave up on life. I went home and watched *Girl, Interrupted* over and over, looking for any hint that might help me. I was (am) a total *ambivalent*. Ambivalent in it's original meaning: that of being torn in two opposing directions.

My Oxford therapist warned me, around this time, that I may find myself with choosing between the choice of a "career" in hospital (as a patient) or living a real life. I dismissed her wise words because by then I did not care – but I never forgot what she said.

The eating disorder that once masked my manic depression and in that way saved me was now killing me in my heart. I was trapped. I felt guilty for not being as strong as the others, and took out this guilt on myself, by slicing my left arm. I started to see with absolute clarity for the first time, the trap that anorexia had me in, and this fact alone made me more depressed. My depression caused me to catastrophise: deciding that for me, recovery was, and always would be impossible. Eating disorders bored me stupid, I just could not find the energy with which to fight my anorexia *or* maintain it.

I can't remember why, but it also dawned on me that my depressive illness was the *major* problem. This revelation did not help me at the time; the world seemed so black and without change. My mood was too low for logical thinking; instead, I believed I would never recover from the depression and death was the only answer. I tried to tell people that the anorexia was *nothing* next to the depression. Clare and I would talk about depression because she recognised it as a major problem for her too. She said, that the bulimia never alleviated her depression except maybe for the first three months she started doing it full time. She also said, "I wasn't drunk to begin with, and any cutting was superficial - it only got worse with the overdoses and coming to Oxford. I was desperately ill when I arrived; Oxford didn't cause my deepening problems, it just highlighted them."

Still I berated myself for destroying my life. My arms reached further out in search of death, which to me signalled the end: oblivion, no more suffering. At first, in order to keep myself free from scars that I knew Dr. MacLennan would see, I had mostly used bloodletting to self-harm: after which I would run in a litre of saline intravenously. I can't exactly explain the logic behind why I felt able to treat my fluid depletion. I suspect there was an element of feeling cleansed: the "ultimate cleansing experience" from inside your own bloodstream. Also, I needed to cycle: being dehydrated and anaemic made that harder. I couldn't bring myself to treat the anaemia (with iron tablets), but the dehydration I could. Dr. MacLennan spotted the anaemia, which was not difficult: I looked like a ghost. Then one day when he asked to check my arm, he rolled my sleeve right up past the elbow, and spotted a puncture wound; and so I told him about the bloodletting. He looked surprised - I never saw him look surprised before.

My therapist and the people running the Program became more and more worried about me. This was despite the fact that they did not know the extent to which my self-harm and suicidal ideation had sunk. I was losing weight without wanting to, and trying harder and harder to follow their advice, and sinking lower each time I failed. But doing as I was advised (regarding food or taking part in group sessions) did not help me either. Nothing worked. I was a mess – overwhelmed. Essentially I was just like you on a really bad day, amplified millions of times over.

I sought reassurance and didn't receive anything I could make use of. The staff promised to support me through eating, groups, and impulses to self-harm: which was all very well except that I was beyond help. (Which doesn't mean they didn't try; it means nothing worked). Also the Day Programme lasted for a measly 7 hours out of the 24 I needed to fill each day. I still feel let down that they were so unable to help me or cope with my eating disordered and mood disordered behaviour – granted I still wasn't diagnosed as bipolar. I don't think people were supposed to act as I did; I know they tried their best, but the fact remained they did not help me – and I felt abandoned and angry because of this. They had, after all, *promised* to help me.

Some examples from my medical notes read:

> *"Katy is very low. She is finding it hard to find any motivation and is feeling hopeless. She said, 'I'll never get over my eating disorder.' She is unable* [note unable rather than unwilling] *to respond to staff and group encouragement."*

> *"Katy was unable to even look at the cake, or smell it, or touch it."*

*"Katy was unable to draw in Art Therapy.
She described herself as having 'too much
in my head, I can't get it all down, I don't
know where to start.'"*

In early December, the beginning of my 5th month in the Day Programme, my therapist asked me to see a psychiatrist. Had anyone else asked me I would have said "No," but I trusted her, and felt able to agree if she came with me the first time. The psychiatrist was nice, although I felt she was a little dismissive about how depressed I was. Once again, my apparent stoicism and "impassive face" did not act in my favour. A plan was made during the Christmas break: when the Day Programme closed for two weeks, I was to be referred to the Warneford Hospital's Day Hospital. A drop-in centre open 365 days a year, with various activities on offer, a wide variety of patients, not just eating disordered people, …and lunch. (Sarcastic "whoopee.") I agreed I would go home to Derby on Christmas Eve, and drive back to Oxford on Christmas Day, to attend the Day Hospital from Boxing Day onwards. I attended for 3 mornings, going home before lunch, and spending the rest of my time researching suicide.

The Day Programme reopened. I'd lost lots of weight, had another review and a couple of extraordinary reviews as well. I began to cut myself more and more seriously: deliriously happy, (in a warped sense) that I could now cut myself seriously deeply. My prior cutting had been reasonably superficial, bad enough to leave scars, but not life threatening or particularly deep. My previous "failure" at cutting myself deeply enough to express my pain to an empty audience had always frustrated me greatly.

(Warning: explicit self-harm details). I had lignocaine (a local anaesthetic, called lidocaine/xylocaine in the US, works like novocaine), syringes, needles and scalpels from my workplace at the Radcliffe Infirmary, meaning I could anaesthetise myself and cut deeply, thus "proving" to myself that I was seriously unhappy. Sometimes I cut for cuttings sake, mesmerised by the cold, precise, clinical form of self-harm I had chosen. Lulled by the visual proof that my life sucked. Such calculated self-harm took a lot of concentration, which "helped" me stop thinking depressing thoughts or be distracted by the Dark-Man-over-my-shoulder. Sometimes I cut to kill myself. Along and across my cephalic vein; close to but not actually reaching the main radial artery or ulnar artery; trying to avoid tendons. Surgically cutting down with precision, learning more each time about my own anatomy. Then I would lie down to die, my arm wrapped very loosely (so as *not* to stem the flow) in several towels, and still the blood would get everywhere: all over my floor, the bed, myself.

I don't know how I survived, but I did, despite doing this over and over again. Night after night, I flirted with Death like this: begging him to take me, excited when I saw and felt the rhythmic spurt of an artery or ooze and drip from a vein. That made me human; which meant I could die. I stood looking into the mirror in my Collage room. Apparently most people who commit suicide by cutting their throat do so whilst looking into a mirror. I held the scalpel at my throat; I pressed hard, but could not make myself move my shaking hand.

"If I commit suicide, it will not be to
destroy myself but to put myself back

together again. Suicide will be for me only
one means of violently reconquering
myself."

❧ Antonin Artaud, written in 1925 in *Le
Disque Vert.*
French playwright, poet, actor and director
(1896 - 1948).

For my 27th Birthday, I treated myself to an Art poster by Scott Lobaido called *Forever 27.*[18] The picture was extremely frightening to me, and yet I hung it on the wall next to my bed. It depicts an unearthly room in the sky, with two people leaning at the bar, a woman leaning against a glassless window. The floor is crumbling, a clock is melting, and in the doorway stands a new figure: a man with tousled, long, blonde hair, and a long shadow. On closer inspection you can see it is Janis Joplin by the window, who died of a heroin overdose *aged 27.* Jim Morrison, who died of a possible heroin overdose *aged just 27,* is sitting at the bar. Also at the bar is Jimi Hendrix who died from choking on his own vomit after a seconal (barbiturate) overdose, not thought to be suicide. *His age: 27.* Kurt Cobain is the willowy figure arriving in the doorway; who died *age 27* from a self-inflicted gunshot wound whilst under the influence of enough heroin to kill a horse.

Though the exact circumstances of these deaths are still disputed by some people, one thing was certain: they were all 27, and drugs killed or part-killed them. I used to stare at this poster; sometimes for hours at a

[18] Scott Lobaido's fine art print *Forever 27* can be found at Art.com

time; I thought (a delusion) that it was a message especially for me; sometimes I'd swear the figures in it smiled at me, calling me to join them. *"How wonderful,"* I thought: *"to never be older than 27."* I didn't believe in heaven or other planes of existence, but if I died, I would be Forever 27 just like them. I got it into my already overcrowded head that I was meant to die at 27.

I remember one good day from this time. Linacre College held a "Heroes Party." (Long before the hit TV series). The idea was to come dressed as your hero, or someone you felt to be a hero – there were prizes at stake. I, being Katy Sara Culling naturally slipped on my Derby Country kit and went dressed as my favourite player of the time – Ravianelli. (I'm blonde you see). The showing off of my long toned legs won me a prize of a free drink. My sister won the Best Costume Award, and rightly so. She came dressed as a New York fire fighter out of respect for 9/11. (Not to take anything away from other heroes on that day).

My cutting got worse and worse until one day, Tuesday February 12th 2002, I decided to have a quick cut one morning before cycling to the Day Programme. This was impulsive and I did not really understand why I chose to do it: just that I had time to spare, and I felt like doing it. With hindsight I think it was also due to feeling under pressure to have regained weight by Thursday (2 days away). I had worked desperately hard in order to gain 2lbs, so as not to be forced to have a week out. I felt angry and manipulated because I did not agree with the whole week-out philosophy when someone needs support. It was unusual of me to cut on impulse; usually it was calculated. Perhaps my angry, impulsive cutting was related to the fact I had just weighed myself and discovered I had succeeded in gaining that oh-so-special 2lbs.

I got a bit "excited" and cut deeper than I should. (Warning: explicit self-harm details). I hit a small artery. Spurt, spurt, spurt went the bright red arterial blood: showing up nicely against my cream painted walls. Because Tuesday's were Art Therapy and the day I got to see my individual therapist, I really wanted to go. So I bound it tightly, and hid my body under a large Derby County fleece, and headed towards the Day Programme. The excitement, the release from the anger, the *relief* at feeling mortal, that I really could seriously damage myself, the image of that spurting, red blood making a huge mess, fired my desire to find arteries. From that day on I never stopped cutting until I did.

At breakfast, the Occupational Therapist asked me "What's that?" "Nothing." I mumbled, moving my arm to cover over where some blood had started to leak on to the table whilst I fake-munched on cardboard tasting cereal. I regret how thoughtless it was of me to not consider the wellbeing of the other patients. However well aware they were that self-harm was happening, even to themselves, they did not want to have it shoved in their faces at breakfast. I later learned that none of the patients even noticed because the staff cleaned up so quickly. I was sent to Accident & Emergency at the John Radcliffe (JR) Hospital, which was on a different site, nearer to Headington, in Oxford. My first JR visit of many. The JR staff seemed kind: I may be cynical, but I think that it was because a member of staff from the Eating Disorders Unit was with me.

Later, when I returned to the Eating Disorders Day Programme, a member of staff asked me to agree to be assessed by a psychiatrist that day. *"Passed the buck,"* was the thought in my head. *"They can't cope with things greater than a bit of crying over eating disorders."* I didn't think the psychiatrist would say anything: my experience of them was that they were dismissive of my problems. As I had a lot of respect for the member of staff who asked me, and because I didn't think cutting my arm would lead to anything much: I agreed. She took me to the Warneford Hospital. That night I found myself, rather alarmingly, in a hospital bed.

I was assessed by the psychiatric SHO ("senior house officer," i.e. a junior doctor specialising in psychiatry). *"He's my age,"* I thought. *"If I'd gone to medical school instead of getting anorexia, maybe I'd be where he is now."* That thought upset me. He was calming and polite, obviously clever, and seemed sympathetic but distant, which I tried to tell myself was tiredness, and nothing personal about me. I decided I liked him, so I answered his questions honestly. When undergoing a psychiatric patient history for a possible emergency admission, there are several areas of your life that are questioned to build up an idea of the risk to your life and determine if you are having a suicide crisis.[19] The highest risk factor for committing suicide is a previous attempt – I admitted to just one because I knew it was in my medical records. The real tally at this point was approximately 90.

I did not offer any additional information, such as proper details of my self-harm, or hallucinations. I did not even recognise my delusion about the Forever 27

---

[19] At imminent risk of actually taking one's own life – more than just thinking or planning suicide, a suicide crisis is when there is a real chance that suicide will be carried out.

poster. My suicidal ideation was obviously worrying, as was my medical knowledge and access to dangerous implements/drugs (via work). I admitted that I wanted to steal insulin to inject an overdose of, but explained that I was too afraid of getting caught and losing my Ph.D. place. *But I could steal cyanide, or potassium chloride for a lethal injection,* I thought to myself. But whilst those thoughts passed through my mind, I just sat there without an expression. Also there was the self-harm they *did* know about, and the fact that I lived an isolated life, even within my Oxford College.

Then came the ultimate questions, "What can you do to help yourself *not* commit suicide? What do you have to cling to, to remember, to pull you through this difficult time?" I sat silently, a blank expression no doubt upon my face: I could think of no answers. Therefore I was admitted to hospital "voluntarily." Voluntary under explicit instructions: if I did not comply, I would be held involuntarily on a Section 5(2) then possibly a Section 2 of the Mental Health Act. I very nearly ran off, but the SHO and other staff blocked my exit and herded me gradually and reluctantly towards the ward: Vaughan Thomas Ward, of the Warneford Hospital, Oxford.

That first admission was just for one night and the following day, but it terrified me. I was admitted at 8pm, unable to get over the feeling of total lack of control about everything. My bag was searched, making me feel dirty; and then I was left alone in a dingy, dirty, smelly bedroom with plastic sheets and nothing to do but feel trapped and alone. I lost it. I cannot bare boredom. I cried, and lay on the sticky bed in the clothes I had worn that day, since I had no others. Fortunately no one saw me going mad that night. I didn't sleep, but I lay very still. I felt like screaming and kicking the place down: but of course, I didn't. I didn't want to cause a fuss to make them keep me in hospital for any longer than necessary. I was still at the stage of thinking: *"I don't have feelings."* Occasionally someone would shine a torch on me to check I was alive and present.

The next day I hid in my room till about 1pm, during which time my favourite nurse specialist and my individual therapist from the Eating Disorder Unit had thankfully visited. They professed to be powerless about my admission, which left me feeling abandoned even though the (small) rational part of me understood the situation. So I turned to the Vaughan Thomas nurses about wanting to go home. I met for the first time, a nurse called Richard Ford, and begged him to help me get the doctor to listen, or at least *arrive* to hear my plea for freedom.

More than anything else I was desperate to cycle. I wrote page after page about how being admitted was a wake up call for me, and that I would be fine back at Linacre College. I found answers (lies) I could give to the questions about how I would survive. I said I'd talk to my College and get extra support so I was not at so much risk. (Of course, I didn't). No one would say how long I would *have* to stay; they just kept repeating that if I tried to leave, I would be detained by force.

The other problem was that I was admitted on a Tuesday night, after dinner and with no offer of dinner. It's true that I probably wouldn't have eaten it, but that is not the point. It was beyond my control and I wasn't even given the option of eating a small amount of it. Why was this issue such a problem? Well although I had gained the 2lbs, time in hospital not eating or drinking, too afraid to leave my room would seriously mess up my plans. Everyone seemed to think was a good idea that I went to the Day Programme in the day, and was kept on the ward at night (*no exercise* meant I refused that option). Essentially this meant that on Thursday, Weighing Group day, *if* I was allowed out to the Day Programme (and had somehow been able to weigh myself), I could be forced to have a dreaded week out. I pleaded with my therapist and the nurse specialist running the Day Programme: surely my mitigating circumstances would be allowed for. I was told they would not. This angered me in its total and utter nonsensicality. I knew that a week out would just mean more time alone to dance my merry dance with Death.

The only thing I had to eat was a cereal bar that I had at the bottom of my bag, and I drank water, which I fetched from the bathroom in a plastic glass. I came out of my room on the acute ward (where there were windows in the doors so that people could watch you), to plead with Richard to get a doctor to come and let me (the hell) out. He did his best despite a buzzing ward. As my despondency increased, I moved and sat on the chair outside the ward's office as if to *will* a doctor to arrive with my desperation and pleading eyes.

The Oxford City Central Mental Health Team doctor I was admitted under was too busy to see me, as was their whole team. Thankfully the SHO from the night before agreed to assess me again, saying it made the most sense since he knew my history. I made my case for release. He agreed I could go soon, but said he wanted me to stay at least another night. *"Oh my god, not another night in this hellhole,"* I thought. I persuaded him to allow me to go that night, based on the fact I needed to eat properly ready for Weighing Group the following morning. He reluctantly and thankfully agreed; but then again, it was _my_ life at stake, not his.

It felt like I had stepped out of one world (the hospital ward), back into the real world. One ethereal world, then the real one: cruel time passing differently in each of these realities. I watched my fellow students, laughing, oblivious, and "normal." I saddened at the reality of *my* world. I rushed into College, up the stairs three at a time, opened my door, and slammed it shut behind me. I sank on to my bed and sobbed. After the shock of hospitalisation, I knew it was unlikely I would make my weight. Still I forced myself to eat dinner, I did not exercise, and I crawled into my own clean bed.

At Weighing Group, I was still in some form of shock from having been hospitalised. I had weighed myself and was two pounds too light (if there is such a concept). So was I to be forced to have a week out, even with these rather extreme mitigating circumstances? There were, it seemed, *no* excuses: I would have been forced out, *if* I had told the truth. I did not think the eating disorder team were "playing" at all fair with *my life*, so lying was not a difficult action to justify. Leaving me all *alone* to ruminate for nine days; self-harming, losing weight beyond all redemption, and powerfully suicidal; would have been, to put it frankly: *fucking ridiculous.*

So I lied. (I was, if you remember, allowed to weigh myself at home). The next day I reset my scales to make them "zero" at +2lbs, thus falsely raising my weight. I then managed to mostly maintain it so I did not have any enforced time out, even though I was unable to actually gain any weight. Fortunately, one option on the day programme was to choose to have a 12-week period at a maintained weight, even if this was underweight.

The Eating Disorder Day Programme that had filled my days for months was, unfortunately, not the right place for me. I became overly dependent on the people (staff and patients) there for comfort, and then couldn't cope at home time. I gave up on recovery, my attendance record dropped, and then practically stopped after Clare finished her nine-month stint, (still bingeing and vomiting 3-5 times a week, still drinking, still troubled with depression, still fighting admirably to survive and get no worse).

By "agreement" I wasn't allowed to turn up at the Day Programme if I was bleeding, or at least if they could *tell* I was bleeding. (Warning: explicit self-harm details). I couldn't stitch my own left arm one-handed, and Dr. MacLennan would check it: so I moved on to my thighs, cutting and then suturing myself (with anaesthetic). I had dreams of cutting deep enough to find my femoral artery... getting through skin was easy, getting through fat was unsettling (because fat = bad), blood vessels were not a problem, but muscle I could not bring myself cut.

With my mood falling lower and lower each day, I couldn't face the Day Programme without Clare, especially when new faces appeared whom I just couldn't cope with. Although the Programme ended at 4pm for the staff, for all patients the support given between members was a twenty-four hour system. Clare was my main support, and I think I was hers. She was having real trouble going to bed, and would often phone me at four in the morning, just as she was going to bed, just as I got up to begin my day with some brutal cycling.

I needed help, but I didn't know it. I don't know how to explain it other than to say it was like some connections in my brain ceased to work, and I simply did not comprehend what was good for me and what was normal. It was no longer a case of telling the world to fuck off: I no longer saw ways to help myself, just ways to hurt myself. I no longer felt such anger towards the staff for trying to help me eat: I was bored, apathetic, didn't care, and just said, "No," or didn't turn up.

For my final weeks in the Eating Disorder Day Programme, I progressively missed more and more days and part-days. I would turn up *after* breakfast and leave *before* lunch. I had a tendency to show up for Art Therapy on Tuesday mornings because I liked expressing myself that way. Usually the images were pretty grim. Ideally my artistic expressions would have alerted people to the fact that things were very seriously wrong, and been more effective than slicing open my arm. But unfortunately we do not live in an ideal world.

My time at the day programme was coming to an end and it terrified me, (even though I was barely present). What would I do with myself? I knew I was too ill to return to work. There was a pre-set limit on the time anyone could stay on the day programme, so I had to leave. Exploding (privately) like a powder keg, I decided that *I* would "choose" to leave early, whilst I was still welcome. I.e. whilst I was still "deserving" and "wanted." Some strange contemplation went on in my head, where I thought it would be easier to leave and therefore show the day programme that *I didn't need them*, rather than use the last months to leave with help, advice and support. I didn't come to the day programme for much of my final month. I remember attending an Art Therapy session one Tuesday, at which I made one of my usual concoctions. I described it as all the things in my life worth living for. Everyone looked pleased and commented that I should notice how much I had to live for. (And in many ways they were right). However, the picture actually meant goodbye. Goodbye to all the good things in my life that I would leave when I died soon.

I left the Programme badly. I left it feeling angry and resentful: because although I recognised that I made all the decisions about what help I accepted, I was not actually in control enough to make any of those decisions – and – *I felt they should have known it and still found ways to help.* They after all, were the experts in whom I had entrusted my life. Then again, you can't help someone who wont let you, and I am a stubborn person, easily capable of out-thinking most people in order to find ways to hurt myself. Whatever we tried, nothing helped me. All in all, there was no one to blame: it was just a situation, a time, and a very ill person who would not open up to anyone. My extreme, external control/anger/denial was a mask for absolute chaos. I trusted them to help me, but they could not. I blamed them for making a promise they could not keep: but it was I who stopped them from keeping it, and unfortunately, I was the one that had the most to lose. A difficult messy situation, with a lot of anger, promises that *felt* shattered: I was a bleeding, thinner, suicidal, fragile, broken person.

I suppose that in retrospection, it was obviously a mistake for me to join the Day Programme; nobody was to blame: it was just the way my life worked out. Of this my therapist said (in 2004):

> "As far as why the day programme did not work for you, my sense is that although we came to an agreement that we would not weigh you, the meal plan represented a tremendous threat to your sense of safety and control, rather than a support in reintroducing solid food into your diet as we had hoped. I do not think we could have foreseen how terrifying it was for you to attempt to follow the plan, although with the benefit of hindsight I would agree with you that it was not helpful.
>
> My sense of what went wrong in day treatment for you is that the programme expectations felt like a re-enactment of the expectations placed on you by your dad, and triggered a complex emotional reaction of anger and despair, culminating in self-harm and intensified depression (you had already been depressed on entering the programme, but this escalated), despite our efforts to reassure you that we were on your side and trying to help."

In 2002, I wept alone, confused. In my depressed and hopeless state I thought I could sense the relief, almost hear the:

"Phew, she's not our responsibility anymore," in my head.

Chapter 6. Sometimes things go beyond Awry.

"I'll not weep.
I have no full cause of weeping; but this heart
Shall break into a hundred thousand flaws
Or ere I'll weep. O fool, I shall go mad."

   ∽ William Shakespeare, *King Lear* (Act IV, scene 1).

It *would* have been nice to have been given a choice. The option to choose between a quiet life of sanity, or a dangerous but raw and honest life of madness; but I got no choice, my reality just started to melt, distort and disappear. Yes it can be possible to come through difficult times strengthened, but I would gladly forgo my depressive illness experiences. (I'd keep the manic times though). Some people may think madness is a matter of choice but it is not. For *some* people there can be an element of responsibility – a subtle but important difference, with no blame attached. Removed from the Eating Disorder Day Programme I entered a period of limbo: an existence that is difficult to explain with any order or clarity. I went for days or weeks without speaking to a single soul except Dr. MacLennan. He warned me that my thinking was "clouded by depression." I lived a trapped and lonely existence in my College room, with just a computer and my secret hallucinations for company.

I no longer felt any need for taking responsibility concerning my life – after all, *I did not matter.* I had lost all (conscious) motivation to give a damn, and my only awareness was deeply depression-influenced. That is a frightening reality in a world where the only person you can truly trust to "always be there," is yourself. I found out how deep the rabbit hole goes, but found that it is always possible to dig deeper. And it's a bumpy, chaotic journey, being dragged downwards, then sideways, then down again, the destination changes, the aims change: everything is a total mess. This chapter is only a small part of that descent into horrific illness: encompassing all-consuming depression, psychosis, mania, dysphoria and death. All of that time, my fingers were desperately trying to grab hold of something with which to earth myself.

I think I probably deserve an award for not appearing as disturbed as I felt. But then again, I still don't know if that was a good thing or bad. *Every* day I thought I'd hit what alcoholics commonly refer to as their "rock bottom." But I was surprised again and again, as every day, I found new depths to sink to. Look how many chapters are yet to come... there's *so* much further to sink, and not enough words to adequately express how it felt. The Dark-Man-over-my-shoulder did not disappear, and my computer continued to float. Maybe it was sheer exhaustion and lack of sleep causing these visions, but as I did not understand what was going on, I did not share any information about them, not even with Dr. MacLennan.

I still saw my therapist, but not often as I had developed an aversion to going near Cotswold House (the part of the Warneford Hospital where the Eating Disorders Service is based). At outpatients I sometimes saw a psychiatrist who was part of the City Central Team: with whom I discussed my low mood and self-harm, and was put onto a new antidepressant that was supposed to also help with anxiety. The venlafaxine XR made me yawn a lot, but did not alleviate my depression or anxiety (and I didn't actually give it chance to, despite fully understanding that antidepressants take time to work). After taking it for less than a month, I deliberately stopped *because* I wanted to kill myself. I made a "clear" judgement call that I was tired of feeling ambivalent about suicide. I thought it would be easier if I felt strongly for or against death, without my cognitions effected by antidepressants: I hoped it would make the decision to die more "simple."

I had to cut my cycling because I was physically weak from weight loss, malnutrition and blood loss. (Warning: explicit self-harm/suicide details). Almost all my cutting was suicidal: using anaesthetic and scalpels, delving for veins and arteries, finding them and then lying down to die. It was at this point I utterly ruined my already stained College carpet and many sheets/towels/clothes. I did the same thing night after night, each time risking my life that bit further; each time hoping to die, believing I would die, and angry that I did not. I learned that (contrary to what Hollywood would have you believe) exsanguination was not a particularly reliable method of suicide, particularly as I could not bring myself to cut my throat; but I still hoped each event, or the cumulative effect would carry me off.

Many suicide methods were beyond my acceptance because of their violence and/or the danger to others. Yes, I realise that slicing an artery is somewhat violent, but I did it in such a clinical fashion that it did not *feel* as brutal as it was. Days were dragging in an unbelievably slow fashion, and so I turned in earnest to find an overdose that would kill.

Meanwhile, as I lived, got bored, hallucinated, but continued to bleed, I only once felt (mentally) strong enough to ask for help with my self-harm, and went to have stitches at the Accident and Emergency department in the John Radcliffe (JR) Hospital. (I could not suture my left arm with one hand). I was not seeking attention or deliberately wasting time: I was ashamed. I know from my friends and working with self-harm victims that despite this being an everyday problem, covered in medical literature with massive insight; malpractice towards self-harm survivors is widespread: which is, in one word, *unacceptable*.

If you work in emergency medicine, and cannot begin to comprehend why someone self-harms: educate yourself. No excuses just do it. Some health professionals are fantastic. Even if you are still inclined to think it is abominable, stupid and/or a waste of your precious time, you should still be professional. That means you are civil, respectful and provide the same standard of care you would anyone else; including consideration of the fact the person is likely to be highly distressed and vulnerable. Treating someone badly will *not* deter further self-harm; rather it will confirm to that person, already filled with self-hatred, that they are as worthless as they feared. And then they will self-harm more, and possibly die from suicide or untreated self-harm.

The one time I decided to get help I had been hallucinating, and, in fear, had harmed myself to quieten my panic and make the Dark Man disappear; breaking my rule of cutting on my legs where I could self-suture. I went to A & E with three large, deep, and either rapidly oozing or pumping wounds on my left arm that I had been unable to stop bleeding. I had hit two arteries and one large vein (plus several small). Now there are arterial bleeds and different arterial bleeds. The two cuts that hit arteries were not large arteries. When I held my arm out for inspection the blood shot about 2 meters (not far really), pulsing across the room. That and the fact that it sprayed bright red up my College wall when I actually did it, is why I described it as arterial.

I was left sitting in the waiting room for a short time, but too long, surrounded by members of the public asking too many questions. I deposited a pool of blood beneath me on the floor. I really don't know where these incredible reserves of blood came from in my body. I began to feel immortal again, and displeased with that worrying, eternal "fact." Waiting patients looked concerned and asked me what I had done. All they could see was a blood soaked towel and floor. I lied and said I had accidentally put my hand through a window; which seemed easier than the truth because I was tired and weak. (I now regret not telling the truth). "Ouch! How awful," they said, and nodded approvingly. Then I pretended to feel faint so that there would be no more questions. Then I really felt faint.

I was called though and seen by an Emergency Room consultant. (I believe that's the same position as an attending doctor in America). I suddenly found it hard to stand or walk. I did not bother to lie about "an accident" because it was bloody obvious to a professional that I had done this to myself, and it was impossible to ignore the multitude of older scars, most perfectly lined across my arm. He looked disapprovingly at me, and didn't speak to me other than a grunt to ask if I could move my fingers. He asked what I had cut myself with, and I replied in a quiet voice, "A sterile scalpel." He shot me a look of disgust.

I know I looked deathly pale, sweaty, unsteady, and I felt cold, dizzy, shaky, tremendously anxious and frightened, but I tried to appear calm. He did not give me any more chances to speak. I couldn't seem to get enough air, and saw shapes moving across the front of my eyes. I had trouble staying focussed. I was fainting/drifting when sitting, I had a woozy head, and my heart felt it was going to explode out of my chest.

It did not occur to me to ask them to check my blood pressure (or lack thereof). I did not ask them to test my haemoglobin. It didn't occur to me to ask for surgery to repair my sliced blood vessels or check I had not cut any nerves – I have never recovered feeling in my lower, left arm. Nor did it occur to me to ask that they should treat my fluid depletion, which must have been quite significant. It should have been abundantly overt that not only was I spraying blood around the clinical room, I had gone into hypovolaemic[20] shock, which needed treatment in the form of 0.9% saline or colloids, and a blood transfusion. But I received no treatment. Nor did anyone check my heart rate or breathing difficulties. My mind did not allow me to ask for their help, I was unable to care for myself properly – that was the job of the professionals.

---

[20] Hypovolaemia refers to a reduced amount of blood and blood components in the circulatory system – which can become life threatening if anoxia – lakc of oxygen – causes organs to fail. *Untreated shock is usually fatal.* According to the National Institute For Clinical Excellence, "If uncorrected, hypovolaemia will initially lead to inadequate perfusion and oxygenation of tissues and will subsequently cause permanent damage to vital organs and multiple organ failure, one of the major causes of death in trauma patients."

The consultant got up and left, and sent a nurse in who stuck about ten packets of steristrips on my arm – she just stuck them anyhow, all incorrectly, with no attempt to close my wounds. Even though the blood just washed them all away, she then proceeded to try to roll a bandage around my arm, which soaked through with blood in moments. Somehow I found the strength to suggest that I needed stitches, and she looked at me like I was fresh dog crap on her best carpet.

I didn't say it, but I knew I was being deliberately mistreated. Deemed unworthy. She ignored my request and proceeded with my blood-soaked bandage, so I pulled away my arm and *demanded* to see the consultant. Where I found the strength to assert myself I do not know. What frightenes me is the question of how many people do not have the conviction to stand their ground, and suffer as a consequence. I suppose I was confident enough that I was right, that they were wrong, that I knew the very least amount of physical medical treatment my wounds required, and that my self-harm didn't make me a bad person.

When, after a twenty-minute wait, the consultant "graced" me again with his presence, I was *rather* pissed off. Fortunately this anger gave me the ability to say that I knew I needed stitches, although my brain was unable to connect with a need for other ways in which I needed to be treated properly. I just wanted the bleeding to stop. I dropped into the conversation I was studying medicine at Oxford; his ears perked up. I already had no respect for this man, who other doctors and nurses would look to, to see how to behave. *"Great role model,"* I thought, *"Respect is earned, not demanded. I wont respect you after this treatment."* So I told him that I needed stitches: soon, where and why, and he just left the room without making eye contact. I spoke firmly but *not* impolitely, suppressing the part of me that wanted slap his face for his haughty disrespect.

The consultant reappeared with a large needle and 20ml syringe filled with anaesthetic, and stabbed me twice, briskly and carelessly, through two of the cuts and into my arm, totally ignoring the third wound, which was bleeding badly. He did not acknowledge me as a person at any juncture, unable to look at my face. I assume he was trying to make a point: whereas I just thought he was an arrogant wanker.

By this point the edges of my wounds were swollen and sore. Now I have been taught how to use the anaesthetic lignocaine (known as lidocaine in the USA). I know he could have used a smaller needle, and should have injected the lignocaine in a few areas, numbing the edges of all my cuts ready for the stitches. And he should have done it much more slowly; I have never seen so much lignocaine injected so fast and carelessly. (The faster it is injected, the more painful it is). The pain woke me up – where I had been floating away. He injected me twice *into* the cuts, which didn't numb the areas around the cuts properly, if at all. There was no suggestion of a psychiatric consultation – technically I was already under the care of the Warneford Hospital, I still had the status of an inpatient even though I was living at home "on leave."

It was another fifteen minutes until a lovely nurse came to do my stitches. I had to ask her to properly numb my arm, which she did, obviously displeased with the consultant and having to suture a wound that actually required surgery herself. Then she closed my skin with many sutures, bandaged it tightly, and we hoped for the best. I know she was uncomfortable with the poor treatment that I received; but she was great, friendly and caring, not at all judgemental. Then I was allowed to walk out.

I should have complained. I *know* doctors are busy. I know Accident and Emergency is busy. Yes, I physically caused my own injuries, but let's not forget that it was under the influence of several mental illnesses battling it out loudly in my head at the time. It was not my "fault" any more than someone who slips with a knife after a few glasses of wine, or who trips through a window when not paying attention, or indeed any other injury in any other circumstance. Self-harm does not make you a second-class citizen. *I was ill:* a fact all Emergency Department staff should know. *I could have died.* People without my medical training, or people less able to speak out about what they needed, would have been shamed, mistreated, scarred physically and mentally, and probably never returned for help again, even if a wound was life threatening. Indeed I never returned to the JR Emergency Department by choice. (Though I did return). I cried alone.

> "There is a sacredness in tears. They are
> not the mark of weakness, but of power.
> They speak more eloquently than ten
> thousand tongues. They are messengers of
> overwhelming grief..."
>
> ❧ Washington Irving (1783-1859).

Far too ill to return to my work, even though I wanted to: the General Adult Psychiatric Department now took over my care. More specifically, the Oxford City Central Mental Health Team. They arranged for me to attend the Day Hospital attached to the Warneford Hospital, as an alternative means of support. I was supposed to arrange to go there as often as I needed, up to 7 days a week. I don't think I went very often. Maybe one or two short mornings a week, that I felt I had to attend else they would assume I was either perfectly fine or in need of psychiatric commitment.

I realised I may end up in hospital (briefly), so I decided I needed to know my legal rights. I was by this point absolutely certain that depression was my main problem, and my anorexia was just a boring digression. I did not understand my manic or psychotic symptoms, and so I kept them to myself. I also realised that I did not seem able to communicate to the mental health staff my distress. They encouraged speaking instead of self-harm, but in reality, only one got their attention. This is what I mean by attention seeking being a necessary form of communication as opposed to manipulative: sometimes it is the only form of expression left. Sometimes in an overcrowded NHS mental healthcare service, it is hard to be heard in any other way.

My short admission weighed heavily on my mind because there was much about the decision processes that I didn't understand. I think a very common problem with mental health care is its lack of consistency and even common sense. How could I be on acute suicide watch, and then just by saying the first thing that came into my head, be allowed out after less than 24 hours? I was bemused. After the Day Programme and my 24 hour stay in hospital I didn't trust anyone to "save" me, but nor did I really care.

Well… more accurately: I *did* care because I wanted to be *worth* saving, I just didn't actually *want* to be saved.

The laws surrounding *involuntary committal* to psychiatric hospital, often called "sectioning" in the UK are actually fairly simple, and devised with the best interest of the patient (and society) at heart. They are about protecting people, be that from hurting themselves or others. The word "section" comes from the fact that the Mental Health Act is basically a very long document split into *sections* covering each piece of law for various situations.

In the UK, an insurance company does not govern the length of a hospital stay; the doctor and hopefully the patient determine it in agreement. It is, unfortunately, governed to some extent by the limited availability of NHS psychiatric beds. I cannot comment much on psychiatric commitment in other countries, but I do know that the process has been described by American friends of mine, and eminent American psychiatrists, as too litigious, with too much emphasis placed on personal freedom, thereby actually harming patients that need protection. I am in favour of personal freedom, but I am glad it was taken from me…as you will soon see.

There are always various interpretations of, for example the terms danger or risk. If the person cannot be proven reasonably (whatever "reasonably" means) unsafe, they cannot be forcibly admitted. It can be difficult to decide whether someone is safe or unsafe, and I have often been both baffled by decisions and surprised at the insight of mental health professionals. Often it is a case of what is *least* dangerous, or what is "acceptable" risk, with, let's face it, the hazard of any gamble being to the patient, not the professionals.

So I learned that there are 136 Sections to the 1983 Mental Health Act[21] in the UK. My reason for learning was to ensure if I were hospitalised, it would be brief. (Warning: switch into law mode now). The one I was most interested in initially was a Section 2, which means that you are compulsorily *admitted* to hospital for *assessment* lasting up to 28 days. It requires three recommendations to enforce, one must be an "approved" doctor, (a senior psychiatrist) and a second doctor, hopefully who has known the patient for a while, such as their GP (general practitioner, i.e. primary care physician). According to Section 12, the "approved doctor" is at least a senior registrar (chief resident) or usually a consultant (attending) in psychiatry, and likely to be the responsible medical officer, (RMO) which means the doctor in charge of your care (who can also order your discharge from the Section and/or hospital at any point – a Section 23). The third person is a specially trained "approved" social worker (ASW). Alternatively a Section 2 can be enforced if the nearest relative makes the application instead of the approved social worker.

After assessment (2) comes treatment (3). Being held under a Section 3 means you are held in hospital for up to six months for *treatment*, <u>and treatment can be enforced</u> if you refuse to agree to it. There are exceptions to enforced treatment, but drug treatment and ECT (electro-convulsive therapy) are permitted without the patient's consent, though a second independent doctor's opinion has to be obtained first. Just like a Section 2, the instigation of a Section 3

---

[21] See recommended website at back of book: *Hyper*Guide to the Mental Health Act.
http://www.hyperguide.co.uk/mha/contents.htm

requires 2 appropriate doctors (one psychiatrist, one doctor who has known the patient for some time) and a social worker. If further treatment is needed, the Section 3 can be repeated at first six-monthly, and then on a yearly basis.

Section 4 covers *emergency admission* to the hospital, and is essentially identical to a Section 2, except that it lasts for just 72 hours, and only requires one doctor's recommendation. That doctor must know the patient or be an "approved" doctor. Section 4 is to cover situations where admission is essential, and there was not enough time to arrange a Section 2 admission. This Section 4 can then be converted to a Section 2, lasting 28 days when a proper application has been made. It is considered bad practice to follow a Section 4 with a second Section 4, or a Section 5, because 72 hours is deemed long enough to arrange a Section 2 or Section 3 if required.

Section 5 was never going to be my friend! It concerns *emergency detention* of people who are *already* in psychiatric hospital "voluntarily." It is threatened or completed if you are a voluntary patient and not cooperating in some manner, though if it does happen to you, there will usually be a good reason. A Section 5 has two parts: a doctor's hold or a nurse's hold. A doctor (your RMO, or a doctor nominated by her/him) can hold you in the hospital for seventy-two hours, which is called a Section 5(2). There is no provision for the period to be extended because it is deemed that 72 hours is long enough to sort out the enforcement of either a Section 2 or 3. It is also deemed bad practice to repeat a Section 5, or to follow it with a Section 4, since 72 hours should be long enough to arrange a Section 2 or 3. (But this rule can be broken, as was threatened in my case). Secondly a nurse can impose a Section 5 to hold you for 6 hours, known as a Section 5(4). This ends when a doctor who is entitled to impose the longer Section 5(2) arrives. If the doctor imposes a Section 5(2), the 72-hour period of the Section starts from the time of the original Section 5(4) reported by the nurse. The doctor can also decide *not* to hold the patient under a Section any further, (thus cancelling the nurses 5(4) hold). "Yes I will stay on the ward," tends to work. But if you repeatedly say this and act otherwise, you don't get away with it.

I used to think it would be better to be a voluntary patient to avoid the stigma of being sectioned. I may be biased by my experiences as the patient-from-hell but I now think that there is little difference between being sectioned to being voluntary other than the name: a psychiatric patient is a psychiatric patient, and all the "voluntary" business can be such bullshit (but not always). You may be admitted "'voluntarily" but you are really having to acquiesce to avoid being sectioned anyway. Pressure can be put on you to comply with suggested treatments; lack of doing so might lead to your being sectioned, *or* even discharged when you want to stay. If you are voluntary, in *theory* you can leave the ward at any time, for as long as you like, including discharging yourself from hospital. But usually this requires you to ask permission, stating how long you will be, and if the decision has been made to keep you on the ward, you will be forced to stay "voluntarily" or be sectioned. It becomes the case that the burden of proof moves (subtly or not so subtly) to lie with you to prove you are safe to be released, instead of the burden of proof lying with your doctor to detain you. That is something many people don't realise until "too late."

There are also a number of interesting Sections including Section 17 regarding permitted and Section 18 non-permitted absence; Section 57 refers to treatment requiring consent and a second opinion; Section 58 refers to treatment requiring consent or a second opinion; Section 135 gives power to enter premises and take someone to a "place of safety" i.e. hospital; and Section 136 covers removal of people from public places by the police. Most of these sections will be important later in this book. Intimidation by threat of a section is common. (I have many misgivings about such coercive treatment). Many people are voluntary for their entire hospitalisation.

Clare and I stayed close, though in fact, apart from making the odd hospital appointment, the only time I left my College room (except to cycle) was to see Dr. MacLennan or Clare and I rarely achieved that. One night she turned up convinced I was going to commit suicide. I refused to let her into the College building because she would try to remove dangerous items that I was in possession of. She knew I'd been on the Internet for pills: I made sure I kept them.

The next time I saw a psychiatrist, having chewed over the communication problem and written pages of essays to explain myself, (that I never showed to anyone), I stressed to him that my *depression* was my worst problem: the primary illness that had plagued me for so long, whilst people focused on the anorexia. He seemed to *hear* that for the first time, (I was gob-smacked). He "liked" it, smiled, the scribbled away in my notes, and copied it in letters to my GP, therapist and the General Adult Day Hospital. I've read my notes, and it reads like an epiphany; which I suppose it was. To help myself, he encouraged that I attend the Day Hospital regularly. I didn't go. He asked how the venlafaxine XR was helping and I said I didn't know. (I had stopped taking my antidepressants for some time by then). So he upped the dose to 375mg, which I still did not take.

The pills I had most interest in at first were those that were sedating. It was legal to buy and import some (*not* all) medications, up to a three-month supply, for yourself; but not to sell them or give away (technically that would be supplying drugs). Laws surrounding possession and importation of certain medications are always changing, and some of what I imported in 2002-3 is no longer legal today. Pharmacies in Mexico, India or the Philippines are happy to help, *for a price*. Plus there is usually a long wait to receive your medication, so you have to plan well ahead, or spend more money. I also bought some nasty painkillers, but freaked out and handed them over to Dr. MacLennan. An eloquent illustration, perhaps: of my unconscious ambivalence regarding death, despite my conscious headlong rush towards suicide.

Sleeping pills are not produced for fun, but I thought they were. I bought generic zolpidem tartrate (known as stilnoct, ambien and many other names). I rarely took them, for I understood that you quickly become tolerant and they loose efficacy. They only made me sleep for a couple of hours anyway. So I saved them for nights when I couldn't face self-harm, and/or the Dark-Man-over-my-shoulder seemed to be particularly malevolent or staring, or I found myself hanging half way out my window mesmerised by the fall and crunch. Even though my insomnia drove me quite literally mad, I usually coped without resulting to pharmacological self-treatment. Just 5mg of zolpidem would get me an hour or two of sleep. I simply did not care if self-medication was sensible.

I cope by seeing the black humour in the following story; most people seem not to find it amusing. One night, working late on my computer, (researching suicide and psychiatry as per usual, also whilst emailing, watching a DVD *and* reading 2 journals), I decided to "give in" and take a sleeping pill that night. Before I even took any medication I was seeing strange colours and movement all around my room. I felt like hanging by my toes upside down out of my window. (I have no explanation as to why). So I took out a strip of zolpidem. I took one 10mg pill, even though I knew half would suffice, and left the strip, now containing nine pills, on my desk where I was working. The Dark-Man-over-my-shoulder was there, but pulsing and fading, he seemed to be stuck across the room, which I preferred. After about twenty minutes, I decided that the pill wasn't working. So I took a second pill and returned to my computer. That is my last lucid memory until the following morning when I woke up to find a friend sleeping on my floor under my spare duvet. Here is an exact copy of the email I sent to her, which I have no memory *at all* of writing:

> From: "Katy Sara Culling <katysara@gmail.com>
> To: ***
> Subject: **excuse m,e whoopdefuckingdoo!**
> Date: Mon, 20 May 2002 11:09:36

Hi ***,,
Everythig is well FUCKed. I did try to
phone my sister Beth earlier, whichhelped
a bit, but there are far 2 many scary
options. Oblivion via sleeping pills miht
save my life for today, untl=il I see my GP
tomottrrow. I am hallucinating, I think.

**ALL THE lines are CURLY And
PURPLE.**

I think I can see Beth sitting behind me,
on my desk? But mydessk is in front and
the bed is behind us. Such a bad day,
several recurrent thoughts to DIE… so to
save myself I am putting myself to sleep
but *should* wake up). My head isn't clear
right now though… I think i can see my
sister sitting on my bed but that is
impossble coz she is in Sheffield.

I am so tired, need help…REFUSE
selfharm (cut(…. want to cry …just going
to   go   to
bed….sleeeeeeeeeeeeeeeeeeeeeeeeeep.   I
have taken pills that will send me to sleep
NOT KILL#

Fuckinh   hell   what   is
yo====goinghon>><<,,,,,,,,,,,,,,,,,

Word for word, typos and expletives included. For a
long time I thought this email was hilarious, now I'm
not so sure. The next morning I tried to piece together

very little memory, what had happened. I had an odd, brief memory of seeing my friend's face at my door, though the image was all stretchy, like looking in one of those funny mirrors in fairgrounds. I also had a fuzzy, dark memory of speaking to someone about how wonderful my D.Phil. was. My friend was fast asleep, so I went out on my bike to get in a quick fifty miles despite being wobbly on my feet, and returned to see if she had woken.

She was awake, so I asked what had happened. Apparently I had emailed her with the strangest email (which you have seen), which had worried her and she came over to check on me. She had managed to get into my College building in the middle of the night, which is a feat in itself, and when she knocked at my door I opened it, smiling, and let her in. Apparently I told her I was going to bed, where I promptly headed, fully clothed, and passed out.

She called an emergency doctor, who was the fuzzy, dark person I vaguely remembered speaking to in the night. Apparently the doctor had trouble waking me up, but when he mentioned my Ph.D. I sat bolt upright, and babbled on about my "fantastic" diabetes research. I told him I'd taken two 10mg zolpidem tablets. He asked why, and my friend told me I had sat up and replied loudly, *"Because I fucking want to fucking-well kill myself and I thought this would shut me the fuck up."*

The emergency doctor said he'd write to Dr. MacLennan, and, content in the knowledge that I would be fine in the short term, he left. I felt guilty for wasting his time but was extremely relieved not to be in "trouble." (Trouble I defined as being forced into hospital). After my friend had left, I searched for the strip of zolpidem. Four pills were missing. I have no memory what so ever of taking the additional two. That kind of behaviour became more common with zolpidem, though I did not really start to "play" with my new toy until my rapidly approaching hospitalisation. This was the first hint I had at enjoyable properties of zolpidem when abused: oblivion, removal of the Dark-Man-over-my-shoulder, and short-term memory loss.

I was surprised but relieved, (wrongly relieved – because I was ill), that no alarm bells rung in the National Health Service because of my depression, eating, cutting, bloodletting, suicidal ideation, physical state (wrecked), overdosing, and now my rather expletive confession to a doctor about wanting to be dead. I began to wonder about the inconsistencies in psychiatric care and *what the bloody hell did someone have to do to get someone to take them seriously?* But I would find out.

Hilary Term at the University had passed without me even noticing. Summer approached and it was Trinity Term; I felt as if I was in some kind of limbo. I had nothing to do and no future was possible. I was not dead, but soon to be dead. Suicide filled my every waking thought. I had several ideas: stolen insulin or potassium chloride intravenously – stolen from my workplace. Alternatively lots of sedatives, serious cutting: or perhaps a mixture of these. I began to philosophise about the consequences of my death: I did not want to hurt people, including my family. I was damn serious about taking my life, my reason was simple: *to make it all just go away.*

I had no gun, nor any way of getting one. I have never been the sort of person able to just from a great high height or jump in front of a train because I thought it unfair to the "spectators," or driver and passengers. I have desperately wished to be that sort of person; but for me, suicide had to be neat and tidy, with absolutely no risk to other people's safety. No one should have to find my body in pieces, minimal blood loss visible, or better, self-poisoning that is invisible. Pain must be minimised, but some is acceptable. My education up to Oxford made my knowledge of human physiology and pharmacology potentially dangerous. But now from my clinical experience in Oxford I knew much more. The Radcliffe Infirmary, the hospital where I worked, provided me with access to lethal means.

Not only was I consumed with planning my own death, I lost another close friend to suicide. A person I had been writing to for years: my San Franciscan, American pen pal who also suffered from anorexia, depression, alcoholism, brutal self-harm and an atypical OCD (obsessive compulsive disorder). For example, her obsession with cleanliness was related to her eating disorder. If she made herself sick she rubbed her skin "clean" until red-raw and bleeding with sandpaper. The viciousness and impulsiveness of her self-harm made even me shudder. We had written several times a day since I was at Nottingham University. Although we were separated by the Atlantic Ocean and all of America, we were so close to each other we were practically co-dependent. I didn't quite realise that until she was gone. At night when I was alone in my College room and phones were usually too scary, my only connection to the outside world was my computer, and my several email friends.

Friends in Oxford were gone once I closed my door, although sometimes I'd call Clare. My other really good email friend, Summer: the ballerina from New York, was very ill in hospital; meaning my friend from San Francisco shared my long nights with me. She warned me about her impending suicide, but so many miles away I was helpless. (Warning: explicit suicide details). I believed her, but I never quite supposed she would go through with it: I cannot explain why. Perhaps I just couldn't fathom the loss of this wonderful person to the world. She committed suicide on the 4th May 2002, in what were the early hours of the morning here in England. I got her goodbye email when I got up later that morning. Her fiancé phoned me the next day: she had cut an artery and died alone.

Her last words to me (via email, giving me no chance to respond) were:

> *"I love you Katy. I can't stay*
> *any longer, need to escape. I*
> *will be closer now though, the*
> *ocean will not separate us*
> *anymore. Just tired Katy, so*
> *tired."*

I was numb for about two weeks, and too upset to go to her funeral. She often used to say that she would pray for me, and I felt guilty because I don't believe in god, but nor did I want to reject her well-meant good wishes. Her fiancé is still a broken man. I am grateful to him for allowing me to include this, and I know he does it because he hopes it will help others in similar distress. He loved and cared for her through difficult, painful times. He and I often spoke of ways to help her, including three times having her committed, and an intervention to help her alcoholism. Their plan was to spend their lives together, married, and then be in heaven in which they both believed.

Obviously this was quite a terrible loss to cope with, even without my non-medicated manic depression, anorexia, self-harm, suicide attempts and plans, and at times, my psychosis. I started to put my affairs in order. I wrote a will (again) and I made a CD of music to play whilst I died. I always thought that I would leave a suicide note, romantically signing myself out from the world. It *is* true that I wrote many suicide notes, but never one I was happy with, or prepared to leave for anyone. I also picked out quotes I would like to leave by my lifeless body. But nothing ever seemed perfect enough. I never left a note. Here are copies of some of my possible suicide notes from 2002; there is nothing "romantic" about them, although I thought so at the time:

જી

"Suicide is the most sincere form of self criticism."
~Anon

And the letters I attempted to write personally as an explanation:

22nd

May 2002 (started).

3rd   June   2002 (cont).

Dear family, Emma, Maggie, Clare, Julius,

I couldn't decide whose name to put first... I love you all very much and I am very sorry that what I am about to do will cause you pain and upset. I was not going to leave a suicide note, but I do not want to leave you pondering the question "why?" I cannot be considered to be in my right mind. (Though I have thought long and hard about this decision).

I am killing myself because I cannot bear the pain any more. I have been struggling with eating disorders and depression for so long that I just cannot take it anymore. I never feel any peace.

I cannot connect with my feelings to tell you how much I love you and am sorry that I will hurt you. Perhaps it is because if I think about all of that I will not be able to do what I am about to do. I am sorry that I am being selfish about this. I do not want to hurt you and I am grateful for your love. However, I cannot continue to live in this pain, just to stop you feeling upset. I have come to the conclusion that you will be better off without me... eventually. It will hurt at first, but then you will be relieved of the burden of worry. You will probably even be glad I am not suffering any more.

I don't know how right any of this is. I know that this is an unforgivable decision in many people's eyes, but I see it differently. I am probably crazy. My thinking is influenced by the depression, I do understand that much. However, since I feel like this all the time, it doesn't seem to matter. I am totally bewildered. I cannot find the words to say what I want to say. I feel so stupid because there are so many things I should be saying as this is my last chance... but no words come... no feelings come... I feel as if I am already dead.

Beth: my sweet sister Beth. When I think of you now I am feeling sad. I am so sorry honey. (Poo-bum). Sorry to hurt you. Sorry not to see you grow older. Thinking about you all makes me want to live, to be with you, because I do love you so very much. However soon the depression will cloud my mind completely and I will not longer be able to remember why I want to live.

Death seems so violent, so final. I wish there were some other way... any other way. But I have been searching for another way for many years now. I do not believe there is another way to be found. Not for me. I simply cannot go on like this. Please know there is nothing,

NOTHING that any of you could or should have done that would have stopped this. Do not blame yourselves, please. I am sorry. Please forgive me.

I love you all.

Yours lovingly forever,

Katy, forever 27 xxx x x x

Dear Dr. M,

Sorry. Sorry. Sorry. Thank you for the time and understanding you gave me. It made me feel less worthless, which was a pretty big deal when you feel as degraded, stupid and valueless as I do. It really mattered. As did your compassion, respect, directness and humanity. I'd say I'll miss you, but of course, I wont because I will be dead.

Thanks for giving me strength enough to carry on as long as this.

With love, Katy x

I was (I feel) rather *blunt*, and full of contradictions. Immediately after writing those letters, I did not act on my suicidal impulses because they made me, for a while, connect and think of the love I have for so many

195

people. Most people think everyone who commits suicide writes a letter of explanation, and I felt I owed one to those I love. But what I have realised is that writing a suicide note can make the act harder to go through with. This may explain, in association with the fact that suicides are often impulsive, why many people's suicides are not accompanied by a note, as none of mine were. Even people who plan suicide for months, or even years, like me, the actual moment that you crack, and do the deed, is an impulsive one for many people. It has to be, it is the only way to do the deed: detached, robotically.

You are about to read about the darkest days of my life, where I repeatedly sank lower and lower. My all-consuming despair would lead me to become a management nightmare for the health professionals. Forced into hospital, absconding from hospital, self-harming and very seriously attempting suicide. All of which I did more frequently than I ever admitted to at the time: in a private, self-destructive mode, unable (*not* unwilling) to accept help, or even recognise it when it was offered. I was seeing things, hallucinating and delusional. Some nurses made me feel worse and act bizarrely by telling me I wasn't depressed or serious about killing myself. Who knew more accurately what was going on inside *my* head: me, or them?

I couldn't understand, control, explain or show my feelings; but I did know that they were genuine. I swung between the anaesthetic of a clouded mind and the acute pain of my angry existence. Nothing was right. My head hurt from all the exhaustion. I was confused: I had given up.

Chapter 7. Touched with Ice.

"Write till your ink be dry, and with your tears
Moist it again, and frame some feeling line
That may discover such integrity."

∿ William Shakespeare, *The Two Gentlemen of Verona* (Act 3, scene 2).

I yielded to boredom and impatience with my life, my depression and my anorexia: I lost myself. I was probably as ill as it is possible to be without being hospitalised, and frankly, I should have been hospitalised. But remember that no one knew of the hallucinations, or the active suicide attempts: daily (at least) by overdose and/or blood loss. (Usually blood loss at that time). I researched every day for a more certain method. I gave up on cleaning my carpet. I bought myself fresh bed linen and bandages/suture kits weekly, and I started keeping a diary. I called my new diary "Touched with Ice," as a tribute to Kay Redfield Jamison (author of "Touched with Fire"). I felt that "Touched with Ice" aptly described my struggle with depression. I felt cold… dead.

Now I tentatively open the cover of the diary, (that actually comprises of three books), filled with my words from not that long ago, my mind poured out onto the paper in many colours and the many peculiar collected items I stuck into it, meaning the book cannot be closed properly. Many of my words are angry. I dread to revisit the life I knew, but I need to see it again. On the inside cover of the first book it reads:

"The darkest moments of your life may carry the seeds of the brightest tomorrow."

Underneath, in (my) blood is written: *"What bollocks."*

The first page has a cartoon picture of a lemming jumping off a cliff whilst simultaneously blowing its brains out. The next page I write all about Derby County being relegated. On 12th May 2002: I wrote a list of reasons to stay alive (many of which I could not enjoy at the time, nor ever will in some instances):

1. My career.
2. My sister Beth.
3. Football.
4. Friends (Clare, my sweet Emma and the boys, Julius, Katie).
5. Art.
6. Music.
7. Because (as Beth reminded me) it would be a shame and a waste to give up now after all the shit I've survived through.
8. My therapist & my GP & my old GP.
9. To find a partner and have a family of my own. A son called Will and a daughter named Beth.
10. To get my own home, a mortgage.

To my eyes today: that list looks as if it is skewed and unbalanced, definitely in the wrong order, and some very important people are missing. But that was the list as I saw it back then, and as you can see my career came top. My Ph.D. or DPhil at Oxford was most important part of my life, as was my possible future work in medicine. *Remember that point for later in this book.*

I knew I was either going to get admitted or die within a matter of weeks. (Warning: explicit suicide details). I fetched concentrated potassium chloride (KCl) from the Radcliffe Infirmary and all the IV equipment, venflons, giving sets, needles, syringes, saline, lignocaine: everything a small country would need for that exact purpose by a variety of methods. A pretty certain (99% certain) death as long as you get a good, large vein, don't dilute it, and whack it into your body, prepared for the sting. The KCl causes the heart to irreversibly stop (for which I imagine you must be conscious at first, no doubt unpleasant and in pain. But there is NO resuscitation from that, no failure as a suicide.

There are a couple of entries, mostly about sitting on my College window sill listening to loud music, helped by the fact Oxford Colleges are fairly solid, and so the loud music didn't travel badly and upset my neighbours. Writing about wanting to die, my thoughts about death, eating poorly, thinking seriously about jumping but never daring. I wanted to be dead but the process of dying scared me. I wish I could say that my fears were on behalf of someone else's pain, but they were purely fears of how much it would hurt, and of losing control. I also still had to cycle, so when had I lost blood, I did keep my fluid levels up using IV saline. I was still cycling about forty miles a day, though it was hard work since losing weight and blood, and my muscles were weaker. This meant I still covered the same distance, but it took me much longer to do so. Buy hey... I had nothing better to do with my time. I had oodles of time.

There's one entry about a meeting I have never forgotten with the locum psychiatrist. My diary reads:

> *"One comment from Dr "Z" is haunting me, making me feel so stupid, worthless, powerless and misunderstood. He said:*
>
> *"If you kill yourself and I have to attend your inquest, I will be able to do so in full confidence that I did everything I could for you."*
>
> *Miserable fuck-head! Does he realise what he is saying? Does he not grasp at all the significance of his words? Does he not see how he is rushing to condemn me; has he no concept that my brain ponders and twists things? He has seen me three times for half an hour, and listened to me tell him I am suicidal and am self-harming extensively. He's done nothing except up the dosage of a medication he didn't bother to ask me if I was taking in the first place. How is that "everything" he could do?*

To me that means I deserve to die, that I will inevitably die, that I am obviously not worth any effort to save. I don't understand. It is inexcusable, but then again, maybe Dr "Z" is simply not clever or empathic enough to see what affect this comment might have. Or was he trying to scare me? Bad move. Cheque mate."

I also wrote about boredom, how much I hate boredom, wanting to self-harm, the Dark-Man-over-my-shoulder, and the belief I would die aged 27. I'd sometimes take sleeping pills or get drunk. I thought of how beautiful my Picasso reprints were, especially when they danced before my eyes. I wished I could fly to New York to the Museum of Modern Art, or go to the Tate Modern in London as a last trip of my life. Instead I spent money I didn't have to purchase more of my favourite Picasso reprints.

I still found myself an unwilling member of the Warneford (general) Day Hospital, this time for depression and not the eating disorder. I was strongly encouraged to attend by the locum consultant psychiatrist I was seeing; but I never stayed for much more than an hour unless I got talking to another patient, which was usually interesting. The idea of the day hospital was to keep patients out of hospital by giving them support seven days a week during the day if they needed it. I turned up now and then, but usually sat in the lounge area rather than joining in the classes or sessions that were put on. (Except the exercise classes which naturally I joined in). I was very underweight but there was no pressure at all to eat the food provided, so I just didn't bother. The notes say:

"Kate avoided lunch."

"Kate only attended after we phoned her."

"Kate has phoned to say she can't make it in."

"Kate phoned to say she feels too low to come in today."

"Kate has not turned up."

Personally I did not find the day hospital useful, although I was too polite to say so. I hated it and it was boring. The only good part was meeting patients with all kinds of psychological illnesses, instead of "just" eating disorders, of which I had become very bored. I couldn't see a reason to go on living. Each day felt like I was trying to run around whilst trapped in a spider's web, pulling me backwards towards death. I do not recall if at this time I saw my eating disorders therapist very often or not. I think I stayed away out of a mixture of anger, depression, hopelessness and fear. I couldn't face Cotswold House or the staff and patients within. My worst fear was meeting the day patients who were welcome where I was not.

One possibility was to go back to my Ph.D., however I felt too distracted and upset to do that. The work was very demanding, and I was a mess. I could not concentrate enough. I'd had nine months off, and knew I could have up to two years if I needed it. Therefore, I decided to try and prepare myself to return, but at my own pace. I found couldn't read papers or even my own work because my mind was so muddled. I couldn't write properly. I began to think I would never be able to work, be useful or happy again. I had always prided myself on being a good academic. Whether I was fat, or anorectic, at least I got A's. I lost all hope. I stopped seeing people. I stopped talking to people. I barely slept.

Planning to kill myself *as per usual*, one Tuesday I told my named nurse at the Day Hospital that I had a possible idea of using potassium chloride. She asked when I thought I might use it, and I said I hadn't made up my mind, maybe Thursday, maybe not. To me, this was not a conversation that abnormal from all the conversations I'd had about suicide over the last year. I wasn't slipping her any different or scandalous information that she hadn't heard from me before – which is one reason why I don't know why she acted on it. I think understanding why professionals suddenly act upon information would save a lot of tears: I know I would have benefited from better explanations from staff when I was in Oxford. Even though lives were at stake, everything seemed so unpredictable; which is even worse when it is *your* life at risk. *You can't trust something that is so unpredictable; you can't feel worthwhile; you can't feel safe.*

That same night I attempted suicide (again), not with the potassium chloride that I had planned to use, because I had reservations about it being very painful. (Warning: explicit suicide details). I anaesthetised my left arm, got a scalpel, and tried very seriously to find my main brachial artery by following its pulse; it is actually unusually deep in my left arm. I certainly did a lot of damage: the cut was huge and gaping, and bled a lot. I went to bed about 3am with my arm laid out down the side of my bed, to encourage bleeding, no IV to replenish fluid, but I woke up the next day. I don't think I have ever admitted to anyone that it was a suicide attempt: not because I am ashamed of attempting suicide, but because I am ashamed for *failing* at what appears to be such an "easy" thing to do.

It always annoys me: in books, films and on TV, how easily people die. They take fifteen paracetamol and die in their sleep within 10 minutes. Oh were it only that simple; I'd have been dead at age 12. On TV people lie "dead" after slitting their wrists, in a pool of blood that constitutes less than half a pint. Why didn't *I* die losing pint after pint? I don't believe in a god, but it felt like some bugger was determined to keep me alive: my only explanation is that it was my own subconscious.

On that Wednesday morning, at about 11am, the nurse from the day hospital phoned me to see how I was. "I don't want to talk. I'm not coming to the hospital today." *"You might try to force me to stay,"* was my thinking. She then asked if I would be keeping my appointment with my GP that evening, which I confirmed I would do, without really thinking much about it. I had decided to keep the appointment I had with my GP, Dr. MacLennan, as a kind of goodbye. I trusted, liked and respected the man, (I still do), and perhaps some ambivalent part of me thought he still might be able to help me, however hopeless I felt. If I wanted anyone in the world to care, to consider me worth saving, it was him. I couldn't understand why he was seeing all the other patients still there, before me. I noticed it happening, but didn't really process the information, or worry what it might mean. I should have worried.

Dr. MacLennan finally called me in: I sat down and he asked to see my arm, which was tightly wrapped. I unwrapped it, it looked a terrible mess, bleeding over his desk from the cuts where I had tried to reach my brachial artery but it had played hide and seek. I'd managed to partly cut the main cephalic vein, and a few tiny arteries, but nothing critically dangerous, and certainly not the brachial artery. The bleeding was not horrific because my arm had been tightly bound for 12 hours by that point. Despite two massive cuts, one deeply into my inside elbow and half way along the inside of my forearm, I admitted only to self-harm, and not a suicide attempt. I find lying hard, especially to people I know. I knew Dr. MacLennan pretty well, and had never previously lied to him. But nor was it a clear-cut lie: I was confused about the events myself, so I told him what I wanted to believe. He looked uncomfortable. My gut instinct made me suspicious; something was about to happen.

Dr. MacLennan asked how I was; I said, "Not good." He replied, "I'm afraid it gets worse: downstairs there's a consultant psychiatrist and a social worker." I panicked momentarily before restoring my emotionless face, and uttered a quiet plea that I not be sectioned. I knew what two doctors and a social worker meant: a Section 2 admission to psychiatric hospital for assessment, lasting 28 days. I didn't want to be sectioned in case it spoiled my career plans of becoming a doctor, (which actually it would not have affected). I also did not want anyone to *control* me. I know I underwent a Mental Health Act (MHA) assessment that evening, but I remember very little about it other than the alarm at my having KCl in my bedroom.

I leaned towards Dr. MacLennan and away from the others. Then I somehow detached myself from everything because I couldn't quite believe what was happening. Ambivalent-Katy had been trying to get people to treat her suicidal ideation seriously for well over a year. She couldn't understand what had altered in their eyes, because for her, nothing had changed for months and months. She was no more or less suicidal than she could remember in a long time. Why now? *Why were they listening now?* She needed to understand the answer to that, mainly *so that she knew how to make people listen in the future*, but also so that she could escape detection if needed. Then she realised (with horror) that they were going to help her today whether she wanted it or not. By force if needed. She felt angry, confused *and relieved.*

It can be an informal "understanding" that you can remain as an *informal* patient, as long as you do exactly as you are told. [Paraphrasing] Dr. T***** said, "Do as we say, or we'll section you and force you to do as we say anyway." However in order to remain as a "voluntary" patient, they insisted I be admitted to hospital immediately, and I was to be restrained and sectioned if I tried to leave. I was crying, and the top half of my body collapsed, partly in anger for my foiled plan, but partly in *relief* that I didn't need to hurt myself anymore. My head fell and hit Dr. MacLennan's solid wooden desk. Ouch. My obligatory, comfort-uniform, black Derby County cap fell off, and my long blonde hair tumbled out from underneath and covered my face in a giant, weepy mess.

I undoubtedly felt dreadful during that long day and timeless meeting, and *would* have gone through with my suicide plan but for this medical intervention (interference). I felt sad that Dr. MacLennan thought he needed to have a psychiatrist and a social worker there. I thought that that meant he thought I didn't trust him. But maybe it wasn't his choice, or he had arranged the least threatening intervention possible, with two doctors I knew, in place that was familiar. (Police knocking down my door to take me to hospital for assessment would have been far worse). Maybe it was just the safest option; I could understand that now.

I was in Dr. MacLennan's room for a long time, suddenly it was after 8pm: all the while being asked questions and asked about going into hospital. I was just so overwhelmed by it all. At first I absolutely believed I was going to drop down dead of shock, and then that lead into thoughts of how to run away. I remember that by the time Dr. "Z" said I would be forced to "volunteer," I hardly heard him. My mind was elsewhere: I was nearest the door, and very fit, certain I could get away if I caught them off guard. But would the doors downstairs be locked?

Then time froze: I stopped momentarily. In slow motion I turned to Dr. MacLennan, ignoring the others, and looked to the man I had come to trust deeply over three years. I asked him, "Neil...Do *you* really think I need to be in hospital?" He nodded and replied, "Yes. I do." That was all I needed to hear, ideas of fighting or running left me, and I accepted his advice. At that point the tension in my body left, and I wilted. I allowed other human beings, (well Dr. Neil MacLennan) to make a decision for me.

Then I challenged Dr. MacLennan on one last point. Since he knew me very well, I questioned the validity of him saving (scum like) me. Dr. MacLennan looked right into my eyes and replied, *"I am always going to do everything in my power to keep you alive."* For those words I was, and am, grateful.

Once the decision to go into hospital had been made, Dr. MacLennan accompanied me to fetch my bike from Beaumont street to lock it in at the surgery. I'd be lying if I said that thoughts of flight did not cross my mind, but it was not something I could do to Dr. MacLennan. Plus I think he would have grabbed me too quickly. Then he saw me to a car and the social worker drove me back to Linacre College to get some clothes and toiletries for my stay, which I had been told would probably be only a few days since I was an informal patient. *Aha!* I thought. *Playing along has already reduced my sentence.* During the assessment the social worker had been very vocal about removing the potassium chloride from my room. We parked in Linacre's car park and I got out. She didn't move, so I asked her if she was coming with me. She said "No," and asked how long I would be. I said five, maybe ten minutes.

Ten minutes later I was still sitting in my room on the top floor of the College. The calm Dr. MacLennan had instilled in me had gone because I was angry at the stupidity of the social worker. I sat on my windowsill, with my legs hanging out and my suicide CD playing. In one hand I had a syringe full of potassium chloride. I knew that once that potassium chloride entered my veins, there would be no medical help that could save me. I slipped the needle expertly into a large vein. I sat, and thought; my hand on the "trigger."

What saved me was blind luck and pig-headedness, together with lingering gratitude that Dr. MacLennan thought *me* worth saving. Luckily I didn't feel "strong" enough to kill myself at that time, but I was very close to it. I thought, *sod you, you stupid, approved social worker - I'm not going to kill myself just to prove you negligent.* I knew the undiluted potassium chloride, once injected intravenously, would interrupt the electrical signalling in my heart leading to cardiac arrest, and that even if I was found by anyone it would be irreversible and I would die within a minute or two.

Fear of pain stopped me too, and at first I couldn't dissociate myself from reality in order to commit the act. I feared the death process, however much I wanted to be dead. The mass of research I had done into pharmacology meant I had read about cases where patients were accidentally given potassium chloride without it being suitably diluted. There were reports of patients writhing in agony "as if their veins were on fire." That description lingered in my brain because it made sense: injecting undiluted KCl would have been injecting concentrated acid into my blood stream. Certainly that would hurt! However I was still very tempted, due to the depression weighing heavily upon me. I started to think that maybe the potassium wouldn't be too painful, and anyhow, it would be over quickly. I began to talk myself into suicide.

With all the time in the world, and my door doubly locked and bolted, I sat on my windowsill, high on the top floor of Linacre College. I could see the towers of New College to my right, and the sports ground to my left. I sat with my legs dangling precariously over the edge of a drop I would never be able to jump, but I thought about it anyway. Too messy and too uncertain; did I want to risk self-induced quadriplegia? But a neat, tidy, quick injection of potassium chloride seemed alluring. After all, it is still used as part of the lethal injection where the death penalty has been incurred in some states of America. No messy body for someone to have to scrape up. No *long* five seconds falling to earth knowing a painful thud was approaching. I refocused on the job in hand. I pressed the needle into my arm again, felt the needle slip into a vein, began to depress the syringe very gently, and then I had a train of horrible thoughts:

People receiving a lethal injection receive potassium chloride as the third and final substance used in the execution. First they are knocked out by a sedating injection of sodium thiopental, which acts as an anaesthetic, rendering them "blissfully" unconscious – at least I hope so. Indeed the barbiturate sodium thiopental is given at such a large dose it would be fatal on its own. The second injection, which is pancuronium bromide, paralyses the subject, stopping their breathing by inhibiting the movement of muscles of the diaphragm. This too is fatal. Yet there is stage three, the potassium chloride. Then subject is *hopefully* unaware of pain, but unable to move or scream even if they did.

I am afraid of pain. Potassium meant pain. I removed the needle and put the syringe away for another day when I had more time and felt strong enough. Fortunately, I did <u>not</u> stop to think that it might be a good idea to anaesthetise the local site of injection in the arm, and as much of the arm as possible to help numb the sting whilst pushing lethal acid into my bloodstream.

All of my deliberation took place in about 15 minutes. Then I packed a few clothes for what obviously was not going to be a 24-hour stay in hospital, and walked down to the social worker still sitting in the car park. She was oblivious (*stupid, stupid woman*) as to what I had just put myself through, which

I should *not* have had the "opportunity" to do. It was a horrendous act of negligence on her part to leave me alone in those circumstances: she'd have been sacked if I'd died, but I wasn't going to kill myself just to make a point. I nearly cycled off on my spare bike – *aha – catch me then*. But, if I ran, I had nowhere to go; then I would end up sectioned and in hospital for longer. At least, those were my fears.

I had hidden in a secret pocket of my cycling rucksack, a large supply of sleeping pills, zolpidem (ambien, stilnoct) to be precise. I made no mention of it to the social worker as she drove me to the hospital in Banbury, where I would have to stay temporarily until a bed in Oxford became available. We arrived at the hospital, Orchard Lodge in Banbury, some time around 9.30pm that night. I made no mention of the pills or razor blades I had on me when questioned during the admitting process to the hospital. I did, however, hand over a plastic carrier bag when they asked if I had any. My actions may seem strange, but I had my own particular reason behind it all. I thought *"if I cooperate with the plastic bag, they are more likely to trust me."* Disturbed reason maybe, but it felt like a great reason to me at the time, since I was hiding plenty. A calming male nurse called Andy took care of the admission process. He told me that I must not try to leave because although I was a voluntary patient, he would immediately section me. Cheers, yes, I got that message already.

When they asked if I had anything else dangerous I lied and they believed me. I was lead to my room, pills and blades safely in my possession. I didn't intend to use them to attempt suicide in the hospital because then I expected they would catch me, section me, search me, and make me stay for a much longer period. Instead I kept them in case the insomnia was bad, or I felt like self-harming, both of which I could remedy in a moment, and keep secret.

I sat in my room, hidden from staff and patients for about two hours, looking at the wall and still taking in the fact that I had been hospitalised by force, even if it did not say that on paper. My arm was still bleeding, requiring stitches, but no one seemed to be bothered about it, and I was so low that I didn't care either. I feel that in the state I was in, the responsibility to medically care for my arm should have been taken out of my hands. But no, I was left to bleed. I still have horrific scars to this day, each about 5 inches long and an inch wide.

Then Andy with his tan and freckles came to fetch me to see the duty doctor. That particular meeting is fairly blurred in my mind so I cannot describe it well. What I remember is that I cried, was angry and claimed I was *not* a risk to myself, I didn't want to die and they could let me go. He didn't even look at my self-mauled arm, which was bleeding, and about which I was asking for help to close and bandage the wounds. I guess he is another doctor from the "Do-not-reward-them-with-attention-brigade."

Then I remember arguing pointlessly for a long time against the duty doctor's decision to put me on one-to-one observations (obs). That meant that there had to be a staff member present with me at all times, but they did not, in my case, have to be within arm's length. It meant that someone sat on a chair at the end of my bed, watching me constantly. Watching me not able to sleep. They always watch, even eating, and as that was a huge issue for me, I didn't eat. They even follow you to the toilet and bathroom. It is not a pleasant way to live. I cried and begged him not to do it to me. I said that it was unnecessary. I was fine, I was a private person, but to no successful purpose.

I was then lead back to my room, where the irony that I had just sat alone in there for two hours was not wasted upon me, and this time I had a nurse shadowing me. I must admit: it was a preferable state to have a real-life, soft-spoken man sat at the end of my bed in bright light, to replace my own scary Dark-Man-over-my-shoulder. I climbed into bed. I tried to sleep but I couldn't. So instead, I sat up in bed, my arms around my knees and my back to the member of staff watching me. I tried to poke out all my spine bones as much as I could or sat there motionless. Time did not exist except when the person watching me would change over from time to time. I didn't bother to look. At some point I wrote the following in my diary:

*"It's about **1.15am on Thursday 6th (I think?) of July.** I am in a hospital ward somewhere in Oxfordshire. OH MY GOD. I can't sleep. I am on level twos, which means someone is watching me right now. Apparently I am at risk. I saw Dr. MacLennan last night, and the end of a long story is that I have been "voluntarily" admitted to psychiatric hospital. Had I not agreed, they told me I would have been sectioned, so it really wasn't a difficult decision. Perhaps they think I am so mad that I couldn't be rational about that. I am sad if Dr M*

thinks that about me. I trust Dr M so I asked him his opinion, and when he said he thought I should be in hospital, I accepted that.

Dr M said he would do anything in his power to keep me alive – I will hold on to those words. *That was nice. Good to be told that I am worthwhile, worth saving, even I don't feel that way about myself.*

I HATE being watched. I am starving but I can't eat the apple in my bag as there is a strange man sat in a chair watching me: a real-life man this time, a nurse with silver coloured hair. Every time I turn around there is someone else sat at the end of my bed. I am SOOOOOOOO tired, but as soon as I close my eyes and try to sleep, my heart starts POUNDING.

There are things I want to write about but I can't in case they try to read my diary."

[The things I could not write about in my diary were the pills, razor blades, and any honest suicidal thoughts].

"Later the same night: I don't know what time it is. I just know I am wide awake and SHATTERED. My arm really hurts – but perhaps they see it as my fault. You'd think they'd clean it or something. Andy, the kind charge nurse is sitting watching

me. His eyes are boring into my back,
even though he is reading a magazine. At
least he isn't scary and dark though."

I sat still a while longer. Finally around 4am I got up
and started walking up and down the corridor, trying to
burn calories. It wasn't long before Andy stopped me
and we sat down for a chat. I told him about my Ph.D.
at Oxford, but I can't remember anything else we talked
about. I had a practiced conversation about my Ph.D.,
the topic, the work, the patients, and the discoveries:
like a security blanket for talking to people. Talking
about anything else seemed too difficult. I complained I
couldn't sleep but was told I couldn't have anything to
help me sleep until a doctor had agreed. I couldn't get
to my personal stash because I was accompanied at all
times. Andy took me back to my room; he sat down on
the chair by the door watching me. It's a very
disconcerting feeling, not threatening, but definitely
invasive. I fell into a light sleep for a couple of hours.
When I woke up, a new pleasant face greeted me.

When I look at what I wrote in my diary the next day,
it seems very muddled to me. On one side I am happy
to be safe, yet at the same time planning death. I have
always been very honest in my diaries, so I can only
assume that I meant what I wrote:

"Thursday 12.30pm. Being on one-to-
one observations (obs) are strange. Very
intrusive, especially when you are a
private person like me. I am
SHATTERED. Utterly shattered. I know I
planned to kill myself (with potassium)
and did try to kill myself (by cutting an

artery with full intent of death). I must be ambivalent. I am, for now, relieved that I cannot hurt myself. I still want to kill myself and am even thinking up ways to do it here...but it would be very difficult to not be stopped. Actually it's impossible right now because there is always someone here.

I am extremely grateful for Dr. MacLennan's words about me being worth saving. Dr. MacLennan was very patient last night, but I think I pissed off the psychiatrist – Ha! I wish I thought there was any point to any of this though. I still seem unable to recover from the fucking anorexia, so I still want to be dead. This is merely a delay in my plans.

I was trying to explain it to them all last night. How I have thought all this through: it is <u>MY</u> life, and <u>I</u> should be able to <u>choose</u> when and how to end it if I want. I don't remember what they said back. I guess they disagree. *"*

The staff and patients were very good to me at Banbury. I remember complaining to their consultant psychiatrist about my mobile phone charger being taken off me, when the (snoring) woman whose room I was sharing was allowed hers. Without thinking through my argument, I suggested that it made no sense because surely I would just help myself to my roommates if I wanted to strangle myself. The result was we both had our phone chargers removed. Oops. I also remember watching the World Cup on the television in the non-smoking TV room. I remember the patients on sedating medication falling asleep in front of the TV whilst I thought I'd never sleep again. Buzz, buzz, mind always active, never resting, and *never* safe.

With the other patients, I enjoyed the camaraderie. Being with people meant no unwelcome, evil hallucinations. However, as I walked the corridor that night again, unable to sleep, reality began to swirl again. I was walking around a dark, lonely place where there was no air, and not a person to be found. I know there must have been people there, they may even have spoken to me: but I could not see or hear them.

I was in Orchard Lodge at Banbury for only two nights before I was transferred, on a Friday evening, back to Oxford, back to Vaughan Thomas ward in the Warneford Hospital, Oxford. I'd telephoned Dr. MacLennan to ask his advice about whether to stay in hospital, and he had told me that I should. (Of course, I didn't really have a choice). At least things were familiar, and my friends and College were nearby. And fortunately Vaughan Thomas had undergone a load of redecorating, with new beds and linen, making it a more acceptable place to be.

I note with a sad smile that in my medical notes it states that *anorexia nervosa* was my diagnosis upon admission to the *general* psychiatric ward. The sad irony was that this happened after my admission to the Eating Disorder Day Programme had been mainly for *depression*. I find it disappointing since I had repeatedly stressed to everyone, that (manic & psychotic) depression were my main problems, and there was no form of treatment for anorexia given on the general ward!

For good or bad, the duty doctor on Vaughan Thomas that night was the same SHO who had admitted me back in February. He looked even more tired. All in all I find him a difficult person to describe as he seemed so detached, but I can describe how he made me feel. I warmed to him as a person, and respected him for choosing the career he had. I think he was trying to strike a balance of being sympathetic but dominant, and the dominant part didn't work. All people, even those that I deeply respect, or people I don't understand, are people I talk to on a human-to-human basis: it's a belief of mine that *no one* is above anyone else. I don't curtsey, I don't bow, generally I don't allow someone to use my first name unless they allow me to use theirs, though titles I feel have been earned I gladly use. Respect can most certainly be earned.

I don't like being told what to do or not do – who does? People may not have thought it, but I *always* listen, and try to respect advice once I recognise reasons why I should. I'll also listen to advice and ignore it if that's my decision. I made a lot of bad decisions that year. I already respected this SHO as he was polite, non-judgemental and took no nonsense, being ever so slightly curt. He spoke to me as an intelligent person who was suffering and in crisis: which was accurate, except that I was *so* much more as well. There was some respect for me there, but not enough, and that displeased me. Whether it was perceived or real: I felt that there was a touch of arrogance in that he was the mighty doctor, and I was the lowly, mad, unhelpful, non-conforming, suicidal, misunderstood mixed manic depressive and anorectic.

I did not think of relationships, even working relationships, in that way; I see them as a partnership.

The less someone listens and the least they appear to respect me, the less I will respect and/or listen to them in return. And I am constantly assessing everyone, all of the time. Nothing about the situation made me think he was a better person than I, and therefore the usual patient-doctor balance was skewed in my favour. I knew that I knew far more about my illnesses than him (and that he knew it). Maybe it pissed him off that *I* was intimidating, when that was his "job." Maybe he was just bored, I don't know. I lied again through my teeth about possessing anything dangerous, certainly no drugs, claimed not to drink at all, and no, I never took laxatives.

Again I was apparently believed and not searched. Perhaps as an articulate, white, young woman, obviously very bright as she was doing a Ph.D. at Oxford, I was the kind of person they felt able to trust. (They shouldn't have trusted me, I am *so* calculating). The first thing I told the SHO that Friday evening, was that I wanted to go home: one area he *did* have power over. He very pointedly and honestly told me I would not be leaving the ward until at least after ward round on Monday afternoon. Apparently the locum consultant psychiatrist's notes stated very clearly that if I attempted to leave I was to be restrained and sectioned: the only person who could make the decision to let me go was Dr. "Z" himself.

I was disappointed but I figured I could make it through three nights. I was also privately a bit relieved because it meant I didn't "need" to self-harm, and the Dark-Man-over-my-shoulder didn't appear to be following me. Of course, I did not admit to anyone these reasons for feeling relieved, especially anything about no longer seeing things that weren't there. If they thought I was seeing things, they would keep me hospitalised. *Most* of me was concerned with getting out and my death; it was just a small, a real, honestly-Katy part of me that felt relief.

The fact that I would be physically restrained to keep me safe was also, in a strange way, comforting. I was moved down to 15-minute observations (checks every 15 minutes as opposed to one-on-one constant supervision). That meant I could take a sleeping pill each night and get some sleep. I did not hide in my room like during my February admission. After years of self-imposed isolation and since I'd soon be dead, I had nothing left to lose, and I felt able to be myself. It is a shame I needed to be on a psychiatric ward for that to happen; but that's the truth of it. I really, hugely loved being around the other patients: I felt connected, human, alive, and we were all compassionate towards each other. Also, my interest in people was reborn as I met some of the most interesting people of my life. I became a member of the human race once again. We all had serious issues, but we all accepted each other without question.

I spent the weekend talking to fellow patients, mostly those few who hung around the non-smoking TV area. (Most psychiatric patients smoke). I remember enjoying the company of these people, sharing their lives with me, treating me as an equal, indeed, treating me as a deserving person. I chatted a lot to a guy called Kevin, an alcoholic who kept putting his arms around me. We mostly watched the World Cup 2002, and whatever else Jeremy decided we would watch, as he controlled the TV! Jeremy was slightly obsessive about food, though his idea of good nutrition was rather warped (four portions of everything). He also needed cleanliness and control of the non-smoking room television. That meant non-stop cop shows, though now and then he'd give in and let me choose something like *Six Feet Under*.

I found myself really enjoying the company of these people, which lifted my mood and made me think. All of us would have been judged by society as mad and/or frightening, but none of them were similarly closed-minded. How many years was it since I had sat on a sofa and talked to people *without* overly straining to put on my happy, successful face? I still tried to appear far happier than I was, but the goalposts had moved, I didn't have to be perfect. How long was it since I had relaxed in the company of others? Had I *ever* relaxed in company? I was desperate to be free again, but being part of the group, even be it a group of mental patients, worked for me. I felt personally valued.

By the time I was admitted to Vaughan Thomas, I had been living alone in Oxford for three years, rarely going out. By rare I mean four memorable times in three years. My twenty-sixth birthday cocktail party; going to see *French and Saunders* at the Oxford Apollo with my sister; seeing a musical at St John's College with my D.Phil. supervisor and his wife; and a trip to Jongleur's, a comedy club with friends. I hadn't been out to a single pub or club. I worked alone apart from on clinical days; I slept alone; I relaxed alone; I cycled alone before most people awoke; I shut myself away in my College room for most of the day and all of the night; and I drove to the football each weekend where I was lost in the anonymity of the huge Derby crowd. Yes: I could *appear* to mix easily and have witty things to say, but the effort this took was unbearable because my low self-esteem was so overwhelming. I did not seek other's company as I was intimidated and depressed. I could not cope with being alone, yet I was forced to accept loneliness, and I *hated* it. I was practically untouchable by other humans, any contact I had meant that they met my mask, not me. Nobody met the *real* Katy, the young woman who for 27 years had cried herself to sleep alone.

I was still fairly cautious about staff, but one nurse, Raymond, with his deep West Indian accent had quickly gained my affection and trust. You just couldn't miss him if he was in the room; and he kept sneaking in the check the football score. I was, I admit, guilty of underestimating him at first. I didn't think he was necessarily that clever, insightful or experienced because he was so laid-back; and I totally over-looked that he was a charge nurse, but I liked him. I spent some time writing in my diary about whether to leave or not on Monday, assuming I would be given the choice. I thought I would be able to convince them to let me go even if they shouldn't. There are pages in my diary, lists of reasons to go and reasons to stay. Many rambling sentences, where I try to convince myself that I will be fine if I go. To be honest, the decision to go was the only option I considered; my mind clouded from rational thought. Looking back at my words I can see that I was trying to convince myself that it was OK to go:

> *Being in hospital is very difficult for me because I can't cycle, can't eat very well, it's so boring, and you know how I hate "boring." I can't sleep in the strange bed in a noisy hospital, and staying here wont help because I will have to leave one day,*

and nothing will have changed. I feel so trapped here, so anxious. If I leave hospital, all those problems will go.

However, I have very definite suicidal plans, and I do not think that the five days I have spent in hospital has changed this. The suicidal plans have been there for months, so why will five days in hospital suddenly make it go away? Then again, I'll die eventually, so why prolong the agony?

Despite all the horror going on inside my head, I am able to put on a face that does not show the torment beneath. Is this ability my friend or foe? Despite all of the reasons for staying in hospital, and despite what I have already written about how comfortable I feel with all the other patients, I am going to try and leave.

As someone was supposed to come and check on me every fifteen minutes or so, I sat in my room like the cantankerous bugger that I am, I closed my door, sat on my bed and timed them. I was testing them to see how safe they made me feel. Such testing of the staff in many ways was to become a major issue for me, and *nowhere* in my medical notes was it recorded that my behaviour might have been that of a frightened girl seeking reassurance, seeing if she was safe, or not worth saving. No, she was seen as a pain in the arse.

On the Monday morning it took two hours and fourteen minutes for my fifteen-minute check. I was, that morning, the only patient on observations. I include this fact not as a criticism of the staff on Vaughan

Thomas ward, rather as an indication of the stress and pressure that all the staff was under. Constantly being called upon for a huge variety of causes, the most vital, perhaps life-saving work has to come first. Therefore, I found myself, a newly admitted, highly suicidal and shaken patient, waiting two hours and fourteen minutes for my fifteen-minute check. Although I didn't say anything, it deeply shook my confidence that they could save me, and made me doubt that they even wanted to; perplexing fears in someone also protesting to be desperate to commit suicide. Little did I know back then, that one day in the not too distant future, a fifteen-minute check would save my life.

On the Monday afternoon I saw the locum consultant, Dr "Z" again for the first time after what seemed like a very long five days. Raymond came to fetch me to the meeting, and I remember climbing the stairs saying nervously to him, "They *will* let me go wont they? Wont they...?" I can't remember his reply.

Dr "Z" seemed quite pleased with himself for saving my life. I naturally encouraging that opinion, so he would think me grateful, and thus safe to release home. (LIE!) Oh how I lied: both directly and also indirectly by being cheerful and calm. *Pompous twit!* I thought quite cruelly. He asked me how I would make sure I was safe with the potassium chloride in my room in College. I told him I'd pour it down the sink. Lie. What about self-harm? I said I didn't want to self-harm. Lie. I said I didn't have anything in my room in College with which to self-harm. Lie. I said I felt better. Lie.

And so I was discharged that very Monday, on the understanding that I would keep an appointment with the SHO (senior house officer) in two days, i.e. on the Wednesday. I agreed with anything, my stuff already packed, called a taxi, and practically legged it out of the hospital door, and got home to Linacre College at about 7pm. I remember walking in to College and seeing all my fellow students, wondering what they would think of me if they knew where I had just been. What if they realised that I had just returned from one world in to the "real" world? A bit like returning to the "normal" world of traditions and mothballs after stepping through the wardrobe from C.S. Lewis's fantastical land of Narnia. That is how peculiar it felt. Surreal.

I then proceeded to go out cycling for four or five hours to make up for being so lazy the last few days. (No allowance being made for myself that it was externally enforced "laziness.") Cycling around the familiar Oxford sites brought be even further back into reality. It never occurred to me that I was hospitalised on a Wednesday, and still hadn't eaten when they let me leave the hospital that Monday night. I took two sleeping pills and went to bed. I didn't want to be in the real world because that required my perpetual torment and ultimate death.

On Tuesday I got up and cycled for three hours. I dropped my bike back at College and then walked into town to try and sneak my bike out from my GP's surgery, not wanting to bother Dr. MacLennan because I felt guilty that he had already given me too much time recently. However he saw me unchaining my bike and came out for a chat. I don't remember very much of what happened. He asked how I was, and I replied, "Not good." Which is my understood code for, *"Aaahhhaaaa fucking terrible."* He asked me if I was going to be OK? So I told him I was seeing the SHO the following day. (Hence letting him know that I planned to live that long). But then I said to him, "It's all very well this hospital business, but nothing really changes and I can't stay in there for long." Dr. MacLennan asked, "Why not?"

Everything else is clouded in my memory. I know I went to the town centre to buy some things to eat. I bought low-fat chocolate mousse, cherries and some asparagus soup. (Amazing that I can recall such stupid minor details years later). I went home to my computer and to read about suicide, ever so aware of the reappearance of the Dark-Man-over-my-shoulder. I know I self-harmed by cutting, but I can't actually remember the details: but I do remember that it didn't help and I felt terrified about something I could not describe then or now properly. It was an intangible fear, and instinctive.

I did *not* throw the potassium down the sink, and it was calling to me to use it. I kept handling the bottles, arranging them, rearranging them. I put the bottles on my desk, then hid them in a cupboard, then under my bed, and finally back on my desk where they called me to them like the Sirens drew men to their deaths in Greek mythology. I lined up all my needles, and picked out a fresh syringe. *"Kill yourself, kill yourself, do it, do it,"* banging on in my head. The Dark-Man-over-my-shoulder just watched whilst hovering.

So in order to save my life, I decided to try and get an early night since I had to see the doctor the next day. I took two sleeping pills (zolpidem) and one 100mg chlorpromazine (thorazine) tablet that I had procured over the Internet. I really wanted to get hold of benzodiazepines such as diazepam (valium), temazepam, nitrazepam; or similar, but these tended to be prescription only, and expensive. (And illegal to import though I didn't think much about that at the time). In months of trying, the only benzodiazepine I ever got hold of (back then) was bentazepam, (tiadepona) used only in Spain, supposedly stronger than temazepam, but I guarantee it is totally useless. Temazepam had worked well for me when I was rather resistant to depressants, but bentazepam never worked, even when I was a rookie. I would say that bentazepam (via the internet), even taken by the boxful, is as effective at sedation as blowing your nose – then again, the pills could well have been fakes.

My drugs of choice are depressants and sedatives, and I will avoid stimulants at all costs, except now, nicotine. I am naturally stimulated quite enough thank you. Hallucinogens have never appealed to me, nor have I tried any. I don't know what made me get the chlorpromazine. I think it was probably because it was cheap and from reading that it tends to have a sedative effect. I was not really well read up on antipsychotics back then (I am now, knowing they are rarely dangerous in overdose). Back then I had no knowledge of how dangerous it could be, or if it interacted with anything else I was taking, what dose was reasonable, or if it would kill me. Nor did I bother to check for interactions, which would have been very easy to do. Checking out chlorpromazine would have taken perhaps a minute of my flicking through the latest BNF.[22]

I did not care that I was playing Russian roulette with an already disturbed mind and a possibly powerful antipsychotic drug, a so-called "major tranquilliser." It certainly wasn't something to take unless prescribed by a doctor. I didn't take my prescribed antidepressant

---

[22] British National Formulary, a handbook used by doctors prescribing drugs and to check for interactions.

venlafaxine XR, just the self-prescribed sleeping pills and chlorpromazine. I don't think I had any alcohol because I didn't have any in my College room. Were these actions suicidal? I don't know for sure, but I think they were more an alternative to suicide, with no care of the consequences.

About an hour after the chlorpromazine I became gradually more and more paralyzed. I couldn't lift my arms, legs, or speak. I felt the presence of the Dark-Man. My phone rang and I couldn't answer it. I lay on my bed, eventually falling into a noisy, broken sleep, and when I awoke the next morning I still couldn't move much. I was distressed that I couldn't go cycling, but I could now lift my arm, slowly. I just managed to call the hospital using my mobile phone to speak to the SHO and request that I come and see him on Thursday, instead of Wednesday. I lied that I had a migraine. By about 8pm that Wednesday evening I was able to move, and what did I do? I went cycling of course, even though I was extremely unsteady and jerky.

The next day I went into the hospital, actually wanting them to tell me I needed to stay there. I was weepy, tired and had had enough. I still wanted to die, but I wanted some peace from the three little bottles of potassium chloride staring at me, drawing me towards their sharp stabbing end of my heart, whenever I was at home. I wanted some protection from the Dark-Dark-Man-over-my-shoulder and other hallucinations. I wanted to be with the patients I had met, who liked the real me. I made it to Vaughan Thomas with my bag packed, including banned items of course. I saw the SHO who after a brief talk with me told me he thought I should some back into hospital.

I can't remember with clarity what I told him. I don't think I mentioned the chlorpromazine, but I do remember saying I had kept the potassium chloride and was still suicidal. I knew he would listen to that. I was not being manipulative, it was merely the only way I had found to make people sit up and listen. I wasn't fucking around; I was *deadly* serious. He actually asked me why I hadn't just poured the potassium down the sink like I said I would in ward round. I was incredulous at the naivety of this question! Wasn't it obvious? I was out of control. I wanted to die. I finally had an almost perfect method sorted out. I wasn't about to throw it away. I needed the potassium chloride for the perfect moment when I felt strong enough to use it.

However, I was definitely ambivalent. I was boldly and very coldly faced with my own mortality: a horrifying experience, even if you do want to be dead. The longer it went on, the worse it felt. I felt scared by the power of my emotions and my inability to help myself. Though in fact, I *did* help myself by returning to the hospital in contradiction to my long-term plan of dying as soon as I had enough courage. The problem with the potassium chloride that kept putting me off was the unknown pain, not any fear I had about an afterlife actually existing just in order to piss me off.

(Thankfully) Ray was on duty and we had a little chat. He said that he was not surprised to see me at all. He said he'd notice me put on a happy face around people, chatting with patients and staff. But he also saw my happy-exterior crumble to pieces momentarily, when he came to fetch me up the stairs to see the locum on Monday. He said he could tell I was deeply troubled. I felt bad that I initially underestimated Ray, who is far more astute and experienced than I gave him credit for.

He said it was OK to be in hospital for a little while, to find my feet, but forcefully warned me against getting too comfortable on the psychiatric ward. "It's not the right place for you," he said. Referring to people like me deteriorating on a psychiatric ward he said, "I've seen it time and time again."

I wish I had heeded his warning about not getting too comfortable, too reliant, and getting out as quickly as I could. But at that stage, I didn't really care. Nor did I think it was possible for me to get worse, more and more ill, and further lose my mind and freedom. I have to admit, Ray is an insightful man, who has my deepest respect, and who was absolutely correct.

Here is what I wrote in my diary the next day.

Friday? It's Friday but I don't know the date. Everything seems pretty pointless, even cycling. I just don't care. Do you know what? I am not even sure what month it is. What I do know is that I went home on Monday night and only survived by cutting and knocking myself out with medication. Bad... I know. I can't cope. Fortunately - I don't know how - I felt able to come back here to Vaughan Thomas and ask for help. They suggested I stay. Although this is a new and fairly unpleasant place to be, I feel I have no choice. If I go home, the feelings, things I see, things I think, my whole life, are all too unbearable and I would want to kill myself. I believe I WOULD kill myself.

I have many very clear memories from the time, a wasted year of my life, spent on Vaughan Thomas Ward, in the Warneford Hospital, Oxford. (Somewhat ironically this hospital is a base for some of the world's best research into self-harm and suicide). Life seemed vivid and yet colourless, always intangible and without privacy. To me the patients were all beautiful and fascinating, even the scary ones. My memories are so clear that I can hear them, smell them, taste them, and even feel them. As crystal clear as these memories are, the sequential order in time at which they took place is somewhat confused. But not quite as confused as the staff were to be by my ill persona! I was *desperate* to be understood, and repeatedly let down. I suppose, in all fairness, that *I* didn't even understand myself that well. My perceived invisibility (to staff) on the ward and sensation of losing my ability to communicate was a major source of further agony and hopelessness: proof of my lack of worth. Fortunately, some people did make contact with the real me.

There are also times I try to forget, and details blur. This "denial" is a very useful survival mechanism of the human brain. Many of these memories are locked in the ink and paper of the detailed diaries I kept at the time. I needed something private to pour my heart in to, and no one else has shared in the contents until now. I only wish I had written down the dates; but those three books crammed full of my scribbling, and bursting with strange keepsakes, were not written with a future book in mind. I truly thought I had no future. In fact they were not written for anyone else to ever see, some pages even removed and burned in case my request for their disposal upon my death was not adhered to.

Armed secretly with tools for self-harm and suicide, and pages to write upon, I voluntarily entered a psychiatric hospital. Whether this was a good or bad decision, I do not know, and never will. I suspect I had very little choice by this point.

Initially afraid and resentful of losing control of my own life, I left the world of normality and embraced the world of the insane.

CHAPTER 8. Clouds Gathering, a Summer in hospital.

"But I don't want to go among mad
people," Alice remarked.
"Oh, you can't help that," said the Cat:
"We're all mad here. I'm mad. You're
mad."
"How do you know I'm mad?" said Alice.
"You must be," said the Cat, "or you
wouldn't have come here."

෴ *Alice in Wonderland*, by Lewis Carroll
in 1865.

I embraced my madness; she became me, I became her, there was nothing but illness about me. I don't know whether it was a personal failure of mine to communicate with the medical professionals, or just the pressure on NHS beds that meant I was so very ill before I was admitted to hospital. But by the time I was finally hospitalised it was very much like the old saying of "closing the barn door after the horse had bolted." I had been screaming for help in every possible way I could think of, and no one seemed able to really hear me, or if they could, they had no power to do anything. When I was admitted I had already lost most of the things people hold dear to life, and most of my reasons for living. I had no self-esteem, no respect for myself, no future I could picture; my family were far away both in mileage and ability to connect with. So I sought the Death with his welcoming scythe. The only way forward seemed to be backwards.

On some level of consciousness I knew that this time, things were different: different from all my eating disorder problems, and different from previous depressive illness. However seriously ill I had been before, I had discovered a whole new level of "low" over the last few months. This time it was beyond serious, and yet I would still continue to decline day-by-day, week-by-week.

I teased Death, and at the same time accepted my madness and surrendered myself more than ever before to be helped. Those people who knew me or treated me at that time might find that statement hard to believe. I was adamant that I was to kill myself. But as empathic, insightful people realised, I was in a state of conscious and unconscious ambivalence: pulled between accepting help, and my death. Ambivalence in its original literal sense: characterised by simultaneous conflicting feelings, torn between two opposites. This must have lead to an outward appearance of an inability to choose or care about the path I took.

I was tired, worn out, my nerves frayed; and torn between living or… not. It was not a pleasant state to exist within, my insides churning, lurching and twisting every second of every minute night and day. I sought sweet oblivion by any means; anything to take away the misery and pain that felt eternal. I just wanted everything to stop, go away, and to find *peace*. I honestly did not know if that would be achieved by recovery or death, and as such, was pulled between the two. Stretched between these two poles so thinly, I felt invisible, and seemed to be voiceless. Whatever message I tried to convey, I failed.

I'd not been in hospital for long before I was told we would be getting a new, permanent consultant psychiatrist. I felt betrayed and anxious. What would the new doctor be like? Would she or he believe me, help me, understand, and empathise? My new consultant was Dr. Alan D. Ogilvie, newly arrived in Oxford from Cambridge. As luck turned out, when I swapped doctors, I received who I now believe to be one of the best psychiatrists in the country, certainly the best I have ever met. (And I have met quite a few!) Dr. Ogilvie was a man with whom I had many battles, but many more conversations. At times I would be angry with him, but I always trusted him and grew to have huge respect and admiration for him.

Trust is a very important thing: lifesaving maybe. As is listening, another of Dr. Ogilvie's qualities. I don't mean just listening or appearing to listen: I mean really *hearing* and *thinking* about what you say, and, importantly, *noticing* what you do not say. His questions were direct and simple, and as such, the English was unable to be manipulated: disabling my ability to *not* answer the questions. I don't know how he did it, but he learned fast when I could be trusted and acted fast when I started to deteriorate. His approach was a humanistic and realistic one; i.e. he pertained to the philosophy of asserting human dignity and using reasoned logic to improve any situation, aiming for attainable, long-term, life fulfilment.

It is one of those memories I have that is very clear. We met, three people, in the musky upstairs conference room, the air filled with dust, the room filled with dozens of chairs, several tables, a fridge and all sorts of odds and ends. As I inched my way through the door, the locum psychiatrist sat opposite me; to my left, in a beige jacket, the sun behind him, sat a man who looked too young to be a consultant. He looked powerful. The whole power balance in the room was wrong: there was little me, and two fuck-off-scary consultant psychiatrists. I was wearing my black Derby County baseball cap, hiding my face behind it. I was well aware they would look at that the clothes I wore, my hat, or the way I sat, (knees to my chest) or even my bag or books, and might well interpret them in some way, but I was past caring. I just wanted to disappear.

Dr. "Z" introduced us, and then fell silent. I looked at Dr. Ogilvie, not really knowing what to say or think. He looked relaxed and calm; neither of which I could mirror, but I felt better that he was relaxed. He is not blonde, but with the sun behind him, he appeared very fair. Then Dr. Ogilvie told me he would be taking over and continuing with my care; saying he would aim to get me home as soon as possible. Dr. Ogilvie would tell me (2 years later) that when I had first been presented to him, it was as someone who'd just come through a suicide crisis, and who could be discharged. I didn't know that at the time: if I had, maybe I would have tried to explain my needs better.

Dr. Ogilvie wanted to hear for himself how I felt. He seemed to listen when I described to him that my impassive face did not reflect the true torment bubbling underneath the surface. People often say they hear me when I say this, but then their notes show me that they do not. Dr. Ogilvie did listen, just like my Oxford therapist had. His voice struck me as soon as he spoke: I liked it. I have to say he has a perfect voice. It is soothing, calming, yet authoritative, and with a soft but distinguishable Scottish accent. I don't know why, but it sounds trustworthy. I always found listening to him easy. Well, perhaps not quite *always*, but usually. He was the only doctor (at that time) that I allowed to prescribe me medication without my questioning it, or researching it for hours on the Internet first. (I'd still look up any medications when an opportune moment presented itself though). I trust and trusted him. He added lithium to my venlafaxine XR (which I had been basically forced to start taking again as soon as I was admitted).

I don't know if it was fortunate or unfortunate, but Dr. Ogilvie was then away for six weeks. Once the handover was complete, it was agreed I would leave the hospital some time that week. I didn't want to leave because I was finally getting some peace from my hallucinations and enjoying the other patients' company, but didn't verbalise my wishes. During the time Dr. Ogilvie was away, the junior doctors made the decision to keep me as a patient, and by the time Dr. Ogilvie returned I had been transformed into a long-term patient (anything over 2 months), after which discharge becomes a hugely complicated issue.

In hospital, life was not nearly as bad as when I was at home. I was prescribed zolpidem to help me sleep; I didn't particularly self-harm because I wanted to show the staff how grateful I was that they cared. I didn't see the Dark-Man-over-my-shoulder very often, although I did seem to wander around at night and suddenly find myself somewhere with no memory as to why. (Which was probably the zolpidem).

I got to know Kevin the old alcoholic who I became very fond of, despite his dirty mind. I got to know Stella who was there because she said men with guns were chasing her – and they ("they" being the staff, "us" being the patients) thought she was delusional. I first began what was to become an intense friendship/relationship with Declan, an Irish fellow, part time drug dealer, and fellow football fan. I watched Ireland get knocked out of the world cup by Spain with him – Declan was gutted, and he refused to support England with me as his second choice.

I soon got to know Ash well: he presented himself as more than fitting the absolute, man-on-street, stereotypical image of "mad."

> "If a man does not keep pace with his
> companions, perhaps it is because he hears
> a different drummer. Let him step to the
> music which he hears, however measured
> or far away."

> ࣁ Henry David Thoreau (1817 – 1862).

Sometimes I wondered how much of his madness was an act for staff, for when he was alone with me he was quiet, affectionate, attentive, intelligent and calm. And yet he dedicated a great deal of effort to be totally loopy and uncontrollable the rest of the time. He'd wander around in a flamboyant fashion, with a headscarf and the most unusual clothes sense: sometimes drunk, sometimes drugged, sometimes in a world of his own. Sometimes he thought he was god, or more specifically an Egyptian god. He used to tell me that I didn't eat because I was sad, and that knowing that made him sad. I'd say that was pretty simply accurate, wouldn't you?

It would have been very easy to underestimate Ash. He's actually an incredibly caring person; he'd do anything to help, he gave respect back where it was given, he knew exactly what to do to get whatever he wanted, and he never forgot anything. Often he would (and still does) surprise me when he recalls events or details that I had (have) forgotten. He has a good heart, cares for people, and listens very well. Even if you don't think he's listening, he is. Sometimes (well, most of the time) he was "off his head," (drugged, delusional, hallucinating) and he'd be the first person to laugh at that and agree. I love him to bits.

Ash tried to get me to eat with him, and with Ray's help I started eating cereal at breakfast on the understanding I could then go out cycling. I didn't care about my weight on any level of consciousness that I was aware of, but cycling still made my days easier to get through, though really I was too weak to do it. I was still depressed; starving and wanting to die, but the other patients were so welcoming, it really picked my mood up. My medical notes do not record me as a depressed person at this stage. I *was* depressed; but I wore a happy face, particularly with staff. However, it *is* true that I felt better than I had been feeling on the out side. Once I had the other patients around for company I was transformed. But deep down this brought home to me the sad fact that when I left (the decision about which was not under my control) I would return to a life of insufferable agony. I was not prepared to go back to a life like that.

Bearing in mind that there was a lot I kept to myself, my notes read:

"Mood objectively dysthymic."

"Cognition and insight intact."

"Pleasant." "Responsive."

"Expressing herself appropriately."

"Settled."

"Euthymic" [euthymic means neither manic or depressed, oh how wrong].

"Dysthymic and reactive." "Dysthymic and not reactive."

"Pleasant." "Pleasant." "Pleasant."

"Out on her bike."

"Denies self-harm."

"Not eating."

"Keeping low profile, only <u>superficially</u> bright. Making an effort to appear happy."

When going through my notes, I was so thankful to reach those last two insightful comments written by Richard Ford who was my named nurse, amidst all the "pleasant" comments. Rich was (is) a lovely guy, a couple of years younger than myself, and yet he maintained an authoritative relationship: possibly because he was stronger (mentally and physically) than me, and partly because I wanted us to be friends. He is a good guy, and a damn good nurse. Caring, experienced, reassuring and helpful. He allowed, even encouraged me to cry and, very professionally, held me to soothe and console me. A caring, decent bloke, tall, kind and strong. Not everything I saw in my notes from him was so easy to read.

Every patient on the ward was given a named nurse, and an associate named nurse. If you had problems, your named nurse was the person to speak to, the idea being you would build up a trusting relationship with someone who got to know you quite well. The associate named nurse was the other nurse you could go to if your named nurse wasn't working that day. But basically it was possible to go to anyone you wanted. I spoke a lot to Ray even though I was not his named or associate named patient. His thick accent was adorable and something I learned pretty quickly to understand. I appreciated his directness and valued his experience.

Ray kept on and on at me to get rid of the potassium chloride: I felt guilty being in hospital when someone else might need the bed. I did not understand the violent noise crashing about in my head, up, down, around, laughing on the outside whilst screaming in agony on the inside. After a relatively short stay, I was afraid of being sent home for being uncooperative. I felt that they all thought I was taking the piss and wasting their valuable time, so I decided to go home and kill myself with the potassium chloride I had previously procured from my work in the Radcliffe Infirmary.

Just like that.

My thoughts went as follows: *I'm feeling scared, there's no point in living, I'm obviously not worth saving, no one thinks I am ill, ... so I'll kill myself.* I just could not see a way of returning to my old life: imprisoned in Linacre College, with all the death, thoughts, emotional pain, endless nights, blood, needles, scalpels, suicide attempts, boredom, overdoses, with an ominous hallucination of a threatening Dark-

Man-over-my-shoulder for constant company, a picture on my wall that talked to me, and a computer that floated above my desk. It *never* occurred to me to just say any of this to someone."

So I left the ward uncharacteristically late one evening, no one stopping me even though I purposely walked past the nurse's office, and slowly unlocked my bike from the railings right under the nurses' station as a test. The fact I had been allowed to freely walk out scared the shit out of me. It made me feel less safe, and proved (to me) that I was not worth saving, since all the staff knew I had the potassium by then. Had I been the professional then, I would have stopped a patient like me.

I cycled home; I felt determined to do it. There were tears in my eyes as I plummeted down Morrell Avenue, the hill taking me from the Warneford Hospital, back towards the city centre. I was determined that this was it. If I wasn't worth saving and was to be forced back into the cruel and lonely world of my own company, death would be better. I got home, ran upstairs, and put my music on. And then, quite out of the blue, I changed my mind. I do not know why I changed my mind, and I regretted that decision *many* times afterwards. Quite often suicidal impulses work against people; mine that day did me a favour instead. Whatever changed my mind saved my life not only that day, but probably ultimately; such was the potential lethality of IV potassium chloride. I had to get rid of the potassium chloride.

I decided that if I collaborated with them, they might let me stay an extra week. Then I panicked and phoned the ward to make sure they wouldn't section me for just leaving like I had. By chance I spoke to my favourite

SHO, the poor guy who had admitted me in February. He reassured me that I would not be sectioned, but I supposed he would have said that anyway. Nonetheless I brought all my remaining bottles (three) of concentrated potassium chloride for clinical use, and handed them over. I felt dreadful, handing over my perfect means of suicide, and as soon as I did it, I regretted it. But it did achieve my aim, as they let me stay in hospital for a while because we were, "making progress."

If I had known then what I know now, I would not have handed it over. Or I would have given them one bottle. What I didn't know was that the Radcliffe Hospital combination-lock to get in to my Ph.D. department would be changed because of a stolen computer, and as I was not at work, I had no reason to ask for the new code. This stopped me getting any more equipment or more potassium chloride. Whoever stole that computer did me a favour because I would surely have been dead had I managed to subsequently get my hands on more of that lethal stuff over the following months. I suppose that technically I could have made myself a potassium chloride solution quite easily: but I didn't think about that – fortunately. Ray was happy and thanked me most vigorously, but *I felt worse*.

An entry in my diary reads:

> *I tell you what... I am AMAZED. People here seem to be doing drugs and drinking EtOH. I always thought you came into places like this to stop that.* [EtOH = ethanol, i.e. alcohol]. *I'm so lucky never to have used street drugs.* [Ah, oh dear, I was

tempting fate[23] there]. *Seeing what it has done to people in here would put anybody off.* [Tempting fate again].

Looking back, I didn't count a bit of weed (pot/marijuana) as a "street drug," (it's a herb), or think prescription drugs could be just as serious. The Vaughan Thomas attitude to drugs and alcohol was clear: a zero tolerance policy. Any illegal substances would be confiscated and the police called. Alcohol would similarly be confiscated, and, in theory, handed back when you were discharged. (But don't expect it back, I had stuff taken every week and didn't get a drop of it back – mainly because the patients knew where the staff kept it and nicked it). The very fact that alcohol was banned made me start sneaking it onto the ward; you always want what you can't have.

Most staff turned a blind eye to alcohol unless you walked up to them with a bottle of vodka going, "Nah nah nah nah nah," which I actually did on more than one occasion. (It was stupid, and no, I cannot offer you an explanation – other than I was manic). The patients stuck together to "beat" the staff. Alcohol, class B and C drugs were always available, and often class A. Occasionally there were room searches, and I was thankful that I had nothing to do with drugs because I didn't want people going through my personal things – this was me tempting fate again. We'd help someone to run away, diverting and/or not tell staff. These things happened all the time. Declan used to climb out of a

---

[23] Note that I mean fate, not Fate: I don't believe in Fate. I use the word "fate" to equal "sods law," bad luck, luck, outcome, life, or life's ironies; Fate equals preordained destiny, of which there is none IMHO.

tiny window in the smoking room that nobody should have been able to reach, let alone get their body through. Later in my hospitalisation I would copy him.

I was allowed out of the ward as much as I wanted, so I was able to go out each day, cycled as much as I needed and return to the hospital loaded with booze (usually just lager) and rice cakes. Where is the logic in that I hear you (silently) cry? I'd also been on the Internet yet again, and used it to get hold of more some sleeping pills, which I bought for the purpose of committing suicide. They meant that instead of the terrible long nights of sleeplessness, I could take a pill or two on top of what I was prescribed, and relax in the knowledge I would fall asleep. This even enabled me to eat in the evenings because I was more relaxed. Life seemed OK with the hospital to support me. I became scared that I would become too well to stay in hospital because I knew I wouldn't cope alone. I felt I needed time. I still had over a year to go before my Ph.D. time limit for time off was over.

Zolpidem (stilnoct, ambien) is open to abuse, and I had a lot of "fun" with it. I did develop some tolerance, but if I didn't have zolpidem for some reason, I didn't get any withdrawal effects. But I *don't* recommend you copy anything I did with it. The advice given when taking zolpidem is to be in bed within fifteen minutes of taking it. My routine became to eat nothing all day, (anything vomited didn't count), take my hospital meds at ten, and then take an additional three zolpidem tablets. Once I had swallowed the tablets, I allowed myself to eat knowing that my eating would be controlled by the fact I would soon pass out. This worked well for me, except for the fact I would apparently wake up and have eaten things I had no memory of eating. I had a huge bag of fresh black cherries, and woke up and they were all gone – including the cherry stones. I had yoghurts, all gone. I wasn't scared by the fact I had eaten food, just pissed off that I hadn't had any enjoyment out of it because I couldn't remember it.

Another thing that started to happen on small doses of zolpidem, was that I started to sleep walk and have no memory of what I had done. Here is an account of one night based on the details from a manic patient, Ivor, the next day. I had told another patient, Ginny about a Picasso print I'd brought for my room. Sometime between eleven and twelve at night, she knocked on my door to see my picture, cigarette draped from her hand as always, despite the ward being non-smoking apart from the smoking room. I have a flash of memory seeing that cigarette in her hand.

Ivor was awake in his room opposite to mine, so he followed her to make sure I was OK and because he always had to know everything that was going on. Apparently I got up, talked about the finer art details of my Picasso print, and then went to sit with them in the smoking room for a bit and I fell asleep in there. Ivor told me that I woke up a bit later, laughed, and swore him to secrecy before telling him about the zolpidem. He walked me back to my room; and did not break my confidence. The "them" and "us" attitude worked in my favour. I have no memory of that evening, except a brief flash, a picture in my head about the layout in the smoking room, which I had never even been to before, because at that time I had never smoked.

I went to look at the room the next day, and it was the same as I had pictured it. I swore Ivor to secrecy again as I was scared my secret would be out. If I had known a patient was secretly taking drugs, and I was thinking clearly, I would probably have told staff. Not because I want to tell tales, but because I would want the patient to be *safe*. Ivor didn't tell anyone. Maybe he thought I would be safe. Maybe he didn't care. Maybe it was what he thought was the right thing to do.

Most of the patients smoked, and I soon started. I didn't do it because I wanted to join in; I clearly remember thinking *"oh well, I'll be dead soon so it doesn't matter about lung cancer and heart disease – smoking will help pass the boring time."* I've read that 60% of psychiatric patients smoke, compared to 40% in the general population, but on Vaughan Thomas it was more like 95% smoked.

I soon met another patient, Caroline, admitted two weeks after me, slightly older than me. We were as similar as two peas in a pod, blonde, wore lots of purple, and became inseparable. I absolutely love her to pieces and have lived with constant fear that she will kill herself from the day we met. Not that seeing suicide from another perspective stemmed my own suicidal aspirations. She was (is) a qualified doctor, an Oxbridge graduate, taking time off from work because she was severely depressed. Fairly soon, she and I would get into a routine of going to the Oxford Brookes Sports bar in the evening to have a couple of drinks, smoke lots and talk. We'd talk about medicine, psychiatry, hospitals, suicide, eating disorders; you know, typical, happy topics.

Talking of routines, being obsessed with routine, I quickly assumed a new one. I was actually quite surprised when George, a nurse, told me that the hospital knew where I was going and how long I would be, so they knew not to worry. He was right that I was in a routine. But oh, if only they had known about my *true* routine. This involved getting up, arguing with Ray or someone about eating two Weetabix for breakfast. Sometimes I'd eat some, especially if Caroline was up. Then I would leave the ward in my cycling kit, vowing to cycle extra miles to make up for the cereal. That's all the staff saw: a "happy" Katy disappearing for a few hours, the idea being that it would help me get out of hospital if I got used to spending more and more time away from the ward. I was cycling between forty and fifty miles a day, nearer to fifty, and telling the staff a much lower number. Then I'd spend the day harming myself in ever more creative ways, but not telling anyone. Then I'd come "home" to the ward and be with people, waiting all day for my 15-minutes of being able to eat.

One night, I didn't have any food in my room, so I just took my zolpidem and went to sleep. However, I must have gotten up, found change in my purse, and walked down to the front of the hospital were there was a vending machine. (At this time I was allowed off the ward to other areas of the hospital). I hope I got dressed – but I can't remember! I have a flash of a memory of Veronica, a patient from our ward being brought in the main hospital door by the police after absconding.

The next thing I remember seeing was Declan when I was heading for my room, with an egg mayonnaise baton. (Something I wouldn't dare eat at that time). I saw Declan on the ward as he was still up; he always stayed up late. I vaguely remember talking to him, but not what about. My next memory was waking up in the morning and finding the sandwich intact, but the egg mayonnaise filling had been eaten. I cycled extra that day. I asked Declan about what had happened, and

248

secretly told him about the zolpidem. He laughed and told me that that explained why I had been so odd last night. He told me he had asked for half the sandwich, and I had laughed, said that it was, "Mine, all mine," then cackled another evil cackle, and dived into my room. It was a very eerie experience, but I continued to self-medicate to spare me from the dreaded insomnia and to allow me to eat.

Of course, the number of zolpidem tablets I took was going to become a problem, especially when I took it with suicidal intentions. Sometimes I'd assume that I'd take two or three, then wake up and find I taken more. I also started to mix zolpidem with zopiclone (imovane), another sleeping pill that, for me, was less potent, but cheaper. I'd often add alcohol to this cocktail, but not much because I was scared of the calories.

If I was suicidal, (and it was a half-hearted kind of suicide attempt at first, though none the less damaging), I would take few pills around ten in the evening to help me find courage, and then take at least 30, up to 50 pills. At the time I thought it would kill me, and again, was very aware of the cumulative affect over time. I assumed that if I died the staff would think I was asleep until it was too late. Not only was this dangerous and extreme, it was also stupidly expensive. You might argue that such overdosing was not suicidal because my thinking was not clear and I would be unlikely to get away with it in hospital, *but the intent was there.*

And today I wonder, would people think my sleeping pill obsession was a form of deliberate self-harm, or me being suicidal. Did I just want oblivion temporarily? Is it an attempted suicide when you do something and are clear in your mind that you are determined to die? Obviously: yes. Is it suicide when you are ambiguous or have clouded judgement, and you still do something so dangerous that might mean that you die, you hope you will die, or probably will die? I am less clear. I think the answer is intent. I had every intention of dying, even if I didn't have the energy to do things that resulted in death, I certainly knew my actions might result in death, and hoped they would. Temporary oblivion was just a bonus.

The *main* reason I picked zolpidem from all the sleeping agents available, was because there are recorded cases of it being lethal in overdose. Although I didn't want to die because of a decision I made when drunk or with no awareness, I *did* want to die, and I continued take small overdoses, completely aware at the time that it *would* lead me to dangerous behaviour and larger overdoses that I would not remember if I woke up. Often I'd take lots straight away. My *main* reason for these overdoses was to *die.* Thus I must class them as suicide attempts. I have only counted my attempts with clear intent, and which I recorded in my diary, as part of the ridiculous 443. The real number if ambiguous attempts are included is way higher.

No wonder I confused the medical staff, I confused myself. All the time I wanted to die, I did very dangerous, life-threatening things without caring about damage or death. All the focus was on death and not what was actually wrong with me in the first place. Because I was so tired and ill, didn't want to make a fuss, and wanted to be able to say I wasn't suicidal when I was, I persuaded myself that what I was doing didn't matter and I didn't care about the consequences. But with hindsight my suicidal intent is blatant. The Katy that I presented to the ward staff was *far* more stable than the real Katy.

The only time I admitted to taking extra sleeping pills, it was treated as a suicide attempt and Vaughan Thomas staff wanted me to go to Accident and Emergency. I refused, stating I knew I would be safe because I had done it hundreds of times. Of course, there is no such thing as a "safe" overdose. I remember later the next day, casually telling Dr Ogilvie that I just took about twenty pills (it was really forty, and then more that I didn't count) to make [in a raised voice] "EVERYTHING IN MY HEAD JUST FUCKING WELL SHUT UP AND GO AWAY." Dr. Ogilvie countered this in a skilfully simplistic fashion. He asked me what I thought the correct dose was. I told him it was, "5 or 10mg." Then he asked me what dosage I had taken; to which I replied, "200mg – about." So he replied that I had taken twenty times the recommended dose, and told me that he considered that to be an overdose. I couldn't really argue with that logic. I knew what I was doing, but wouldn't face up to it at the time. I didn't care if I ever woke up.

One day, I wrote a letter to Dr. Ogilvie who was encouraging me to get out and about in preparation for going home. This letter was written after a ward-round (weekly meetings of the consultant, ward staff and the patient) I had with Dr. Ogilvie that I stood up, violently kicked the door and walked out, slamming the door behind me. Such self-expression was unlike me, but I thought they were fucking with my head. What I really wanted to say was: *"Please let me stay on the ward because if I go home I will badly hurt myself, I'll see things that aren't there, then I'll die, and I really don't want to. I don't understand what is going on; please help me."* Of course, that was not how I put it, or even the situation as I was aware of at the time. I was overwhelmed.

Dear Dr. Ogilvie,

I have decided to write you a letter because it is the clearest way that I can think of to communicate. I do not want to fall into the trap of acting like a controlled child who rebels angrily from time to time. I seem to allow myself to be controlled (good/ unemotional/ quiet), or, when I can't take it any more, I rebel, get upset and angry. I get very angry about being controlled.

With people I see as authoritative, (which includes doctors, especially men), I will normally do as I am told. I will not express my wishes because I have been taught (by my father) that they are not valid and will be ignored. I am learning this is not always true now, but it is still the automatic response that I have. I learned that people aren't "allowed" emotions. I am amazed I cried in the ward round because I hardly ever show my emotions.

I see that you have my best interests at heart and are trying to balance keeping me safe with not disabling me by being in hospital too long. I can see you are right, but I am also very scared. I have spent the last few months living right on the edge of death and it is a huge relief to feel safer. Yet at the same time I hate it here. It is confusing and I do not know what to do. Yesterday I was going to rush home and kill myself and it scares me how close I came.

One thing I need you to explain to me is how it is possible that one minute I am being threatened with being sectioned, then next I am being told I should go home? I do not understand it – the inconsistency. My feelings about suicide have not changed.

Actually, I suppose that there is a subtle difference because I now feel scared that I might kill myself, whereas a couple of weeks ago I didn't care. Is that it? I need to understand this, so I know how to tell you if I need help again in the future. I cannot ask for help when I need it.

Every day my face hurts because I put on a fake happy face.

Telling him about my hallucinations would have been a good idea – but telling anyone would have made them more "real." Telling him about the money I was spending as freely as if I had millions would have been a good idea too. Not a mention of the drugs I was getting through – I didn't want them to spoil my suicide plans. My silence didn't help the professionals trying to diagnose my problems.

My diary of the early days in hospital, are mainly filled with me swearing and writing angrily about my anorexia. I was after all still technically classed as having anorexia, and after more than ten years of the illness I was at the end of my tether. It is certainly true, that in *my* case, manic depression has always been the more serious problem, and indeed was the major cause of the eating disorder. The problem now was that the anorexia was adding to my depression, whereas in the past the anorexia had alleviated the symptoms. This was all mounting up to a seriously ill person, unable to cope or see a future. For some reason I felt overwhelmingly angry and upset about the anorexia.

Ivor told me that he thought I was in hospital for the anorexia, which implied I must have looked quite ill and thin. Yet on the ward, there was no direct help or treatment for the anorexia. Ray would cajole me into eating sometimes. He even wrote in my diary, "You have to take it step by step."

What I am trying to say is not that the anorexia was ignored, but that the ward was not set up for people with anorexia. Nor was I even there for my anorexia, I was there for depression. Sometimes Ray would sit with me so that I would eat some cereal; I was rewarded by his company. The nurses working on that acute psychiatric ward were not trained to deal with eating disorders, which often require long-term treatment. The staff were always busy, but would try to help you if you asked. Some knew the basics about anorexia, but I noticed bulimia was pretty much ignored. I was aware other patients were vomiting. I would agree to eat, take food to my room and throw it away. No eating disorders unit would trust an anorectic to eat food whilst left alone! I also refused to be weighed, in fact I refused a physical examination all together since I hated my body so much. Thankfully I was not forced.

As there was no enforcement of eating or weight maintenance, I could have become very ill as some grandiose "fuck you" to everyone trying to help; whilst only hurting myself in the process. I suspect that had I chosen this option I would have been shipped to some eating disorders unit somewhere eventually, which would certainly have been the end of me. It would also have had to have been as a sectioned patient, for nothing would make me choose to go. Fortunately I chose to eat enough to maintain my weight. Why? Not because I had the foresight to recognise the possibility of being stuck in an eating disorders unit. I did it out of choice. I did it because I was tired to the bones (literally) with anorexia, so bored and angry, that I ate, even though this was still in a restricted manner. I didn't want the label as "ward anorectic." I was 8st 6lbs and 5'11'' (118lbs with a BMI[24] of 16.5, so technically anorectic at a BMI < 17.5).

My sense of humour saved me too. I thought the inexperienced, blunt "coaxing" from staff and patients into making me eat was funny, they were saying *all* the things that eating disorder units have learned not to say! Somehow, I preferred this direct approach, as it seemed more honest and well intentioned. I wasn't so low in weight that people with no knowledge of eating disorders could pick me out. (But that's because people

---

[24] BMI = Body Mass Index. It is a weight to height ratio, weight in kg divided by height in metres squared, 19-25 = "normal." Under 17.5 is anorectic.

expect a walking skeleton). I got a lot of comments about being too skinny, but that I could cope with. Nearly everyone with an eating disorder welcomes such comments, even if they claim not to. But I did not want to play the anorectic patient anymore. I wanted help for the depression because that was what had subjugated my whole life, tearing away my hopes, dreams, ambitions and health. I was finally beginning to realise that whatever form of depression I had was ignored too much for years, whilst the anorexia was pounced upon eagerly. I suppose anorexia is more "interesting."

The acceptance from other patients continued to keep me going. Their unquestioning tolerance was not only a relief, it was like a powerful drug rush after feeling so misplaced for years. I often sat in the garden with Declan, watched the footy, or spent hours talking with Caroline. Declan once sat in a garden with me, stoned, and stuck a post-it on his forehead. It was a well-known advertisement slogan regarding the colour orange and the future.

I remember thinking it was quite odd because neither of us felt like we wanted a future. So who cared what colour it would be. Who cared about a future? Then for some reason, I pointed out to him, that I hate the colour orange. I wanted it to be purple! Declan promptly made a new post-it, 'The future's bright, the future is purple!' He wore it for hours, whilst we laughed, smoking cannabis in sunshine of the hospital garden, right under the nurses' noses. I still have that little post-it with his messy handwriting on, stuck in one of my diaries. A few days later, at two in the afternoon, he jumped off the hospital fire escape.

Declan didn't die, but he broke his back. It was the end of July; I went out cycling as per usual, and whilst in town I bought a birthday card and present Declan. I got back to Vaughan Thomas in the late afternoon, only to be told he had jumped from the fire escape. Time stopped as I waited to hear if he was dead or alive. Then I heard the words "he broke his back" and thought *"oh no, oh no, he's dead, or if he's not dead he'll never walk."* Declan was not dead, and he did walk again – eventually. He was twenty that day. I never dreamed that he wouldn't make it to 21.

And now I really was stuck in a difficult place. I hated needing hospital, being in hospital, being condescendingly handed my pills at various times of the day; yet I could not see an existence within which I could survive without Vaughan Thomas. I was still ambivalent regarding suicide, amazed I was allowed to roam free and unsearched. I was attempting suicide and self-harming in secret; nobody really knew what was going on. I felt like they were trying to shove me out of the door, and so, to "prove" I needed their help I began to show my self-harm (only a small amount of the total), and tried to tell people how serious I was about killing myself. There is nothing more frustrating than telling someone *honestly* how you *want to die*, how *you want help*, only to be told you *aren't* depressed, and you *aren't suicidal* because if you were, you would already be dead. This fired my already overly present anger: not good.

Everyday, if I had a lie in, I was up at 4am. Before most patients were awake I'd be off to cycle how ever many miles I felt I had to that day. Then I'd go to Oxford town centre, buy healthy food and drink for Caroline and I, and head towards my other home, Linacre College. I'd check my mail, usually waiting for boxes of sleeping pills, go to my room, eat lunch, throw up, have a shower and then take a deep breath: the rest of the day my own. I would surf the Internet for hours about medications, drugs, suicide, and psychiatry. Or if I couldn't concentrate, I'd sit on my windowsill, dangling my cycling-toned legs out of the window at the students on the sports ground. Whilst sitting on the windowsill I'd play blaring music, smoking cigarettes and dropping them, watching their impact on the ground. Minimal damage. If I stayed long enough for fellow Linacre students to get home, we'd sit in my room smoking, listening to music. Then I'd cycle back to the ward.

Optional afternoon self-harming/suicidal activities before returning to the ward included dissolving lorazepam and/or zolpidem in a little alcohol and water, and injecting them. (Highly dangerous, do <u>not</u> do it). I knew this was dangerous and thought it might kill me. Was it suicidal? My intent was to satisfy curiosity, maybe sleep, and die if it happened: in other words, I do not know. Other activities were cutting, usually the tops of my legs so that I could stitch them myself and not get caught. I was not interested in pain: I anaesthetised my leg with lignocaine. I was doing it because the act of slicing open my body excited and fascinated me; and it used up Time, the adversary whom I constantly battled with.

Cutting also provided me with something to occasionally show the staff and say, "Look, you can't send me home yet." This, I admit, was a form of getting people's attention, but not in the deliberately manipulative fashion people misjudge it to be: it was sheer desperation. I needed help, nobody was taking notice, it made people listen. It didn't make people sympathetic, caring or kind: quite the opposite in fact.

Self-harm resulted in a variety of unpleasant, critical, pissed off, disempowering, and belittling treatment – making me want to self-harm more not less. But at least it stopped me from being ignored or labelled as "fine."

If I could have found a more effective means of communication, trust me, I would. Caroline was always taken very seriously, and I used to wonder what she said to enable that to happen. Whatever I did, I couldn't communicate what I needed. They always said, "Don't self-harm, tell us when you feel bad and we'll help you and not discharge you before you are ready." But then they break that promise: they don't listen. They break it because if you are able to stop self-harming you are "improved," you "obviously" must need less help to cope with emotions/life, and they have to make room to treat the most ill people: i.e. the people who are harming themselves. However much they try not to "reward" you with attention for self-harm, sometimes it is the only way to communicate. I felt forced to prove I was in danger; I know there are people out there doing exactly the same right now. That could be changed if people kept their promises about paying positive attention (and making sure the attention is obvious) to other forms of communication. Rant over.

I did not count any of these self-harm events in my suicidal 443; indeed they are still quite puzzling to me. The cutting was partly a misdirected "fuck you" to the world for the events preventing me from being a medical doctor. I think I just hated myself and felt I needed punishing. I also think I felt I had to do things like that (privately) in order for *me* to feel I *deserved* the help I was receiving from the hospital. Now when I look back, that seems rather illogical.

Sometimes I blood-let, using white needles or a blood giving set, but I didn't do this much or remove much blood at this time, it was purely for self-harm. Such equipment is available on any high street if you know where to look. The most I would blood-let was half a pint. Basically this meant that I inserted the largest needle I could find into a vein, and drained some of my own blood. This has been recorded many times in eating disordered medical professionals, and I am sure there will be depressed medical personnel who've done it. I did not do it to lose weight or as a method of purging, knowing that after the immediate fluid loss, bloodletting slows the metabolism and is therefore more likely to result in weight gain than weight loss.

I always drained my blood into a measuring jug, to keep track of what I was doing. What were my reasons for bloodletting? Morbid fascination, a fuck-it-why-not attitude, wanting to feel weak and ill, a need to feel punished, a what-if-I-die desire, a pissed-off-that-I'm-not-a-doctor feeling, and a feeling that I must do crazy things to prove I needed help. (Though I didn't actually tell anyone about the bloodletting).

On one occasion late that summer I self-harmed for the first time on the ward. That was a mistake, because the point of being on the ward was to feel safe. If I didn't feel safe, and if the staff did not think I was benefiting from hospitalisation, I would be sent home. Usually this sort of behaviour by patients resulted in a trip to the John Radcliffe Hospital emergency department, but on this occasion I was stitched by my favourite SHO, in the clinical room on Vaughan Thomas ward. I see that it was noted that they saw the many unreported cuts, some still with my own sutures in, on my legs that day.

They tried to stop me leaving the ward to cycle the next day, but I left anyway. I asked the nurse blocking my exit if they would section me if I left, she said no, so I left. The only concern in my mind at that time was going cycling. And as I cycled for miles and miles I thought to myself: *"Obviously I'm not seen as that ill, why don't they see it? What do I have to do? Or perhaps they have given up. Yes, that's it, they've given up: I'm worthless."* When cycling, the SHO's stitches broke, but my own stitches from a day earlier stayed in. I took this as proof I'd make a good doctor. Illogical: even by my standards. I'd just had more recent practice, and lots of it. I did get a royal bollocking when I got back to the ward about "accepting medical advice" and the gravity of having a low haemoglobin (Hb) of 7.6 g/dl. (Normal female Hb are 11.5-15.5g/dl, male values are 13.5-17.5g/dl. Emergency blood transfusions are normally given to people under 7g/dl; anything under 10 to 11g/dl is classed as anaemic).

When I returned from my daily explorations, it meant smuggling in substances that were banned. I achieved this because no one stopped me to ask what was in my giant cycling rucksack. There were always sleeping pills, anorectic "safe" food for me to pick at between taking my pills and passing out. Including some of the following, usually in a ritualistic fashion, fat-free yoghurt, the filling of low-fat sandwiches, cereal bars, fruit, and alcohol. I'd always eat the nicest thing first, because I usually wouldn't remember (or eat) anything else. I'd bring alcohol for other ward members too: occasionally Ash and Declan (when he was there), but usually just for Caroline and myself. She would also bring alcohol for the two of us. I wouldn't have brought back booze for anyone if they had not had the ability to get it freely anyway. It never entered my head that my actions could be harmful to the other patients, or myself. I will never know if it did any harm.

Just after ten o'clock night-meds, Caroline and I would sit in the large meeting room upstairs where I'd first met Dr. Ogilvie. It was now abandoned, but usefully had a fridge for booze and yoghurts! This was a typical anorectic-who-drinks fridge, low calorie food, and alcohol whose calories do not count. This was before all the rebuilding, when Vaughan Thomas ward still had an upstairs, and Caroline and I were on the female corridor, right next to the abandoned meeting room. We'd have a little wine, or a few shots of this apple flavoured schnapps, before heading to bed. It was not ever a large amount of alcohol; it was just our wind-down time together before bed, getting away with something "naughty." What Caroline did not know, was that sometimes the Dark-Man-over-my-shoulder was with us in the room. But with Caroline there, his power over me was reduced.

There were two problems with my friendship with Caroline, both of which I felt were far less important than spending time with such a fantastic person and did not allow them to spoil what was and is a great friendship. The first most frightening problem was that I was afraid she would kill herself and I would lose her too. The second was heightened jealously that she was a qualified medical doctor. I did not want to take anything away from her; it just made me reflect on what I perceived to be a massive failure of mine. I remember feeling upset that I got ill before I even got into university, whereas Caroline didn't get noticeably ill until she was in med school. What happened to me is in no way Caroline's fault, and I do not wish to imply she has not suffered terribly herself: she has. My failure was something I struggled to live with, and I know I always will.

Talking to Caroline was eerie. We had so much in common, right down to our suicide method, (for clarity, I mean the insulin overdose method, since I had several prepared methods). It was a relief to find someone with whom I could relate: someone warm and clever, someone else who was up at 4am, someone with similar access to lethal means. Both of us passionately wanted to work in the health field, hopefully psychiatry, helping people. Caroline and I would often talk medicine. We never spoke about our specific patients, but I soon got an understanding of the stresses of life as a house officer (or as they are affectionately termed by senior house officers: house-plants!). Caroline was bright, and diligent, good at her job; but the stress of the job as she progressed up the career-ladder was obviously immense. I loved her stories; I listened intensely, all the while burning with envy despite beginning to see the down sides to the job.

Caroline and I also shared the fact that we were depressed *and* sufferers of eating disorders. I know we are not alone. Caroline was a bulimic, though she told me she was pretty much back in control of that part of her life, but still had "slips." Like me, Caroline was a veteran of eating disorders, and decidedly pissed off about having one. We tended to hang out as a pair, but sometimes Ivor joined us, always smelling of pot. He said he was forced to be a psychiatric patient to avoid prison, preferring hospital. He'd been in and out of psychiatric wards all his life, and claimed he could talk about psychiatric illnesses as if he was a psychiatrist.

(He couldn't actually do it, but was convincingly knowledgeable at a basic level).

I first met Ivor when Clare (Baker) and I were sitting in the lounge area of the day hospital prior to my admission. For some reason he started ranting about how he couldn't understand people with eating disorders. He'd met plenty during his time in hospital and so was obviously an expert on the subject. I looked at Clare and we smiled at each other. I was underweight (118lbs, 5'11'' BMI 16.5) at the time. Clare was purging more or less daily. I think many people wouldn't have said much back when faced with this butch, loudly opinionated man, but not us. Ivor said something along the line of his cure for eating disorders would be to "feed the anorexic to the bulimic." My reply was that he had better feed me to Clare then because I had anorexia and she was bulimic.

Silence.

Then we laughed. Clare and I were so sick and tired of our eating disorders, and too bored with them to feel ashamed. We had learned the hard lesson, that knowledge about why you are behaving in a destructive, eating disordered fashion will not cure you. Even knowing what you should be doing will not save you from doing the exact opposite. So much had happened to us both that we were passed caring what people thought about us having an eating disorder. However, we both cared that people *knew* we weren't ashamed. And I guess we saw the funny side, so we laughed.

So when Ivor arrived on Vaughan Thomas that summer, he apologised for what he had previously said, and told me I was the "most normal, down-to-earth anorexic" he had ever met. I think he would find that true of many anorectics if he took the time to get to know them. I thanked him for the heartfelt apology, and reassured him that I had seen the funny side of things. I hoped that he would think differently about rapidly judging people with eating disorders in the future, but I was only partly right. He decided to tell Caroline the hilarious story of how he and I had met, not expecting for one moment for her to turn around and say with a perfectly straight, innocently sweet face that she was bulimic too.

You should have seen his face! I suppose that laughing at Ivor is probably unfair, because eating disorders are baffling to outsiders. Then again, it is such stereotypical behaviour that I have sworn to fight against, whilst trying to maintain my dignity and sense of humour. Humour seemed to be the best way to cope with Ivor, and I actually spent a lot of time talking with him.

Caroline being a bulimic fascinated Ivor, and one night, he came to the TV room and plonked a load of chocolate bars down on the table. He told Caroline to eat them all because he wanted to see what it was like. So Caroline, bless her, with her perfected, chaste face, graciously ate one bar and said, "Thank you, that was nice." I smiled, and, of course, ate nothing. We returned to watching whatever crap police programme Jeremy had chosen for us. Ivor tried to make Caroline eat more, and continued to be fascinated by our eating disorders, but Caroline and I didn't take the bait. We just coped, talking to each other helped, but mostly we just didn't give a shit. Depression was our concern at the time.

Anyone who knows about bulimia knows that you don't do it to put on a show for someone. It's private and hidden, though bulimics may sometimes binge and

Katy Sara Culling

purge together, it's not something I have done or even considered doing. It happened on Vaughan Thomas, but not with Caroline or myself. Many bulimics, particularly anorexic bulimics will binge in a very controlled situation, where subsequent purging cannot possibly be interrupted. Bulimics like Clare describe bingeing at parties, or overeating in a restaurant, and vomiting in public toilets or even streets. That was something I could never do. I also know that no bulimic will binge for the benefit of someone else's curiosity. It's not precisely something you really want to share.

Caroline and I decided to keep a record of the funny, "mad" things that some patients said; being fair, we included ourselves. I couldn't make these up if I tried to; each is a genuine quote, word for word. My favourites are Ash's classics!

Ash: [To a male patient]. "I hear voices and they don't like you."

Ash: "Fucking hell! Who turned the sun on?"

Caroline: "We're allowed to be mad, we're mental patients."

Me: "It's OK, we're safe. Ivor says he only kills people on Thursdays."
Caroline: "It's Thursday today Katy!"
Me: "Oh fuck."

Ash: "If I didn't know what I wanted to know I'd be confused."

266

Joanna: "Katy be good, and if you can't be good be careful, and if you can't be careful, get a job as a doctor."

Zee to Ginny: "Stop being so fucking abusive!"
Ginny to Zee: "Fuck off!"

Ivor: "Some spells don't work on sane people."

Ash: "FUCK sex!"

Ash: "Hi how are ya? I'm safe as fuck."

Caroline: "It's not rocket science!" (Regarding psychiatry, medicine, staff behaviour, patient behaviour, Tottenham winning, Derby losing, smoking, drinking and pretty much everything).

Ash Power is not the first or last schizophrenic patient I have known, but he is certainly the most charismatic. I was fascinated by his behaviour, which seemed so… inexplicable. I assumed he had his reasons. We talked a lot, and he regularly asked me to be his girlfriend, to kiss him, and sometimes he was overly forward. Other times he would prefer men, or think he was a woman. He'd ignore the ward rules and just walk into my bedroom on the female corridor. But he was harmless. Usually he seemed stoned, but I couldn't tell if that was Ash himself, or the drugs.

Ash continued to be very fond of drugs. He particularly liked nutmeg; or so he claimed. I was a little baffled at the idea of nutmeg being a drug, and when Ash returned from the hospital gardens with what looked to me like small pinecones, my bewilderment grew. He claimed he had eaten twenty and they were nutmeg, which clearly they were not, since nutmeg is a spice that is derived from the stone of a fruit in the West Indies. However, he described the feelings he had, first complaining of stomach ache, and laughing he'd get diarrhoea soon. Ouch - he must have felt so ill afterwards. He walked about for hours with a dopey grin on his face. The power of the mind is an unusual thing.

I've since done some reading about nutmeg; it can be used as a drug, and is a hallucinogen producing some of the symptoms that Ash appeared to be experiencing. However, in his case it was not down to the pinecones, (which contain no nutmeg), it must have been the placebo effect. When the upstairs of Vaughan Thomas was rearranged, and the women moved on to a corridor downstairs. Ash was given what had been my room. He came down giggling, and claimed to be high. He told me he'd found some tablets, and showed me a handful of my sweeteners. He was giggling all day, I didn't have the heart to tell him.

If all of this makes you think that being in hospital was a party, it wasn't. Underneath my calm, happy exterior still burned a soul filled with anger and despair. I was able to be myself more so than in most places, but much was still hidden. The evenings on the ward with the other patients were when I was at my most relaxed. Most of my day was hell. I thought a lot about death. If I had to write about what I did during my hospitalisation that summer, that terrible period of my life, it would not only be about the wonderful friends that I made, it would be that I though a lot about the experience of death, which lead on to philosophising about religion. An obsession with death was not unusual for me, but the intensity with which I sought oblivion via suicide was stronger than ever.

I moved on to the whole philosophy what of suicide means. I wondered what I would feel the moment I died, and if it would be as poetic and calm as described by Kevin Spacey (as Leicester Burnham) in *American Beauty*. Poetic and calm despite the fact he had just had his brains blown out. I was beyond caring if it would be painful, but it had to be "tidy." I was attempting suicide erratically at this time, and I assumed my death by suicide was a sure bet eventually; and so I moved beyond suicide planning, to thinking about the *meaning* of my death, both to me, and those I would leave behind. Did I want to be a statistic, my life and potential extinguished forever? Of course, I believed that for me, my suicide was the end of suffering, peace and absolute nothingness. And peace for those I would leave behind.

Naturally I worried about hurting people, but I was, at that time, almost incapable of being aware or in touch with the actual pain that I would cause. To an extent I was unable to see their suffering. I am horrified at those thoughts now, with my renewed awareness of the desolation suicide brings, now able to see it clearly with a lucid mind. I don't know if understanding that people might well have been unable to comprehend the pain their suicide would cause will help people (those of you) who have lost someone to suicide. I know it helps me cope with those I have lost.

Selfish as it will sound, the thought of hurting other people was not always enough to stop me trying to kill myself during those times I could connect with the pain I might cause. Leading up to suicide, people suffer great torment about the pain they will cause. However, my view of other people's torment became detached or minimised compared to the utter misery of my existence. I sometimes convinced myself that everyone would be better off, happier, or gratefully celebrate my departure. I used to imagine them popping the cork on champagne. I don't know if that was delusional or low self-esteem: I suspect a bit of both.

I also thought that a short sharp pain would be better than years of watching and supporting me through more years of illness. My thinking was always clouded, and sometimes, the pain of existence was just so great, that all other thoughts were lost. I agonised about the repercussions of my suicide one moment; then (unconsciously) somehow detached myself and could not see any direction other than towards death.

I would like to be able to argue the point that suicide after many years of psychiatric disorders could be a rational decision, but I would struggle to do so. I have believed my suicide to be the only rational option in the past. The stumbling block for me is that no matter how passionately, how often, and how long I have wanted to end my life, I subsequently experienced times when I have been *so glad to be a failed suicide*. I am grateful to be alive. Grateful for things I have not missed, grateful for pain I have not caused, grateful to those who have helped me, thankful for the people in my life, thankful to be able to help others. Whether or not that will always be true for me, I do not know.

I am an atheist. I am a scientist by profession and an artist at heart. I am sceptical. They don't always come together, but they do in my case. I basically believe that we are all atoms that come together to form cells that form life, and our awareness of that life is our consciousness, which in turn is due to our neurobiology. To me, "death" fundamentally means an end to our consciousness, and that those atoms that are part of us will eventually move on to become parts of the sea, the sky, new creatures, or something. Essentially we are all dust.

Such beliefs can sometimes make suicide "easier" because of the lack of after death possibilities, or rather penalties, compared with other people's beliefs. I believe everyone is entitled to their own opinion as long as they do not try to force it on to others. I am happy for someone if their faith gives them comfort, relief, support and happiness. It just doesn't work for me because I have no faith. Personally, even ignoring all science and just concentrating on what I feel to be true in my heart, I feel *nothing*. Occasionally in my life, I have wanted to believe in order to belong and feel comfort, but I cannot make myself feel what I do not.

I do not believe in god because of all the suffering in the world. What "god" would look over us with supreme power, and allow such pain? If there is a god, she is cruel, sick and unworthy, and I am not afraid to have that opinion because I do not fear that I will be held to account. I am a good person, which is enough for me.

But all this debate does not mean that I think people who believe in god cannot be close to me, or that I think their opinion is less worthy than mine. Yes, I disagree, but it's just a belief. I am happy for suffering friends who find solace when turning to the church. If spirituality helps or cures people, then halleluiah with whipped cream and cherries on top! I know that Christianity helped Ayeesha when recovering from anorexia. I know that Caroline's faith helped her to not attempt suicide because she saw it as a sin. I know my mum feels comfort from believing her parents are in heaven and she will see them again.

I also know that Ash thinks he *is* god; and frankly I'd worship Ash before I'd worship something I cannot feel or believe. If that makes me an idolater – so what! What works for one will not work for another; religion just doesn't work for me.

I do not believe in karma or reincarnation, or any other afterlife belief accompanying a faith. I do not believe suicide is a mortal sin. I do not believe in heaven, though I do believe that people should try to live "good" lives, and be responsible, helpful, loving and caring. If humans have souls, to me this describes something that represents our collective thoughts, our consciousness of self and others, and the sum of our good and bad experiences in life. I believe that this soul (consciousness) dies with the body because it is built up of neurons and neurotransmitters: essentially living biology and chemistry that ultimately breaks down into atoms. Nobody understands how the neurons in our brain and their various connections give rise to consciousness, awareness of self, functionality and our personality. But I do believe it is a biological process, and death, which is always ultimately due to lack of oxygen to the brain, is the end of a biological process for each of us. This does not give me much comfort when someone dies, perhaps that is why religion is so popular: I can understand that. Who doesn't want to believe in a continuing happy existence for those we love.

And yet when I thought this over during the long spring and summer in the Warneford, I struggled. I struggled to understand. It is a very difficult thing to be faced with your own mortality and try to understand it, particularly if you are like me, thinking and dissecting every aspect. I think like that about everything, not just death and suicide. I analyse everything to extinction in my head. Sometimes it is good, it means I listen, consider, understand and do not judge; but too often it has been turned in on myself unhelpfully.

Few people know when or how they are going to die, a luxury that a suicide is not afforded. Despite my personal, strong, logical and emotional beliefs about life and death, described just above, my feelings left me with doubt. My beliefs are logical to me, but a person cannot so easily switch off their emotions, which are not always so rational. My beliefs were not always strong enough to overcome the small doubt I felt. I cannot think about death and separate it from emotion; or rather, I cannot *usually*. I have done so at least 443 times.

Fundamentally, *I was afraid that death was not the end*, when most people fear the reverse. Although my beliefs about the finality of death are very strong, I used to worry about possibility my consciousness might continue after my suicide, and that I would not be able to cope with this, nor have the power to change the situation. This was morbid and obsessive philosophising that did not fit in with my actual beliefs, and probably saved my life a number of times. I was also trying to kill myself or at least weaken myself every single day, i.e. I was ambivalent, and usually certain in my belief that death equals oblivion. A scientific approach to any situation requires open mindedness, in order to deal with the results without bias: which meant I was susceptible to doubt. Not very much doubt, but some, and sometimes that is all it takes.

"To believe is very dull.
To doubt is intensely engrossing."

❧ Oscar Wilde (1854 – 1900)

I was engrossed with death. My fears angered me because I did not understand them, and it felt like my overactive imagination was tricking me in order to keep me alive. Against my beliefs I worried that I may remain on the Earth, conscious but without a body; or if I had a body I would be like a ghost, unseen, and lonely. I imagined my ghostly experience to be exactly the same as my experience of being alive: depressed, anxious, still in hospital, but unable to speak to anyone, take medication to help, eat, or sleep. In other words, it might be worse than staying alive.

The other fear I had is probably unusual, and I have not met anyone else who has considered it. Limited to those of you who have seen the film *Beetlejuice*: a Tim Burton film. In it, all people who committed suicide ended up spending eternity as civil servants. A secretary, a file clerk, a councillor and so on, reels of paper and piles of paperwork everywhere. Plus the body you are left with for eternity is the same as what is left after you die. If you jump under a truck, you are a flattened mess with one hand and half a head, and you still have to be a civil servant. For some reason, emotion, i.e. fear often won; no logic was required, and all of this stuck in my brain and kept me alive on a number of occasions.

Please don't misunderstand me. I do not believe in an afterlife. I do not believe in any god, and not in the possibility of being a ghost, nor a punished civil servant. But when ill, I was not entirely rational! All I wanted to make everything stop and go away by dying. Thinking about suicide (seriously) is far harder than carrying out the act once you have made a decision. But I was afraid. I was afraid because I was absolutely resolute that I wanted to die; at least that desire was all I was conscious of. I think fear at your own extinction is perfectly normal. Sometimes my fear was manifested as doubting my own beliefs, and imagining horrible alternatives to the nothingness that I believe death brings. I notice that I did not ever believe in a happy afterlife, I was afraid of a fate worse than death. As Clare put it, "Most people are scared to die because there might be no afterlife, you are scared to die in case there is."

Looking at my medical notes from this time is upsetting. It is difficult to accept how badly I was misunderstood – then again, I wasn't very open. There were no mentions of hallucinations, so I must have looked normal whilst they were going on. I told John that I had to die before I was no longer 27, but saw no sign that this had been recognised. It is also hard to see your days summarised in a neat, cheery fashion, when you know that all of that time, you were clinging to life by a rope you were simultaneously cutting through:

"Pleasant."

"Claims to feel low." [The "claims" implies that I was lying?]

"Has gone walking with Caroline." [To the pub].

"Katy seems to be writing to the staff instead of speaking to them." [The point being?]

"Issues of transference."

[George, a nurse who made a point of talking with me wrote]: *"Will inadvertently mention a topic, go quiet, then change topic."* [Oh dear, no, no, never. Do you really think I EVER "inadvertently" mentioned anything?]

"Sleep OK." "Sleep poor." "Not sleeping."

"Appears bright and cheery." [<u>Appears</u> being the operative word].

"Katy has two deep cuts to her legs, but has refused to go to Accident and Emergency, and so was given steristrips and dressings to look after her own wounds. Returned with sutured wounds." [I wasn't ever going to go to A & E again whilst conscious].

"Katy returned from a football match seeming low. Derby lost." [Come on; that's normal].

Dr. Ogilvie started me on buspirone for anxiety, discussed me moving out of College to get a "fresh start," and decided to refer me to Dr. Steve Pearce, consultant psychiatrist and consultant psychotherapist based at the Warneford Hospital, Oxford and the University of Oxford, an expert in "difficult cases" and personality disorders: to get a second opinion about my diagnosis. I had always hidden manic symptoms, afraid of what they meant. He explained he felt I had a very severe depression that was treatment resistant, but wanted another expert to confirm I did not have borderline personality disorder. My recollection of that meeting was that Dr. Ogilvie was almost completely certain about my diagnosis, and that this referral was just tying up loose ends. It took five months for that referral to take place; and even then it was hurried up as desperately urgent because I had …well… died.

I would find out later that it is quite common in rapid cycling or mixed bipolar sufferers, especially, in women, that a diagnosis of borderline personality disorder is often made in error.

Richard, my named nurse, was on holiday – and expecting me to be discharged before he got back. I passed a letter to the staff:

I am afraid. I am afraid to be alone.
[Explaining about my hallucinations would have been sensible, but I did not].

I am afraid that if I do go I will never be admitted again, however suicidal I feel, because I have taken so long to leave this time, and have been given "my chance." I know you reassure me that that is not true, but I don't believe you; and forgive me for being cautious when it is my life on the line.

When I talk about suicide it is not meant as a threat. It just "is." It's how I feel.

I believe you don't care whether I live or die, and that I do not deserve help.

I do not know why I push people away.

That letter was, I believe, a perfectly clear way of expressing my feelings and asking for help. I received no response – the letter was not even kept in my medical notes. This is just one example of why self-harm became a necessary form of communication: they couldn't ignore self-harm. A few days later George was on duty and found some time to spend with me; for which I wished to express my thanks. All the staff was busy so I leaned into the office and said, "Can I just say one word?" They all looked at me, and I said, "Thank you." The three nurses in the office, George, John-the-Hippie and Simon (the boss), all said in unison, "That's two words!" I laughed and swore. I liked all of those nurses, especially John who was a bit of an intellectual and would talk to me for hours. They all gave me their time, even after their shifts, which made them good in my opinion.

It seemed obvious to me that when in a social situation, even a fake-social situation like in hospital, I was mostly incapable of showing my sadness due to my constant crusade to be funny and liked. They were the experts, wasn't it obvious to them?

&

Ash paid Ginny one pound each for any lorazepam tablets she could get him. This would now be illegal, but at the time it happened lorazepam was one of the benzodiazepines that it was not illegal to possess without a prescription. (I'm unclear whether selling it was illegal). I hadn't ever had lorazepam, and told Declan about this scam going on. That night he palmed a lorazepam tablet in order to give it to me. I took it, no regard for consequences, hoping it would make me sleep. It didn't.

How did Ash fund all his drugs and booze when his income was eleven pounds a week? He often borrowed money from me, but gave it back faithfully every time he received his benefit, always accurate to the penny. Whatever went on in his busy head he could remember about money owed or due. I soon learned how Ash managed to fund his lifestyle. Many patients were confined to the ward, but as Ash was not considered a threat to himself or anyone else, he was allowed out during the day. He would buy things for patients confined on the ward, in return for them buying his requirements.

The basic rule of thumb went like this: whatever you wanted Ash to fetch would cost you twice its actual retail or street value. If you wanted a bottle of vodka, fine, he'd smuggle it in, but you had to buy him a bottle too, cash up front. Drugs, fine, just buy him the same and there was no problem. Of course, Ash was in fact very ill, and cannot justly be held responsible for these actions. I am amazed that staff didn't catch on, perhaps they did? A blind eye was turned for booze or marijuana. I was once asked for a urine test, and I refused. I claimed this was because I sat in the smoking room and therefore probably inhaled enough dope to give a positive result, even though I never touched the stuff. Of course I did really, though rarely. My actual reason for not wanting to pee in a cup was that I was embarrassed to give it to either of the male nurses who asked.

Ash decided that I was an Egyptian princess. I picture Egyptian woman as olive-skinned with black hair cut in a severe bob. I have long, light blonde hair, lightly wavy unless I straighten it, and was so pale from poor nutrition, self-medication and blood-loss that I don't really understand how Ash's brain made this leap, but he did. He said I had hair like the sun. And the beautiful thing was that I knew he really meant it.

He used to kick up a fuss about side effects from his antipsychotics in order to get procyclidine. I asked him why, and he told me it got him high. He told me it was his favourite drug. Ash was already a patient on Vaughan Thomas when I was admitted. I remember thinking clearly that Summer, that *as long as I was released before Ash, things couldn't be so terrible, I couldn't be that ill.*

My diary reads:

> *"I wonder if they would stop me if I tried to leave today? I can see Ray in the hall sometimes. They wouldn't stop me; I'm not worth saving. I don't know where to go, what to do, or what would help.*

Nothing helps. I don't fucking know what the fuck to do. Do I need to immolate myself in order to get taken seriously? [Obviously I was being taken seriously, or else I would have been discharged]. *What fucking mess have I got myself into? What the fuck am I doing? They don't get what's going on in my head. I don't fucking get what's going on in my head. I help myself; I hurt myself. I don't know what I am writing this for."*

I couldn't understand why, when I wanted death as much as I did, I could be allowed to roam freely in and out of the hospital – unless I didn't matter. When I was out, I self-harmed, with a gradually escalating severity – was I trying to make a point in a very inarticulate way? Maybe it was the only means I had to communicate. Often it was communication with myself; proof that I needed help, and not something the ward staff ever knew about.

One self-harm event really upset me because of the response of Dr. Ogilvie and because it was, for me, abnormal self-harm. It happened one night when I was sitting up in the smoking room; seeing how many fags I could smoke between the sun setting and the sun rising. I'd been in hospital for almost three months, and for the first time with any clarity, I saw the-Dark-Man-over-my shoulder. He was sitting in the corner of room and I could see him out of the corner of my eye. I did not dare look right at him, so I turned my back. But that didn't help; I could feel his eyes burning into my back.

And so, I took the cigarette in my hand and started to burn my left hand. Burning is extremely painful, and as such, not a form of self-harm I would choose. But it seemed rational that night. The room was swimming, the pain intense, and as long as it hurt, I felt safe: grounded. And so I sat there for hours, gradually working my way over my left hand and up my left arm burning circular holes into my skin. I detached myself from reality, where reality with a Dark-Man-over-my-shoulder was mad and made of cobwebs that she slowly burned away. As the rest of the ward slept, content that they were safe, Katy Sara saw a Dark-Man-over-her-shoulder and burned him away.

A few day's later, I was called into ward round as per usual on a Monday. One of the nurses brought up the fact I had burn marks that were becoming infected. I didn't really know what to say because I had not deliberately shown anyone what I had done. For a split second I thought to myself, *"I could tell Dr. Ogilvie about the Dark-Man-over-my-shoulder; what would he think? I think he'd understand."* But my thoughts were cut short when Dr. Ogilvie said dismissively, "I don't think we need to worry much about a couple of burn marks." *"Ah,"* I thought, my defences rising. *"You are from the school of I-do-not-'reward'-self-harm and I-do-not-need-to-understand-WHY-in-each-case."* If someone paints a picture of an apple, it is easy to decipher. Self-harm is a picture that should always be investigated, unravelling the various layers contained within. Who knows how beneficial it would have been for me to admit to having hallucinations or delusions? I was saddened. It was one of only two events with Dr. Ogilvie that I wish had gone differently. I certainly wish I had told him about my hallucinations: a rather important part of my manic depressive pathology. As a result of how I felt (i.e. it was my poor choice) that day, no one found out about my terrifying hallucinations, indeed no one will until they read this book.

The summer droned on. The weather was good and many of us spent time in the ward's garden, soaking up the sun. Caroline and I walked over to the Brooke's University Sports Bar most days, where we drank, talked and smoked. We did mad things because we were mental patients and we were supposed to. We met for a fag at 4am, we ate trifle at 11pm, one day I decided to get a tattoo, and went to the best Tattoo artist on Cowley Road to get a Derby Ram tattooed on my lower back! Another day Caroline had her hair put into purple plaits that lasted almost a week. Whilst she was mid-plaits, Caroline borrowed my precious Derby County baseball cap – which made me smile because she is an Tottenham fan. Kevin left, Stella left, and Ash never left me alone.

One week for ward round, Caroline and I, the suicidal twins, wore matching black T-shirts that said, "Fuck it" in white on the front. We were making a serious statement, but doing with a smile. Caroline went in first, so I was nearly crapping myself when I went in. Dr. Ogilvie later said to me that he didn't even notice!

Declan came back from the John Radcliffe Hospital in a body cast, and he and I would sit on the grass under the nurses station whilst he smoked a different sort of grass; talking the many hours away. Playing the counsellor and trusted friend made me feel worthwhile. Declan's life had been a sad one.

One night at 9pm, the end of the late shift, an unnamed member of the nursing staff took Caroline and I to the pub, where we drank the night away and were snuck back onto the ward after midnight. That was fun. Those memories are not so bad.

One day, a friend of mine with manic depression who was visiting, peeled a "Warning, may contain nuts" sticker off the piece of carrot cake she had brought in for me. She stuck it on the front door of the Warneford Hospital, and we collapsed in giggles at the hilarity. All the patients thought it highly amusing; for some reason the staff did not.

Probably the best moment was one evening at around 9pm; I was still fairly free to come and go as I chose within the hospital. Caroline and I went down to the patients' smoking room at the front of the hospital. It was usually empty and we wanted the chance to have a private chat, including details about our suicide plans and a possible suicide pact.

For this special occasion I had bought two mini bottles of champagne from Marks and Spencer. We sat there, in our matching fluffy purple dressing gowns, Caroline in slippers and pyjamas, me in shorts and bare feet, and sucked champagne through straws whilst chain smoking. A security guard came in and caught us with our drinks in our hand. Alcohol was prohibited anywhere in the hospital, not just on the ward, and he started to tell us he would have to take it away, so I said, "Don't worry, *we're doctors.*" He humbly apologised and grovelled backwards, out of the room. Caroline and I crumpled with fits of laughter. Well it wasn't a complete lie... but it was 9pm and we were dressed for bed!

That was a good moment; and the last time I would genuinely laugh for a long, long time.

Chapter 9. A Colourful Autumn where I did not Exist.

"To be, or not to be: that is the question:
Whether 'tis nobler in the mind to suffer
The slings and arrows of outrageous
fortune,
Or to take arms against a sea of troubles,
And by opposing end them? To die: to
sleep;
No more; and, by a sleep to say we end
The heartache and the thousand natural
shocks
That flesh is heir to, 'tis a consummation
Devoutly to be wished."

&~ William Shakespeare (1564-1616).
Hamlet, (Act III, scene 1, written 1600-
01).

Autumn is actually my favourite season. I think it is the colours that I love best. Forever fond of trees and nature, the colours of the leaves remind me of a more innocent, care-free time: smelling the bonfires and kicking the leaves that lined the fields and streets in Derbyshire. And whilst it is true, that Autumn is a period of dying; I do not think that that is a reason why I love it so. But the Autumn of 2002 was different: it was supposed to be my last.

It was early Autumn when I prepared to move out of Linacre College (where I had lived for three years), and into a new, small flat, on the Iffley Road, Oxford. Clare lived in the same house, having a small room near the front. I had the penthouse (OK, a converted attic flat).

The advice, that seemed entirely sensible at the time, was to give me a fresh start, in a new Oxford home, away from my home of manic, angry, psychotic, depressive, anorexic, self-harming, (and at the time, the vast number of undisclosed suicide attempts and hallucinations).

If had been thinking clearly, I would have remembered that moving home did not ever make these memories, visions or impulses go away. In fact, room 34, in the Bamborough Building, Linacre College had become my shelter, if a somewhat precarious one. It was the best home I had ever had. I realised too late, how much comfort I felt my Oxford College room, with students and staff around. In College I could talk to fellow students and get lost in intellectualisation and feel the desire to return to my own research. In College I could have a cigarette in my room, play music loudly, sit on my windowsill, and be joined (not on the windowsill) by other students, from all around the world. (Linacre College is a truly cosmopolitan College). However, I was ready to try anything, even moving, if it might ease my depressive state. It is only possible to say this in retrospect: it was the wrong choice.

Initially I kept up with my cycling and kept my weight low. The Dark-Man-over-my-shoulder was waiting to greet me in my new home, and now all of my art prints or film posters were talking to me. I was often sick during my day trips out from the hospital, though I was desperate to stop that particular behaviour. It wasn't as compelling or upsetting as it had been when I was in my early twenties, probably because now I had my own flat; so I didn't have to deal with the guilt of other people knowing, and I kept my flat spotless. I didn't eat binge foods, I ate healthy foods, usually smoked salmon; paid for by the £3,000 grant Oxford University had given me.

I began to wish I wasn't allowed out so much, but only so that I didn't have to be sick. A big part of me now wonders if I hurt myself more and more just to make the hospital staff keep me in hospital to stop the bulimia from returning. All I know is, I felt out of control and wanted (needed?) someone to take the control from me. Yet I remained as a voluntary patient, which meant that control rested with me. Dr. Ogilvie always resisted taking over any aspects of control. I realise now, that he did that for my own benefit, to maintain my autonomy and in theory, aid a speedier recovery. At the time, I was still torn between wanting people to tell me what to do, and wanting to remain voluntary, avoiding the stigma of being sectioned.

In my diary, I wrote:

> *"FAILURE. FAILURE. FAILURE. I want to die. I want to live – but only if it is worth it. I wish Rich or George were working tonight. NIGHTS ARE THE WORST. I am alone. I am so alone. I hate myself. I am so fucking stupid and am more of a mess than anyone could possibly imagine. I want to die right now.*
>
> *I can't believe I am still here. I have been here too long and nothing is getting any better. Gained friends, gained scars, lost blood, lost money, will I lose my career? Gained hope, lost hope, been*

*lonely, been alone, been sad, been angry,
wanted to cry but I couldn't."*

On the 25th of September, Prof. Keith Frayn (my
D.Phil. supervisor) and my Linacre College Tutor
visited me in hospital with only a matter of hours
warning. It was to prove a most unproductive and
upsetting meeting. With a bored nurse beside me for
support, I sat and listened to Keith tell me I had lost my
studentship place, "because in such a rapidly advancing
field, your research will soon lose its value." (That was
thankfully bullshit as we later collaborated to get my
research published – for which I thank Keith). My
College tutor was decidedly unhappy and wanted me to
keep my studentship; she fought Keith, trying to
suggest many ways to work through the problem, but
Keith had the last say. I was crying; I couldn't believe
what was happening. I was allowed to have 2 years off
and I still had 10 months to get back on my feet – in
theory. It wasn't actually the end of my career at
Oxford, but on that day, and for days to come, I though
I had lost everything that mattered. I was strangely
numb.

When I read my medical notes I discovered that all
the ward staff knew what was going to happen a whole
day before I did:

"Katy's tutor [Prof Frayn] *has withdrawn
funding and is not prepared to support a
further application for postponement."*

This, of course, took from me the most important
thing in my life. Rightly or wrongly I cannot calm
feelings of anger towards Keith for what happened,

despite his genuinely expressed concern for my wellbeing. You do not tell a student who has worked her guts out for 2 years on a Ph.D. that she is canned whilst she is in hospital on suicide watch. Since my work was my love and future, he broke my heart and my dreams all in one go, and with that, he removed my remaining slivers of hope.

I felt as if I had been erased. I didn't jump around screaming or crying; I swallowed all my feelings. All of the anger, all of the sadness, consumed in massive quantities, added to the overrunning quantities I had already had lost control of deep inside me, spreading like cancer, infecting every part of my body, mind and soul. From then on, I no longer felt ambivalent: I wanted to die. Full stop. However, I was so down that I couldn't really put a plan together. I continued to overdose with greater and greater amounts. I continued to cut and bloodlet, with death being my aim. But I didn't seem immediately able to put a "good" plan into action. I wrote in my diary:

"I am so tired.
But when I lie down I do not sleep.
I just hear my heart.
Lub dub, lub dub.
Fast.
Heavy.
Tired.
I have no strength.
I don't believe what I have done.
I don't believe what I am doing.
I am tired.
Alone.

In the end we are all alone.
I am lost.
Lost.
Lost?
This is not a fucking poem."

So what did I do? Well, after I had put up bulletins on several walls of the hospital saying "OXFORD CAN FUCK OFF." I started to overdose on zolpidem, zopiclone and any central nervous system (CNS) depressants that I could get my hands on. This was an expensive adventure. I would often take twenty, thirty, forty, fifty, a hundred pills or more, sometimes I'd take every pill I had in the room, which would be two hundred at *minimum*. I seriously wanted to die, expected to die, but didn't know for certain if I would die. I knew the cumulative affect of the medication was dangerous, as was the ever-increasing dosage. I wished for death. On occasions I took 500-1000 pills, a mixture of sedatives, always with alcohol to increase the chances of death. I really should have died, but I didn't. My whole mind was so clouded and muddled by depression that I was not thinking or acting clearly.

Please heed my warning that *no overdose is ever safe;* most people would die if they copied my example: please don't. Nor have I escaped from that behaviour without a heavy penalty. I expected to die in 2002, but now that I want to live, I am told my liver is already in retirement, waiting to fail. Eventually I will pay the highest ultimate price for those muddled, clouded suicide attempts.

I never had any money of course, as I was in debt and everything I had went on sleeping pills and regurgitated smoked salmon. Pills arrived weekly, with two or three packages always on the way. Some arrive in a week, but they cost more. Planning ahead saved money. Even at massive doses at night, I would be up early in the morning. The comments in my medical notes are conflicting:

> *"Katy seems drugged up." "Katy is bright and fresh."*

I was still allowed to leave the ward to cycle, although I had to be more specific about what I would be doing and when I would be back. I had to state clearly that I would not self-harm or put myself in danger – but of course, I lied. A "no sharps rule" was implemented, whereby I was supposed to keep myself safe on the ward by not bringing scalpels or needles in to hurt myself with. This worked on a trust basis, and I was supposed to hand in anything dangerous to staff. It was prohibited at all times for any patient to have a razor, glass, a knife or anything sharp: but this was supposed to help me by setting boundaries and reinforcing rules. Of course being the sod that I am, I thought of a way of bending that rule.

One day, whilst home from the ward, I put a venflon into my cephalic vein. A venflon (catheter) is a plastic tube that has a needle within it, and which is used to insert the plastic tube into a vein, and then the needle can be removed, leaving behind the tubing *but no sharps*. I secured it, and kept it flushed to prevent clogs, using tap water, since I had no sterile water/saline. (Mmm – now there's a "good" idea for you *not* to copy). I then kept going, all afternoon to let out a little blood, flushed the venflon, put the cap back on, watch TV, then let some more blood out. I prided myself at my skill, and being able to pour blood down the sink whenever I felt like it. When I was called for night meds shortly after 10pm I didn't go; I just stared at the TV without really watching it. Then a guy, a night assistant, not a nurse, came over to see how I was. I showed him my arm. I cannot explain my actions: that's just what happened.

Nothing big happened. The duty psychiatrist was called, and it was none other than my favourite SHO, who was probably decidedly pissed off with my shenanigans, not helped by the fact it was nearly 1am. Then, one nursing assistant stood outside, and three male nurses surrounded me, together with the SHO, in the tiny treatment room. That meant I could hardly move an inch with five strong men crowding me – which I think was intentional pressurization? It *was* intimidating. I expected them to just hold down my arm and take it out: which I could have coped with. But instead, my favourite SHO told me to take it out myself. I said "No." How polite of me; and very brave, very ill, or very stupid depending on your point of view.

He then said, "If you don't remove it you are not behaving in way that is compatible to inpatient treatment: remove it." *"He's a clever one, threatening me with discharge,"* I thought. *"Well go ahead my friend because I don't give a shit anymore."* So I replied "No. I'll leave it until morning; I'd prefer to leave it until then." I moved as to walk away and the bodies blocked my way. He said it had to be removed, "Immediately." So, as I knew it was a battle I couldn't win, in an arrogant, misunderstood, pissed off fashion: I yanked it out, pushed my thumb over the hole, and walked off, leaving five members of staff all staring after me like I was deranged... I suppose they had a point!

The sum of this event was that due to my own behaviour (which I accept as unacceptable) I was left feeling like a complete idiot, not worthy of attention, just to be spoken down to as a child. I assume they were trying-not-to-reward me by treating my self-imposed form of danger. However making a suicidal patient hate herself even more is hardly good patient care. Medical professionals really should learn how terrible people who self-harm feel when they are condescended to and/or bullied.

They then told me to go to bed, but I refused citing insomnia as my reason. I wished that they would give me something to knock me out, but no such luck. And so I tested boundaries: seeing if they could make me feel safe. The SHO's orders were that I not leave the ward, so that was the first thing I went to do. To my amazement, the nurse assistant came over and said to me that he strongly recommended I did no try and leave the ward. I asked, "Why not?" His response was that the doctor had "recommended" that I remain on the ward; and so, in my pyjamas, I opened the door and left.

I was testing them, desperately wanting to feel safe. No one restrained me, and there was no threat or imposition of a Mental Health Act Section. I spent some time wandering around the rest of the Warneford hospital; there is not much to see. I went from door to door, seeing if any were unlocked, and found two that were. I nearly left, but even I recognised that would be taking things too far; and anyway, I was in pyjamas with bare feet. I was not thinking at all clearly.

Surely I am not the first patient to test boundaries to feel safe; and surely when a patient does do this, people realise that that person needs reassurance and clear boundaries. Many patients are totally perplexed by the inconsistencies in mental health treatment. One minute someone has to watch you pee, the next you are free to go. Often decisions are made that seem to make no sense, and certainly there seemed no constancy, no common sense.

I walked back onto Vaughan Thomas ward, ignored the nursing assistant, and went to my room. That was at 5am. Someone checked on me every 10 minutes, and I spent an hour writing in my diary: I wrote a lot of swear words. At 6am I had a shower and got dressed, and hovered around the main corridor waiting anxiously for the morning shift to arrive at 7am; waiting to be allowed out to cycle (…and self-harm). The notes from that night and morning do not mention that I had not slept (for nights in a row). They say:

> *"Patient was observed writing in her diary last night on all room checks."*

> Rich (who arrived at 7am) wrote, *"Cheerful and reactive to fellow patients."* Later he added, *"Tearful at times."*

Other notes from around the same period say:

> *"Flat mood."*

"Claimed she would never overdose as it's 'not my style.'"
[Ahem, that was not strictly true].

"Pleasant."

"Lethargic."

"Quiet."

"Minimal eye contact."

"Katy has gone to church with Caroline."
[I think he meant pub, not church].

"Subdued."

"Compliant."

"Katy slept well. Was observed sleeping from 23.30 to 00.30."

"Happy because Derby won yesterday."

Dr. Ogilvie wrote: *"Remains objectively low in mood."*

Rich told me: *"You are not cooperating with respect to self-harm."*

Another night I went to bed, stuck a new needle into a vein in my arm, and went to sleep allowing it to bleed down the side of the bed between me and the wall: I cannot explain my motive, I just did it. I have not counted it as a suicide attempt as I remember that I knew I would not die. I also thought nobody would see. Jean who was on staff that night spotted what I had done, I'm not sure how quickly, but it was within a couple of hours. The staff checked my blood pressure, and let me go back to sleep. They asked if I had more needles, and I lied. At this stage, people were treating me with a lot of trust, far more than was safe; but that was how things worked out at the time. Obviously it was nice to be trusted; but in my case, it was the wrong choice. But then again, there is only so much that staff can do. They can have a brief or detailed examination of your room, against your will, (even if you are a voluntary patient), but there is no way that they can work miracles or find everything. No one tossed my room that day, or indeed stopped me going out cycling the next morning.

Every night I would have people coming into my room and checking under the bed with flashlights to make sure I was not bloodletting. That's not greatly helpful for someone with insomnia, but I accept that *I* caused it to be necessary. A few times when it was a male nurse/assistant and not a regular member of staff that I knew, I was totally freaked out by suddenly having a man in my room, by my bed, under my bed, or basically anywhere near me. At first I thought I was hallucinating, then I thought I was about to be attacked. Thankfully the staff immediately took this into account, and made sure it was a female member of staff, or at least someone I knew like dear Harry, that came into my room at night.

There was a meeting about planning my care, which was originally supposed to be a discharge-planning meeting. However, it was decided that, "discharge would be premature." It was also decided that I would not be allowed to leave the ward so freely; my safety to leave would be assessed by the nurse in charge on a day-by-day basis and I was put back onto checks every 15 minutes. I thought, *"Screw you guys: I'm going home."* Straight after the meeting I cycled off, and fetched a load of needles from home. I didn't do anything with them; I just wanted them with me.

By this point I had really handed all responsibility for my safety over to the hospital but they had not taken it on board. They would tell me to be responsible for myself; and I would tell them that I could not be because more of me wanted to die than wanted to live. I could not (still cannot) understand how I could tell them what I did: *"I want to die, I will kill myself, I want to self-harm, I don't want to live, I am out of control, I need help, please stop me hurting myself;"* and yet be allowed to roam quite freely. I didn't want responsibility for my safety, because I knew that if I had it, I would die. Maybe the fact that I *did* want to die meant that I didn't explain my fears and desires for help well enough. So after I had been told they would "assess my safety to leave on a daily basis," I was grateful. I was also cantankerous, and put it to the test. As I was about to leave to cycle, I was asked if I would be safe. I replied, "No, I am going home to bloodlet." And they let me go…!

It's hard not to assume people think you are lying and worthless after a situation like that. It's also impossible to feel safe. I did go home and bloodlet: angry that I was not believed, but not attempting suicide. I carried on until I'd lost over a litre of blood. (Exceedingly dangerous, especially as I was regularly losing blood: *please* do not copy me). I then had to make it from my flat on Iffley Road, across south Oxford, up Divinity Road, which is very steep, and back to the Warneford. I decided not to bother, at which point I passed out. My phone woke me up. It was Vaughan Thomas wanting to know why I had been gone for so long. (My time out was limited at this point). I said I was fine and hung up. They called back and I ignored it, my heart was racing, my head swimming, then I passed out once again: I was in hypovolaemic shock from the blood loss.

Once again my phone woke me; it was late afternoon. This time it was John (the Hippie) and I liked John a great deal. He didn't take any crap from anyone, and that I respected. He asked me when I would be back on the ward, and I said I didn't know. He then told me in a matter of fact way (not threateningly) that I had to come back straight away or someone (i.e. the police) would have to fetch me, and I might find myself sectioned. Because it was John asking, and nothing to do with the possibility of being sectioned, I agreed to set off straight away. I warned John said I might take a little while because I felt ill and would have to walk.

I set off on my bike: Iffley Road, Cowley Road, Divinity Road. At the bottom of Divinity Road I passed out and fell off my bike. Had it happened a moment earlier I would probably have been crushed on the main Cowley Road. A couple of people kindly helped me up, and I laughed about losing my balance. They looked worried and asked me if I was OK: I looked pale (apparently). I smiled and said it had been a bit of a shock, and then set off up the hill, walking slowly, leaning on my bike for support.

Half way up the world was losing its focus and shapes flashed in front of my eyes. I stopped, sat on the garden wall of someone's house, and put my head between my legs. I don't know how long I sat there, but I knew I couldn't go on and couldn't think straight. Then the man on whose wall I had sat came out to see if I was OK. I told him I had to get to the Warneford but felt dizzy. And so, that kind stranger helped me up Divinity Road and right to the hospital door, carrying my bag, pushing my bike, and pulling me. I went straight to my room and passed out. I didn't tell anyone what had happened.

One night, the film Clockwork Orange was on, and the patients decided to watch it. I was having a bad day in general: hallucinating in a frightening way. I couldn't seem to make myself "real." What I mean by that is that I felt like I was floating from room to room, not-quite invisible, but not actually there in body. Everything was very colourful. I would reach out to steady myself, to touch someone or something, and I couldn't feel anything. I don't mean like a ghost, I could move objects and people could feel me: I just couldn't feel anything, as if all my nerves had shrivelled and died. And so I floated at the edge of the TV area whilst the film started and patients crowded around. I don't know how much of the film I saw. It felt like a minute, but could have been an hour. The images distressed me; though I am not certain that I actually saw was what was really there. I went to my room crying.

George was on duty that night. He saw me and stopped me to talk to me; I must have looked distressed (for a change). I told him that the film had upset me, but nothing about the hallucinations, and I told him I wanted to hurt myself. He told me I was safe on the ward, to which I replied that I wasn't. He asked me if I had any forbidden items and I told him that I had several needles. (I didn't mention the sleeping pills I had). George told me he would give me 15 minutes to go and collect them and hand them over to him.

I went straight back to my room, found the biggest needle I had, used my dressing gown belt as a tourniquet, and stuck it straight into a large vein, allowing the blood to collect in a plastic jug and the floor. I was very low on blood reserves before I started; and I promptly passed out. The next thing I remember was waking up in the treatment room with blood all over me, the duty doctor had been to see me, and I was put to bed. My room was searched, although I did not find that out until I saw my medical notes. It must have been a superficial search because all they took were the needles that were obvious. They didn't even spot the bottle of wine on my windowsill.

The thing with hiding items in hospital is spread things out, be original, be creative, and be prepared to lose everything. I say that because I am going to reveal all my secrets, with the hope that people will read this and keep others safe. Of course, I could be giving people ideas... Posters are excellent for taping razors, needles, strips of medication behind – anything flat and light. Draws in cabinets tend to have spaces behind them for anything; wardrobes on wheels almost never get looked under. The bin is a great place to hide almost anything, either under rubbish, or under the plastic bin liner filled with rubbish. Beds tend to be checked, but small items can be hidden in cloth. I had a bottle of vitamins that had substances that were *not* vitamins within it. I had bottles of coke that had vodka in them. Larger items such as bottles of booze are harder – I wrapped several up as Christmas presents. That got me through one search, but a later search resulted in them all being confiscated. On your windowsill can be good, as can in the cistern of a toilet; but with caution in case another patient finds it. Hiding things on your body usually works, in pockets, sock, or your bra (gentlemen). My all time favourite hiding place was my Rammie teddy – who has now gone to teddy bear heaven. He was really a furry hot water bottle holder, but trust me when I say, it was never a hot water bottle inside. I got away with that one until very near the end.

At 5am I got up, George was still on duty and he informed me I was ward-based. That meant I was not allowed to leave the ward, and if I tried to, I was to be detained and sectioned, and if I left without permission, they would AWOL me, thus involving the police to bring me back to hospital. (AWOL = Absent With Out Leave). They checked my haemoglobin and it was 6g/dl; a blood transfusion was advised but I refused it.

Ray was working the next morning – and I tested the boundaries to see what would happen if I tried to leave. At first I tried to walk out, but Ray ran around me and blocked the exit. He was angry that I was following the path he predicted back in June, when I was admitted (i.e. I was getting more ill in hospital, not better). He reminded me that he told me not to get comfortable; and said that now I was well and truly institutionalised. He said if I tried to hurt myself I would be sectioned. I was truly saddened that I had let Ray down, and that made me angry with myself. Anger meant I had to hurt myself, because I didn't want to be an angry person and because my emotions were so *intense*: it made me realise how similar I am to my dad when he lost his temper – except my anger felt so extreme I don't think it possible to be more angry. I didn't want to be like that.

"For we are the same that our fathers have
been;
We see the same sights that our fathers
have seen;
We drink the same stream, we feel the
same sun,
And run the same course that our fathers
have run.

      ∂ William Knox, Scotsman (1789-1825).
From the poem entitled *Mortality.*

My anger was bubbling away under the surface that people saw, and I was afraid of my anger. *In my mind*, my dad got angry, not me. If I did not show the anger, I fitted his stoic philosophy; if I was angry, I was weak or cruel – and a disappointment to him. I couldn't win. My anger was extreme – dysphoric mania – more angry than words can describe. And so what did I do with my anger, trapped on Vaughan Thomas with no way to express it? Well, I took out a screwdriver that I had in my rucksack for bike-maintenance; and I used it to start unscrewing my bedroom window to get the hell out of there. I was on the ground floor, and the windows were safety windows; but with a screwdriver... Three nurses landed on top of me as I tried to get away. That was interesting; and a terrible relief, because it meant that I was safe. Ray told me that if I did ANYTHING else I would be sectioned and put on one-to-one level observations. I believed him: and that made me feel safe.

∂

After a while, I was allowed to go out again in a time-limited fashion. I was supposed to go cycling and nowhere else. Of course, I was unable to do as I was told: and soon would be found on the Internet ordering more zolpidem, cutting my thighs and suturing them myself, and bloodletting. I also brought fresh supplies back to the ward. Rich was working nights, and I was pleased because I hated nights the most because they were so lonely. The only advantage was that if you seek help from staff at night, there is usually more time available for staff to spend with a patient as most people are asleep.

It was another floating night. I hadn't slept for 4 days and nights, and wandered around the empty TV area and smoking room that seemed too large with no one else there. All the furniture would float, the doors moved, and lines of the hospital corridors wobbled. I'd flop on one sofa by the TV, curl myself up and lie still until I could bear it no longer. Then I'd move somewhere else, probably to have yet another cigarette. I'd sit there, motionless, trying not to look over my shoulder, scared of what would be there. Nights were broken up with speaking to other people; company brought me slap back into reality. Rich and I spent hours talking and smoking, but I can't remember a word we said. From looking in my diary I am reminded of what happened one night.

I sat at one of the dining room tables late into the night. I was extremely rare for me to sit in the dining area, but it just seemed like the right place at the time. It meant I could see into the main corridor where some of the staff were standing guard. I had previously denied ownership of any dangerous items; telling myself it wasn't a lie because it depended on the definition of "dangerous," and I could think of some pretty radical definitions. (Compare a needle to the danger of an armed thermonuclear device: and the needle isn't that dangerous).

I must have been sitting there for a long time, not moving, a green needle (not very big, but the biggest I had left), palmed in my hand. I remember that I was trying to stop myself from self-harming, trying to make myself hand over the stupid bit of metal. Rich came over to see how I was; and I don't know why, but I whipped the needle out and told him I wanted to self-harm. It was a sterile needle, opened right in front of him. He reached to take it; but I wasn't offering it, and I moved backward. The result was that Rich stabbed himself/was stabbed by me with the needle. It was not intentional. He ran off.

I blamed myself for him being stuck by the needle. True, it was an accident; but I deserved and took the ultimate responsibility. I knew it was a clean needle, but needle-sticks are obviously the sort of thing medical professionals want to avoid. Consumed with guilt, I proceeded to stick the same (no longer sterile) needle into my arm, and begun to bloodlet: at least, until the nurses restrained me. If I'd had a gun or knife I would have used it on myself. The notes from that night record those events as I have just described, and detail my not-so-high quality/quantity of sleep:

> *"Katy went to bed at 5am." "Katy was up at 6am."*

The first serious, coherent suicide plan that came together was a suicide pact with Caroline. We had dreams of just running away together; we wanted to disappear. My plan, which we called most originally called "Plan A," was to just leave the hospital, go back to my new flat, and get pissed. "Plan B" is something that I cannot describe as either of our inventions, it was a 50:50 suicide plan. The mechanics of the plan were Caroline's creation: she'd stored up amitriptyline, enough to kill us both, and we would go somewhere together to do that. We talked about going to my flat or her house, but thought we'd get caught. Caroline was very insistent that we have enough time to die so that we did not get rescued and end up brain damaged. I was in full agreement. We thought about going to The Bear in Woodstock; then we planned to go abroad and do it there, where Caroline's family have a Summer home. I made sure I had my passport; ready to go whenever Caroline decided the time was right. The amitriptyline sat in her car on the road outside the hospital, so that we were ready to go.

I did not want Caroline to die, or ever to pressure Caroline into anything; and she, I know, would never want to hurt or pressurise me. It was not a case of either of us leading the other: we simply shared a common goal. But I sat there thinking to myself, *"how can this beautiful, intelligent, amazing, fantastic person die. It would be such a waste. She is far too good to die, far too valuable."* We both understood something that only a person who has suffered and been ill enough to want to die can understand: life alone was of no value; it was quality of life that counted. So whilst we were both very aware people who cared for and valued other people highly, we were (are) also people who understand that sometimes, valuing someone means letting them go.

Somehow, I don't know how, Dr. Ogilvie got to hear that there was some kind of pact. He came to the ward to see us both – separately. Caroline and I had already agreed to not answer any questions on the subject; and to avoid sectioning, not give any details that could be used in order to section us. We agreed to say, "I'm not prepared to discuss it." Caroline went in first (as always). She came out and I was whisked in, without the chance to talk to her. I don't actually remember the conversation I had with Dr. Ogilvie that well. I do remember that I was very, very scared; Dr. Ogilvie seemed very, very big; and also rather pissed off. I didn't know what Caroline said to him, or whether she stuck to the agreed response, "I'm not prepared to discuss it."

I do know that I let one thing slip. I told Dr. Ogilvie that I thought Caroline was the most amazing person, and that theoretically speaking; her suicide would be a terrible loss to the world. I also told him I was frightened for her, frightened that she was not competent to make the decision to end her life. Of course, I didn't care or question whether *I* was similarly competent – I wasn't competent, but the fact I worried about Caroline made me look more competent than I actually was. To me, it then seemed as if Dr. Ogilvie was personally very angry with me, although I do not know how objectively I recall this event. Perhaps the anger that I perceived in him was anger that I felt at myself? I felt like he totally blamed me, and Caroline was the victim. I thought he felt that I was leading Caroline astray; that the whole thing was my fault, and that I was *so low* as to risk her life, just to get what I wanted. I thought he meant I was unimportant, but

Caroline (as a person and a medical doctor) was important.

Those feelings of perceived anger, rejection and unimportance from Dr. Ogilvie due to the suicide pact stayed with me for years. It probably would not have hurt me so much had I not cared what Dr. Ogilvie though of me. The idea of myself preying without conscience on other patients, of even being judged capable of such disregard for others tortured me. Our pact was not one-sided, it really wasn't. Caroline and I were good friends, intelligent, depressed women, with a common aim, shared understandings regarding dignity and quality of life, no peer pressure was involved, and neither of us were competent.

Being completely honest, at the time I did not think I would ever have been able to go through with our suicide pact because I loved Caroline too much. I simply could not have watched her die; I cared too much for that to happen.

So for entering a suicide pact with a highly intelligent, young doctor and friend; who conceived the plan, had saved up the medication to use, fetched it, and stored it, *I* was to blame for everything, after expressing concern that Caroline was too good to die. It was "my fault" because she had never attempted suicide before, and *I* said that she was incompetent. Whether or not that was the intended message, that was the one I walked away with and simmered with self-hatred over. I felt like scum. I felt (note I felt, it was *not* what I was told) that Dr. Ogilvie wanted to help Caroline and found me disgusting. I found that hard to live with; who wouldn't?

In my medical notes I find an unambiguous and accurate description. With a clearer mind now, I note there was *no* actual assignment of blame. Dr. Ogilvie wrote:

> *"Katy couldn't gauge severity of suicidal intent. She appeared much more distressed about this ideation as it involved someone else's death. Mood remains objectively low. Katy expressed fear that Caroline is too ill to be objective about choosing to commit suicide. Loss of her Ph.D. is exacerbating her depressive state and dysfunctional personality traits."*

I think it was then that I started to notice a pattern. I started to notice that whenever I saw Dr. Ogilvie I would end up self-harming and attempting suicide more voraciously than "normal." I say this not as a criticism of him, but more as a compliment. I was an angry person, desperate to explode: Dr. Ogilvie undeservedly bore the brunt of my wrath, although most of it was contained within me. The truth of the matter was that when I saw Dr. Ogilvie, I told him a lot of painful "stuff." He became my confidant, I respected his insight, and I liked him. In my own way, I put him on a pedestal, a powerful pedestal. It was always hard to hear difficult truths from someone I liked (like) and whom I didn't want to think I was disgusting. (I do not mean he thought that I was disgusting, just that *I* feared it – in fact, I know for a fact that he did not think badly of me). I was a management nightmare: nobody knew what to do to help me, including me.

The notes about me at that time say:

"Tearful."   *"Low."*   *"Anxious."*
"Worried."

Dr. Ogilvie wrote that I needed to *"address past events and address current perceived rejection."*

"Katy went cycling as agreed but has not returned to the ward. She was contacted via her mobile phone and said she was at home and did not want to come back. Upon strong persuasion she was persuaded to return."

"Patient's zolpidem was doubled from 10mg nocte to 20mg nocte. Sleep improved. Patient slept from midnight until 1am." [Yeah: a really great improvement - not].

"Katy slept from 1am to 4am."

"Patient was given 20mg zolpidem with good effect. Went to sleep at 1am. Patient up at 2.30am." [Mmm – *sarcastically* good effect].

Rich told me that Dr. Ogilvie had me listed as an acute suicide risk. He also told me that if I didn't stop self-harming, I'd still be there in two years time. He told me that I was "pushing help away." I wish I had cared, but it was impossible because I planned to be dead soon. But being a long-term patient was really beginning to become an established fact. Ironically I was no longer scared about being sent home because I was determined to die: and so I suppose it was for the best. I was asked to write about ways I thought the staff could help me. What I needed to say was "*Keep me safe by...*" All I could do was write this message:

I feel terrible that I am being offered help but not using it. That is a pattern that repeats itself over and over in my life. I don't expect help and I certainly don't deserve it. I didn't realise I was "pushing help away."

I feel I can't work out how to communicate how badly I feel without self-harming. You all say, "Don't self-harm just come and tell us when you feel bad and we will support you." Then you don't hold up your end of the bargain.

I will hate myself for saying this, but you really shouldn't let me leave the ward so easily.

Understand that sometimes I don't even realise that my behaviour is less than ideal/dangerous/unhelpful/mad. Unless you point it out to me, I don't know it.

I am verbally impotent; self-harm is my means of expression. I deserve punishment for losing my D.Phil., for endangering Caroline, for not getting into medical school when I was 18, for eating instead of starving, for being 27 and wasting so much of my life, for being a fucking disaster, being unemployed now, forever unmarriable, for not being perfect, nowhere near perfect in fact. That's without even going near childhood events...

I just want to go self-destruct.

This is bollocks. It is impossible.

There is still lower to sink, and far, far worse to come.

Chapter 10. So I Died with Galloping Horses in my ears: $C_{21}H_{23}NO_5$

"There is in this (melancholic) humour, the very seeds of fire. In the day-time they are affrighted still by some terrible object, and torn in pieces with suspicion, fear, sorrow, discontents, cares, shame, anguish, etc., as so many wild horses, that they cannot be quiet an hour, a minute of time, but even against their wills they are intent, and still thinking of it, they cannot forget it, it grinds their soul day and night, they are perpetually tormented.

In the midst of these squalid, ugly, and such irksome days, they seek at last, finding no comfort, no remedy in this wretched life, to be eased of all by death, to be their own butchers, and execute themselves."

❧ Excerpt from *The Anatomy of Melancholy* by Robert Burton.
(1577–1640). Clergyman and scholar.
Born in Leicestershire, educated at Oxford.

(Warning: this chapter contains explicit details of suicide).

One day in 1999, I left the same region of England; bound, I thought, for greatness at Oxford, so this quote fits this particular chapter, in which I effectively died. Though my feet were planted firmly in Oxford soil, I was running from two things: academic "failure" at

Oxford and allowing oxygen to reach my brain. The best way I can describe it is that I died with horses galloping in my ears. This unequivocal attempt at suicide was executed with no hesitation, no ambivalence, and a high chance of lethality. The usual overdoses and bloodthirsty self-harm continued too, at an elevated level.

Written in 1621, the above quote describes perfectly, how after a long period of illness, such as depressive illness, it is possible to reach breaking point, and therefore choose death. Everyone has a breaking point, no matter how much they do not want to hurt those left behind. In my case I was well beyond that point, which meant putting into practice plans I already had prepared, with as much determination, dedication and precision that I could muster.

At the beginning of November, Ray (charge nurse) came back to Oxford after a long trip back home to Trinidad. I was glad to have him back because he always made me feel safe. Rich was good, we laughed, he was supportive, he often kept me safe; but Ray *always* kept me safe. Hippy John was fun, clever, and able to put positive thoughts inside my head; but Ray pinned me to the floor to keep me safe. At that time in my life, I needed all of those things, but on a basic level, before anything else, I needed to be kept safe. George also kept me safe. Well actually they all tried to keep me safe, but I made it difficult; Ray always kept me safe, and George usually kept me safe – neither afraid to search my room or restrain me. Other people had a more humanistic approach (which I admire and in an ideal world would have preferred), but I needed something simple like *"You will not go out. If you hurt yourself you will be placed on constant observations."* I had reduced myself to that level.

One evening, with Caroline for company, (both of us fairly shocked that we were still allowed out together) we went to church. This was obviously something very unusual for me – I have never been in a church other than at weddings or funerals. Caroline was going and I thought I'd give it a shot. Why not? I'd nothing left to lose. And so we went to St. Andrew's in North Oxford. I sat down. When the first hymn was sung, I stayed in my seat: I couldn't sing it. When the prayers were uttered and heads were bowed, I looked straight ahead, feeling nothing. When people took communion, I sat still throughout. When there was more singing, I sat there feeling a fraud and very much out of place. I left thinking: *"Well you can't say I didn't give it a chance. I felt nothing, there is nothing, I am secure in my beliefs, but that means I am alone with them too. It would be easier to have faith in something: comforting, warming, reassuring, but I can't make myself feel something that I don't."*

We got back to the ward, and John approached – I must have looked upset. I asked if I could talk to him because we had shared a number of philosophical debates about life, death, life-after-death and lack thereof, religion, illness, suicide... and much, much more. I think I actually cried. John had often told me that I did not really want to die. At the time I took this as a personal criticism and an indication that everyone thought I was lying about wanting to commit suicide: and so I felt I had to prove myself. However, despite elevated suicidal cutting/bloodletting and overdoses to "prove myself," I didn't actually tell anybody about the "proof."

That evening John explained clearly what he meant by describing me as ambivalent. I still struggled to understand. He pointed out that despite powerfully wishing for death, I had asked for help, and why did I remain a patient if I wanted to die? Why did I not just get on with it? He had a point with the first one – I did want help. I did want someone to find an alternative route from suicide for me; but no one else could do it. I remained a patient, frankly, because I didn't know what else to do, and because I liked the company of the other patients. Why did I not just get on with it? Well of course, I was getting on with it: overdosing, cutting, and bloodletting. It just hadn't worked yet (defying medical sense); and none of the staff knew about it. A better question would have been: why did I keep on testing boundaries and forcing them to clamp down harder and harder on my freedom? That, definitely, is one reason why I am alive today.

And so I found myself talking to John about my horrific experience in church. He knew I was an atheist, and was surprised to hear where I had been. I told him how I had hated it, how I felt nothing, how I felt so *empty*. I questioned why all those other people felt contentment and not me? I am not a bad person. Then I said to John, *looking him directly in the eyes and meaning every word of it,* "I *am* going to kill myself. Soon. Very soon." He looked at me and nodded sadly. I know he believed me; and that was a relief. Then he said to me, "Hold on." I must have looked puzzled. He said, "You know, when you feel really low, know that it will pass, so just grit your teeth [John gritted his teeth and clenched his fist], and HOLD ON."

Some patients had gone since I arrived, but there seemed to be a core few long-term patients: Ash, me,

Caroline, Wayne, Jean, and some people who must have spent 23 hours and 30 minutes of the day in their room, only coming down for medication and food. Stella had gone, Kevin had gone, Declan was back – in a body cast. One new patient was a guy called Tony (Anthony) Carrick: a manic depressive/alcoholic. We talked a lot and he was clever, attractive, confident and charming: more about him later.

There was a schizophrenic lady in her early fifties (I'm guessing), who had the room next to mine. Sometimes she would throw plates at people who weren't there. Once I sat with her to have a smoke, and she started having a conversation with me and three other people who weren't there. It's a bit hard to answer questions if you can't hear them. She wasn't getting any better, and then I noticed she was vomiting straight after meds. After a few weeks of supervised medication she was fine and went home. She soon came back again though; she didn't keep taking her prescribed medication.

There was another new guy who I am going to call Achilles. Achilles was a first-rate guitar player: sometimes confrontational but more usually puppy-soft, at least with me. And he was addicted to heroin. When I was a kid I thought drug users were stupid; but I'd long since realised that it is just an illness like any other – the drug is a form of self-medication. I started to spend quite a lot of time with Achilles, I wanted him to get well. I could see the sadness in his eyes and I wanted to protect him, although I was in no position to be able to that emotionally. He was on the heroin-substitute methadone; a substantial dose that he told me would kill me if I drank it. *"Oh, kill me would it? That sounds good,"* I thought. *"I can't get hold of any though."*

Dr. Ogilvie wanted to work with me to make me feel safer, so if I felt like self-harming I would be strictly ward-based, i.e. prevented from leaving by force, but congratulated for my honesty. If I didn't tell them I felt like self-harming and then self-harmed (at home or on the ward) I would be strictly ward-based for a longer period. If I self-harmed on the ward my room would be subject to a detailed search. (At least that's what they thought). Of course, this whole plan rested on me being honest. John shrewdly pointed out that I would either self-harm less or lie, and he was spot on with the latter: I lied.

A few days later I found myself ward-based after being unable to lie to direct questions from Rich:

"Why are you limping Katy?"

"Am I?"

"Yes – Is there something you should be telling me?"

"I don't think I'm limping Rich."

"Well you are Katy. Why? What have you done?"

"Maybe I twisted my ankle or something Rich."

"Or..."

"Maybe it's a bit stiff from all the cycling. It'll be fine."

"Or…"

"Really Rich, I'm fine. I just banged it I think."

"Or…"

"Or… [Under my breath with anger and sarcasm] *maybe I sliced open my thigh, tapped out 'Fur Elise' on my femur, then stitched it back together myself, and now it hurts **just a little**."*

I sat down on one of the hall chairs waiting to have my leg checked, and pulled a glum face as I was told I was ward-based until further notice. I dropped my head and slumped in the chair; Rich pulled up my head and pushed back my shoulders. We talked, but I can't remember what about. I was probably trying to convince him to let me out as soon as possible. Then Achilles got back to the ward and I went to smoke with him in the smoking room. He was on the wacky-baccy and gave me some. It was the best I ever tried in my life. Ash was extremely upset when he saw that I had cut my own leg; he threw a chair through a window and caused a great deal of mess – and trouble for himself. That made me feel really guilty, and rightly so.

By this time Achilles knew I was basically in hospital for being suicidal. He told me he had tried to kill himself many times with a heroin overdose; then explained it was hard for him to OD because he was a regular user. He told me it would be "easy" for me because I had no tolerance. This sparked through my brain: what a great idea, what better way could there possibly be than going out feeling high and then unconscious? I asked Achilles what it felt like when he took heroin and OD'd on it: he told me that it was "beautiful." So I asked him to get me some heroin, and he did.

A few days later we sat down together in the dining area so that he could give me step-by-step instructions on how to cook heroin in order to prepare it for injection. I am looking at that page in my diary right now; it is rather frightening. (And obviously *not* going to be reproduced here). The title is "Heroin Overdose Instructions," and it has a skull and crossbones drawn underneath, in nail polish, and no, I don't know why I drew it in nail polish. The next page in my diary is a list of things to do before I die, so many uncompleted.

As it happened, Rich and Ray were working nights that week. As usual I would swan around Vaughan Thomas at night, whilst my compatriots slept. Sometimes I wore a tiara – gaining me the pet name "Princess" or "Princess Vaughan Thomas." Hey, if you are labelled as mad you might as well do mad things! This insomnia was despite the fact I took regular, secret overdoses of zolpidem – only "small" (under 50) ones because I didn't have much. Rich would often join me in the smoking room since he was also a smoker, and we were supposed to be working on ways to help me get back in control: it made sense to use the night hours whilst all was quiet. One night I was groggy from the zolpidem, and in the same way that people say things they regret when they are drunk, I said something about planning to OD on heroin. Consciously I did not want anyone to know my plan, and have no idea why I said what I did.

Suddenly I was being marched to my bedroom, and told to hand over the drug. I refused, and they started ripping my room up. The heroin was safe in my furry Derby County hot water bottle Rammie, which they missed, but something told me they weren't going to stop until they had found it. I had to be present in my room whilst they searched, so I sat on my bed and cuddled Rammie. When I thought they weren't looking, I sneaked the heroin out from him, so as not to lose my hiding place. Then I made a run for it...

I didn't get far. Ray and Rich were far stronger than I was – just one of them was stronger than I was. Planning to flush it away, (not even sure that it was heroin, because I never opened the packet), I said, "Look I just want to go to the loo. OK?" But obviously it was *not* OK. Ray told me to hand it over. I didn't move. Then Ray said, "Look, if you cooperate and hand it over 'voluntarily' it will look a lot better for you." I thought, *"Look better to whom? What's he on about? Who gives a flying fuck?"* But I saw there was no way other than "cooperation."

The ward policy was to call the police if someone is caught in possession of drugs. I can honestly say that it never once crossed my mind that I was in possession of a Class A drug, for which I could get a criminal record, or maybe even go to prison for 7 years. I really did not comprehend that anything was wrong about my actions. That may seem unbelievable, but it is the truth. Unfortunately the police did not see it that way initially.

You've all seen it on TV or in films: when police play "good cop, bad cop" when interviewing the "evil" criminal. Well, it was kind of like that, except they played "bad cop" and "very bad cop."

Without any warning, totally uncomprehending of why the police were asking to speak to me, I was taken to a room on the ward to be interviewed. Because I was classed as a "vulnerable adult" I needed to have someone with me, and a strange social worker I did not know was given that job. She was asked if it was OK that she was with me, I replied that it was not, and said I needed someone who knew me. I was ignored. The social worker didn't ever say another word to me, nor support me, nor stop the police when they got heavy.

The very bad cop then shouted that they were going to question me about possessing heroin and that I was in serious trouble. She read me my rights. In my head things suddenly clicked and I thought: *"Holy fuck! Shit! Bugger! What? Fuck! What the fuck is happening? I don't get it? What? What? What? Prison? Possession of a Class A drugs? Lawyer?"* And so I responded in the way all the clever people do on CSI (Crime Scene Investigation) or various other cop shows I'd seen, *especially as I was guilty*: I said I needed a lawyer before speaking to them.

Bear in mind that I had hardly been able to walk from my bedroom to the interview room – a matter of perhaps 20 metres. I had only made it by leaning on a nurse. The very bad cop then made loud tutting sounds and scowled at me. She growled threateningly, "Well, OK. But if *you* say you want a lawyer then we are going to *arrest* you now and do this down at the station."

Now I don't know whether my description of this intimidation will inspire sympathy, or if people think I got what I deserved. I expect views will be mixed. The fact remained that I felt so physically ill, weak and depressed: I agreed to be interviewed on the ward, waiving my right to legal representation in a way I would never have done were I well. There was no way I could walk far, or mentally confront leaving the safety of the ward that day, certainly not in handcuffs and a fluffy dressing gown. *"Plus,"* I thought, *"I'll be dead soon, so it doesn't matter if they charge me: I'll be dead before it gets to court."*

The bad cop sat and took notes. The very bad cop talked/shouted at me. She held up a small polythene bag containing a syringe, a spoon, a lighter and the unopened packet of heroin that Achilles had given me. She asked me what it was. I replied, "That's my suicide kit." So then she asked me what each individual object was, and I said, "A syringe, a spoon, a lighter, a packet I was given." She asked me what was it a packet of? I replied, "I am not sure, I never looked in it." She then said, "We have it from the hospital records that you handed this over to the staff claiming it to be heroin." I said, "Well I say a lot of things after I take my night meds and don't really remember." She asked, "What do you believe the package to contain." And... ... I capitulated, "It might be heroin, but I'm not sure if it is, and my mind is very muddled; I'm ill, I don't really understand what is going on."

Then of course, they wanted to know where, who, why, when and how I had procured the said illegal substance. I told them that a friend gave it to me, I hadn't bought it or looked at it, and that I didn't know where or how he got it. "Ah, so it was from a man then," said very bad cop, pouncing on my words like I had stupidly admitted something. I said, "Yes, but you already know that because I know I admitted that much to my doctor, the nurses, and it will be in my notes." She looked pissed off. I decided further clever-dick behaviour would be highly stupid. They wanted to know "who." I refused to answer. Was he a patient? I refused to answer. It was suggested it would be helpful to my cause to cooperate. I refused to answer.

I was not about to get Achilles sent to prison with a life-sentence for possession of heroin with intent to supply. What had happened was *my* responsibility and he was trying to claw his life back together. He was depressed and suicidal himself; you know, there are good reasons why people turn to drugs in the first place. (Although it has been said to me that him helping me showed him to have questionable morals – I know he understood the desire to die). Without my testimony they could not do anything about it, even though every single member of the hospital staff knew exactly how I got it. Both cops looked pissed off. Achilles was moved to another ward, and was not allowed onto Vaughan Thomas even to visit. But of course, we both had a mobile phone.

Bad cop scribbled away and very bad cop continued to glare. I was informed that the package would be taken away for analysis, and if it turned out to be heroin I might very well end up in prison. *"But I didn't understand what I was doing,"* I thought: *"I'm ill, really ill. This is my first offence. Bloody hell Katy, that's one heck of a first offence to pick, let alone get caught for. You stupid cow! It is heroin. Flipping typical."*

I realised that there was absolutely no way I could ever deny that I did possess that package; however I suspect I could have pleaded insanity. Fortunately they took it no further, although I did not find out I was "off the hook" until mid-2004 when I read in my medical notes that the police had phoned the ward to inform us they would not press charges only shortly after that interview. I still cannot believe I was left to worry, not informed that I had been declared unfit to be charged – I asked regularly if there was any information. It was obviously an added stress factor. One person took the call from the police, and then it got missed in the volume of my notes – Still, that is unacceptable. The fact that I was looking at up to 7 years in prison only gave me one more reason to kill myself. It also meant that with my ill mind, and no logic, I thought: *"Fuck it! Who cares anymore if I get some more heroin to try again? I've well and truly screwed up my medical career when anyone hears that I possessed heroin. Fuck it. Fuck you all."*

Of course it was some time before I was allowed to leave the ward again. Clare helped out by bringing me some food that I was prepared to eat, and shared her invaluable company. I didn't help myself by abusing Rich's trust when he allowed me into the nurses' office to use the computer to "check my email." He caught me on the "thank you for your purchase" page, just after I'd ordered some more zolpidem – although I still denied having ever taken it as a suicide attempt. I had it sent to my pigeon-hole at Linacre College because otherwise Clare (who lived in the same house as me on Iffley Road) would have intercepted the pills.

Eventually I was allowed out to cycle – but I wasn't supposed to do anything else. I wasn't allowed to go home in case I self-harmed (cut/bloodlet) or used my computer to buy pills. I wasn't supposed to go to into town because I could buy needles or various self-harm paraphernalia. I agreed to these rules, and bent, rather than broke them. I went to an Internet café on Cowley Road to buy zolpidem. I went to Boots on Cowley Road to get needles. I also bought booze – which I was not supposed to bring back to the ward, but did. I had to have it because I wasn't "allowed" it!

Almost immediately Achilles and I met up outside the hospital in order to buy heroin. He wanted us to kill ourselves together, I explained I wanted to do it alone, but obviously I needed his help to get the heroin, and I promised not to warn anyone of his own suicide plans. Before I left the ward that day, John stopped me and asked if I would be OK. I replied honestly and said that I wasn't really sure. I said I did not intend to hurt myself in any way, but I asked him to call me on my mobile in an hour to make sure. I soon regretted asking him to do that.

John first called me as Achilles and I walked towards the Westgate Centre to meet the heroin dealer just behind it. Achilles was using my mobile phone to call the dealer, so I had to get rid of John quickly. I said I was fine, and John asked how long it would take for me to get back. I said, "Perhaps an hour?" He commanded, "No longer." An hour later and I was sat in my flat on Iffley Road, with Achilles, drinking wine whilst he cooked up heroin for us both – to try, *not* OD on. I was well aware of the dangers of street heroin and its impurities, the risk of an OD or poisoning, and that injecting it was the most dangerous way to take it for a variety of reasons. Did I proceed cautiously and snort it the first time? (Not that I recommend that either). Did I try smoking it? What about chasing the dragon? Nah, that was for pussies who actually cared if they lived or died.

Yes, straight to an intravenous injection of heroin – probably the drug most people fear more than any other. John called just after I'd injected a substantial dose. I felt really ill: all shaky, sick, dizzy, the world was swimming away from me, I couldn't focus – in a similar way to some of my non-drug-induced hallucinations of the previous year. I wondered why on earth anybody took heroin! Then Achilles told me the first time you take it, it can make you feel ill.

We both lay on the floor for a bit and I dropped my phone unanswered because I couldn't coordinate my body. We had bought £100 worth of heroin, in 5 little balls that looked so innocuous. £20 was to test it, and Achilles had most of that. Then I had one £20 ball; he took the rest. That was supposed to be enough for each of us to OD, alone if I had my way, together if he had his. But I didn't want to get into a suicide pact ever again – I always intended to go alone.

John called again. I put on my best happy voice and said I was fine, I was at my flat and really feeling fine, no need to worry. John didn't buy my lie for a moment, and told me to get straight back to Vaughan Thomas. Time seemed to have gone by really quickly; it was suddenly 8pm and John asked me to get back in time for him to see me before the end of his shift at 9pm. I just made it. I couldn't really walk, so had to call a taxi, which all took time.

As it happens, John was busy, which meant I didn't see him. If I had, I have no doubt whatsoever that he would have known at a glance that I had taken heroin. George was on duty that night, a recent convert from general nursing, and whilst he was concerned, he didn't spot the tell-tail signs. He wrote in my notes:

"Unsteady on her feet when returned to ward. Refused to have her rucksack checked but informed staff that she had no implements to self-harm. [Actually true].

Unable to collect thoughts, giddy, carotid pulse visible, query lorazepam taken recently? Duty doctor called."

I laughed when I read the "query lorazepam taken recently." I laughed a lot less when I read what the duty doctor wrote about me – a curt, junior doctor I had never met before. She put:

"Reviewed patient's notes. Impression of <u>severe personality disorder.</u>"

I've read my notes. The only mention of personality disorder prior to this entry was Dr. Ogilvie telling me I did *not* have one. Dr. Ogilvie had also written that losing my Ph.D. studentship had "exacerbated dysfunctional personality traits," which I cannot deny, but it is quite a leap to then diagnose a "*<u>severe personality disorder</u>*" before even meeting me. Maybe it came from a nurse's opinion that was voiced and not recorded?

Don't misinterpret me: people with personality disorders are not people I condemn or think badly of. I know some wonderful people with personality disorders. I just object to a whimsical diagnosis by someone who had never even met me. After her non-evidence-based "diagnosis" (that fortunately I was blissfully unaware of) she actually examined me. The notes say:

"Outwardly settled and appropriate. Willing to engage in conversation. Euthymic. Apsychotic. [Not psychotic] *The patient denies any ODs in the last 48 hours. Refused blood tests. Responding to cues. Adequate gesticulation. History strongly suggestible of a PD – borderline type?"*

Not depressed or manic? In fact I was *both*. Apsychotic? In fact I was psychotic. Where did the borderline personality disorder (BPD) come from? It was hardly a detailed history that she took – lasting maybe 5 minutes. My eyes were so pinned[25] you could spot it across a large room. But this was missed, as was the fresh puncture mark on my arm. Obviously I refused blood tests because I had just injected heroin…(!)

The following ward round, the events of the previous week were considered. I was not told I might have BPD, or that anyone had considered it. But I was ward-based and told if I tried to leave I would be detained under the Mental Health Act, which is as good as being sectioned without the paperwork. Dr. Ogilvie had also spotted that I often responded to the weekly ward round by finding ways to hurt myself even more, and therefore ordered that if I did anything harmful I was to be put onto one-to-one level observations – which he knew I hated and would avoid. I was ordered to have blood tests and told my room could and would be

---

[25] "Pinned" is a colloquial term to describe the main closing of the iris or the eye to result in pin-point looking pupils that occurs after taking heroin and some other drugs.

searched as often as the staff felt it appropriate. I considered trying to run there and then, but I did not.

Two days later I had another meeting with Dr. Ogilvie, and other people, but I only remember Rich. Unbeknownst to me, Achilles had phoned my ward and told them I had heroin at home that I intended to use to kill myself - it's entered in my notes. Dr. Ogilvie reminded me that I was going to be assessed by an expert regarding not having/having a personality disorder, as we had discussed many months ago. However at the time I remember feeling that his position seemed to have changed from that of thinking I did *not* have one, to him considering that I might. It says in my notes:

> *"Borderline personality disorder could be contributing to management problems."*

I was then told I would remain ward-based, and be sectioned if I tried to leave, for a minimum period of 2 weeks. It's then I have one of those really clear memories. I remember hearing Dr. Ogilvie's words, then switching off all sound entering my brain, and looking out of the window at the rippling leaves of the trees outside. Everything around me slowed down and I remember thinking that 2 weeks was an eternity. I felt as if the sentence of a personality disorder had been passed, and I moved (outwardly calmly) into "fuck-it" mode. I thought; *if I have a personality disorder, I'd rather be dead than carry on.* That afternoon I tried to leave the ward but I was prevented at an early stage (but not sectioned).

I didn't remember that Rich and I spent some time discussing BPD that afternoon, until I read his report in my notes. I do remember feeling that (for me) this extra label felt particularly hopeless. I challenged Rich on every single diagnostic criterion, except those describing a low mood – in other words, I had manic depression and we all knew that anyway. I told him BPD couldn't be diagnosed if another major illness such as depression or manic depression explained the depressive symptoms. I also explained that my self-harm was due to my depression, and that it was a mistake to diagnose anyone with BPD "just" because they self-harm. I then added that I had anorexia to further complicate things.

Remember that at the time I was very ill and hardly thinking with clarity. At that stage the only person I had met with BPD was also a psychopath - I feared they thought I was like her. It deeply insulted that they thought me promiscuous or that I had a lack of conscience, (just two of many possible BPD symptoms that I happened to remember at the time). *Nothing* **could be further from the truth about the person that I am.** Of course, without my knowledge, but evident in my medical notes, there were *lies* and overheard *lies* from male patients about me having various amounts of contact with them, *lies* about me dealing dope, *lies* about me being in suicide pacts and *lies* about teaching people how to self-harm or kill themselves. I dread to think that all those things were believed when they were so untrue. Was it not obvious from talking to me that I wasn't a bad person? And as for men and sex… It's not really my thing. I'm a bit naïve. (But when manic/mixed I seem to be out of control re this issue, at times).

Since that time I have met many people with BPD and count 2 amongst my close friends – Lin and Chris (who is recovered). I no longer see it as a hopeless illness and I no longer fear it. Indeed, People with BPD who come through it are the most amazing people you will ever meet. They have suffered more than is imaginable and yet they have survived. When they achieve wellness, they are well-placed to turn their experiences around and help others.

I spent the rest of the day keeping a low profile and being cooperative. Whilst I did that I got clear in my head, for once and for certain, that I wanted to die. The personality disorder business finally did it for me; it tipped the balance. I wanted death more than ever. In my diary I wrote:

> *"Dr. O thinks I may have borderline personality disorder. Fuck that. FUCK THAT. There's no hope now. He told me before I didn't have it. I've screwed up completely. Goodbye World."*

At 10pm, clad in pyjamas, all the patients slowly gathered to collect their night meds from the clinic room. I joined the line wearing trainers, socks, purple and black cycling shorts, my bright, luminous yellow cycling jacket, cycling gloves, detachable bike lights, keys (hidden in my pocket) and my purple cycling helmet, strapped securely in place on my head. I had a plan: though not such a good one as to think less obvious clothing might have been sensible. I stood tapping my feet impatiently. I said, "Hi," to Neil, the nurse handing out the meds, quickly downed the concoction, and then walked to the garden door to leave.

One of the night nurses asked me, "Princess, where are you going?" "Just for a quiet fag on the step, I can't face the smoking room," I replied, showing her my lighter and menthols. And she let me go... against Dr. Ogilvie's orders! Jean, another patient came with me to have a cigarette too – which I had not planned.

I immediately started getting onto my bike. I said to Jean, "Look I'm sorry to do this to you, but I didn't know you'd come outside. Please don't tell anyone I'm gone, hopefully they won't notice for ages." Jean nodded, and (amazingly) kept that promise. And that was how I found myself heading straight for my flat on Iffley Road at about 10.30pm on the 13th November 2002: the night I died.

When I arrived home I knew I had to get on with things immediately because at some point I would be missed. I locked and bolted my door, and was grateful that my home address was probably quite hard to find. I pushed my huge antique dressing table across the door – it was so heavy I could hardly move it. I looked for alcohol, but all I had was the bottle of Gordon's gin I kept for my sister's visits. I started to swig it neat from the bottle, expecting to hate it, but not actually tasting anything at all. I knelt in front of my tiny attic window, and began to prepare the entire £20 ball of heroin for injection.

Someone missed me: Tony. He called me on my mobile to ask were I was. I told him I was fine and to go away. He asked me if I was going to "do something stupid." I replied that I was fine, but that I was busy and couldn't talk. I hung up and ignored my phone. I filled a 5ml syringe with what I knew was a concentrated and lethal dose many times over, and, without pausing or hesitation, pushed the needle into a vein. There were no thoughts about upsetting people I left behind; I could not connect with the world or those I love. I just wanted all the thoughts in my head to stop. So, after checking I was in a vein, I started to push the murky brown heroin solution into my body. I thought I could hear the sound of horses galloping in the distance, quickly getting closer and closer.

I continued to force the lethal mixture into my vein, all of this taking less than 10 seconds. I felt a calm unlike ever before in my life, and pictured horses galloping in the English countryside through the pouring rain. At first they were far away, but their gambolling hooves became louder and louder. Perfectly serene, I waited for their smack against my skull, spilling my life force from within. Then everything went black...

...And I died.

Chapter. 11. Overcast: Winter in hospital, dancing with the devil once more.

"No green leaves in that forest, only black;
no branches straight and smooth, but
knotted, gnarled;
no fruits were there, but briars bearing
poison."

❧ Dante (1265 – 1321), *Dante's Inferno*,
Canto XIII, where the poet and Virgil
enter a forest where the trees are the souls
of suicides.

I had always hoped that the process of my death could be peaceful and poetic – despite having seen the reality. Death is never beautiful. When I was briefly conscious, I heard galloping horses; but once I was dying and dead there was no life-flashing-before-my-eyes, no bright-lights, no colours, no hallucinations, no memories, no friendly and welcoming voices, no bright tunnels, no angels to take me to heaven, and no devils to drag me to the depths of hell. Nothing. There wasn't even that slight sense of time passing, which you can feel when you sleep. One minute I was depressing the syringe plunger, the concentrated liquid with a brownish twinge entering my bloodstream, for a second I heard the galloping horses (blood pulsing in my ear), then blankness. Nothingness. Sweet oblivion.

The oblivion was *so* sweet that I would dream about it day and night for months – I still dream about it with some regularity, although it frightens me more these days. Whilst I accept that it may be true that as you die you "see" what you expect to see, my death reaffirmed my atheism. It made my previous doubts of no value. I know that death equals oblivion, and content in that knowledge, crossing the line between being alive or dead no longer holds any fear for me. I can cross it without even being particularly low-mood; and I will certainly cross it if depression re-enters my life with any force.

At about 4.30am, I woke up half naked in the John Radcliffe (JR) Hospital emergency ward; Clare was curled up beside me on the single hospital bed. Police were at my bedside asking for the keys to my flat so as to secure my home. I had no comprehension of what had transpired; initially I couldn't work out why or how I ended up in a hospital bed, I didn't even remember what I had done, but very quickly I felt shock and anger that I was still breathing. It was confusing and overwhelming: I knew I deserved to be dead, and that I was now living on borrowed time. I had to piece together the following description of events from that night from other peoples' accounts and my medical notes.

After I hung up on Tony, he had run back up the hill to the Warneford from wherever he was heading, straight to the Vaughan Thomas ward office and told them I had run away. I also know that *immediately* after I hung up on him, I injected the massive OD of heroin – which rendered me almost immediately unconscious and stopped my breathing. Until that point, nobody had missed me. I had foreseen the eventuality of escaping to my Iffley road flat, and, unappreciative of any intervention, had deliberately given minimal/confusing details of my address to the hospital. Even with a good knowledge of Oxford, it was not an easy place to find – there were twenty addresses within the property. My flat was hidden in the attic on the 4th floor, there was no way of climbing in through the high, tiny window; and the huge, shared house needed a security code just to get in.

By the time the alert was raised, the heroin had been working in my body for too long for me to be able to sit here writing these words – yet here I am. As I do not believe in God or Fate, I must presume my unconscious body fought for its life and I took a few shallow breaths during that time. *Usually just 5 minutes of oxygen starvation (anoxia) results in brain death.* Three minutes results in brain damage.

Tony later told me, "My guess is that it was just under five minutes for me to peg it back and alert the staff, and they responded PDQ." (<u>P</u>retty <u>D</u>amn <u>Q</u>uick). I don't, and won't ever know the response time that amalgamated from the time taken for the ward staff to mobilise, and then a response time for the ambulance and police – all heading for some obscure location on the charismatic but crammed Iffley road. They would have reached my (solid, wooden) door to find it locked, bolted and barricaded from within. The police took my whole door off by its hinges to get into my flat quickly: finding me all but dead.

The Vaughan Thomas night staff must have stressed to the police and ambulance service the jeopardy to my life. A response I did not expect, because I felt like I had been pushing people to take me seriously for many months – *without* effect. I didn't expect any interruption. The time between self-injection, to them responding and actually getting into my flat, could not have been less than 20 minutes, and no more than 30 minutes. Whichever: I should still be dead. I *should* have been *irrefutably dead* after less than 10 minutes; I *should* have *stayed* dead, and am lucky not to be brain damaged. When they found me, any breathing had long stopped: I was in arrest and blue in colour. But the paramedics still scooped and ran with me to the John Radcliffe (JR) Emergency Department. It was at this point, Clare saw exactly who was being carried into the ambulance outside our home, and climbed in with the dead-me.

Then I take note of a lie in my medical notes, but I suspect it was a "good" lie, used so that the hospital could send the police round to break into my home. I wonder who thought it up at the time? It states that the ward phoned me and I told them I had "done something." I am 100% positive I did not answer my phone to them, partly because I remember everything up to the injection, and mostly because I was *immediately* incapacitated by the heroin: therefore completely unable to answer my phone and claim… well… anything at all. This suicide attempt was unequivocal and deathly serious: I remember it all so clearly right down to the last detail – until the heroin went in, after which: I was unconscious, dying, then dead.

My favourite SHO was on duty in the Warneford that night – though I did not see him. He wrote a letter for the JR Emergency Department in which he stated that I had borderline personality disorder – again prior to any proper assessment for that disorder. The doctors at the JR had to maintain artificial respiration because I had been in respiratory arrest (I had stopped breathing). I had been given intravenous narcan (also known as naloxone), which blocks the action of opioids like heroin. It is used in the treatment of respiratory depression caused by overdose. Then, in time, I began to breathe on my own. I vaguely remember ripping out a drip (a narcan infusion) when I awoke. I was still hooked up to an ECG machine and it's very slow, "blip" noise, wearing just a pair of jeans. I had to ask for a gown because the JR staff had just dumped me on top of a bed, naked from the hips up, lying in an open ward. I guess I wasn't their favourite patient.

It was a life altering experience, one that removed my fear of the beyond, and something that (back then) I felt was beautiful and perfect. This, as I describe it to you, was not a rational response: it was intensely emotional and disturbed. It was as if I fell passionately in love with the idea/beauty/certainty/cleanliness of death by heroin. After all my suicide attempts I had finally found something that could remove life from my body; the relief I felt within was powerful and warped. Previously I had (grandiosely and disappointingly) felt immortal: eternity was a concept that scared the willies out of me.

I was *furious* that "they" had taken my "perfect" death away from me. It was *my right* to choose my own time to die. It had taken time, money, circumstance, effort and determination to go through with my plan, and I was *distraught* at its failure. They might have just succeeded in restoring the life to my body; but that had not restored any meaningful life to my mind.

All I could think about was when I would be able to do exactly the same thing again. Clare told that they had worked on me in the emergency "crash-room" (for critically ill patients) for a very long time, about 30 minutes, trying to restore life to my body. She told me that I had then sworn rather viscously at the hospital staff for reviving me. I don't remember doing that; it is very unusual to my normal character (but normal when dysphoric). I later sent them a card apologising.

Apparently I had kept saying, "I want to die," and "I'm dead." Not able to accept I was alive. I dreamed of the syringe with its murky contents entering my vein: a picture that would not leave my head.

There are an awful lot of "what ifs," about that night. What if Achilles hadn't warned the ward I had heroin at home? What if Dr. Ogilvie hadn't given the order to AWOL me immediately if I left the ward that I was not supposed to leave anyway? What if I had waited until I was allowed out to cycle, and done it then, when I was not going to be missed? What if Tony hadn't noticed my absence, or run to the alert the ward staff? What if he hadn't phoned me at all? What if the staff that night hadn't taken it seriously? What if the police and ambulance had been 30 seconds or a minute later? What if I had managed to inject the entire dose of heroin that I had prepared, instead of passing out with ¼ of the syringe left full? What if the ambulance staff had pronounced me dead? What if my Oxford-student neighbour hadn't heard the noise, and lent the police a screwdriver to removed my door from its hinges? What if the staff in the Emergency Department had given up?

The answer to all of the above is: neither this book, nor I would exist. I would be a statistic by now. Another heroin user found dead at home after an OD. Dust. For months and months all I could do was dream of this, my "perfect suicide," re-enacting it in my head, and desperately wanting to do it again. A large part of me still wishes that that overdose was how this (my) story ends.

Instead, there is more pain to come: the horror of surviving death, the pain of continued illness, further attempts, and the bittersweet sting of recovery and a compromised life. I'm sure recovery is brighter for most people: don't (as Dr. Ogilvie once said he did) "buy into my depressive nihilism too much." I have days when I am so glad to be alive, days when I grind my teeth with fear as to how close the end came.

The following day, two nurses were sent to fetch me back to Vaughan Thomas at the Warneford. I was to be on constant observations, but no mention of sectioning was made. They made me go in a wheelchair, which was not a bad decision because I was very unsteady. Whilst still quietly furious at people foiling my plan, I found one hope to cling to: I hoped that never again would the nurses be able to fuck-with-my-head and say [paraphrasing/summarising with how I heard it at the time] that I was *not* depressed, *not* ill, *not* normal, *not* worthy, *not* suicidal and *not* capable of taking my life.

My knowledge of my secret, repeated and serious bloodletting/sedative overdosing meant those words from staff hit me low – I had been attempting suicide seriously prior to this event – but I couldn't correct them without giving away what had really been going on. I couldn't explain that I had to *shut up the noise in my head*; the noise of a million TVs all on static at full volume: sounds, visions, thoughts and activity that I did not understand. I felt like a fraud and time-waster; I didn't want to admit to failing at suicide a couple of hundred times or more, what sort of medical professional would that make me? I was already furious enough with myself for surviving. *Intensely* angry with everyone and everything, but most especially, with myself.

It had not been easy to hide all of my previous suicide attempts. Hundreds of attempts at death had gone unrecorded; information I was burdened with, and yet unable to share out of fear. I couldn't hide the heroin overdose in the same way could I? *"But now,"* I thought: *"who would, who could be so <u>arrogant</u> as to argue that this nearly fatal suicide attempt was 'not serious.'"*

At the time I felt sick of feeling disbelieved; I assumed that would no longer be an issue. I had *never* said I wanted to be dead or die without meaning it – and yet I felt I was not believed by many nurses, or my death and suffering were unimportant: just another depressive, another job, difficult to manage, opinionated, a person who may or may not die. I projected my self-hatred onto every person who saw me. The notes say:

> *"Does not express remorse or regret for attempting suicide or for it failing."*

> [A nursing assistant I was very fond of wrote]. *"Katy is wearing her suicide attempt like a badge on her arm."*

> *"Katy doesn't trust people."* [Is it any wonder]?

I didn't express remorse or regret for attempting suicide because I had none. I didn't express regret at it failing (despite bitterly regretting the failure) because I wanted to get out of hospital as soon as possible. As soon as I realised I might get out quicker if I expressed regret, I lied. I started to say to people that I regretted this suicide attempt, that I was "lucky," but I didn't mean a word of it, not for years. If I wore my "suicide like a badge" it was because I felt hopeful that people would finally understand me better. But no, the staff seemed angry more than anything else. (Was that projected anger?) There was no empathy; there was not even pity.

"FORGODSSAKE. I wasn't pissing about here," I thought. *"I fucking died. I hurt inside. I fucking died. Died = dead, and I should have been left that way: at peace. I don't want to be here any more that you obviously don't want to have me here to deal with. So let me go. Just let me go. Please? Please? Easier lives for you without that reluctant responsibility to 'contain' me… And the ultimate emancipation for me. I just want to be dead; it's not much to ask. You're the ones that 'saved' me, and now YOU'RE ANGRY?"*

Clare (bless her) went home to sleep and to clear my room of any drug paraphernalia. It was not a request I made, it was something she told me she was going to do. I felt guilty: stress from me was something she could do without. I later learned that she took an opportunity to self-harm with equipment in my room – the old myth of injecting air into one's veins. She threw away my little bag of innocuous citric acid that was not illegal or dangerous on it's own. The hospital had asked the police to clear my room, but they refused, saying it was not part of their job – despite the presence of a class A drug. Apparently it's *not* illegal to possess heroin if it is in your bloodstream.

Other patients seemed to know what was going on – I assume that was because Jean saw me cycle off and Tony knew I had some smack (heroin) at home. All the patients knew I was suicidal and had disappeared. Then I reappeared, looking ill, with a nurse on each side of me. The facts were requested, I told them simply that I had tried to kill myself using heroin. A few people looked shocked, but my word was never questioned. No patient doubted my pain. Their response was warm, understanding, and someone said: "They stopped you then? Well, now you get to join the Vaughan Thomas suicide club properly." They were glad I had failed, but in a twisted way they were "proud" of me for getting so far. *"Nobody else here has actually died,"* they reminded me.

I didn't feel proud. I didn't speak to Caroline about what happened; she couldn't cope at the time. Ash shouted at me, upset that I had nearly died, and then hugged me, saying he was never going to let go. Tony was (rightly) proud of his part in saving my life, and curiously I never felt angry towards him. He had done what I would have done had our roles been reversed. There followed a long debate about situations where others had attempted suicide – there were similarities amongst feelings, but methods were wildly different, some reckless and dangerous. Of all the experiences I heard, nothing were like mine. Some made me think: *"Ooh, ouch, madness, holy fuck, you gotta be kidding, how on earth???"* For other stories I just thought: *"Well, that won't ever work."*

I stuck the ECG pads I removed from my chest into my diary; in a big lump meaning it will never close properly again. Underneath I wrote:

I DIED. I REALLY DIED.
...But I came back.
Now I must go again.
How boring.

Inside I was so relieved to have found a way to die, and to know that death was the end of everything. Everyone and everything ends. I have an end. I was waiting to find it again. Then came the obligatory assessment by Dr. Ogilvie: I don't remember it. In my mind was a picture of a syringe with the murky-brown solution entering my veins; the rest of the world happened only in shadows, which I could only half-see. I can remember that Dr. Ogilvie was concerned, straightforward and thankfully non-judgemental, but I don't remember anything we said. I don't even remember if I told him it was a suicide attempt: I didn't need to. All I have to go by are his notes in my file:

[Before I entered the room, and remembering that I had always denied any manic symptoms and had not divulged my hallucinations].

Assess major depressive disorder. Assess borderline traits.
Consider possible Axis 3 diagnosis.
[Physical illness].
Get urgent 2nd opinion from Dr. Pearce.

[Whilst I was in the room].

↑↑ VERY HIGH SUICIDE RISK. Could be from:

- *Impulsivity?*
- *Mania, dysphoric, mixed episode evident?* [This was actually what was mainly wrong]. *Atypical presentation, unclear.*
- *Major depressive disorder is present with severe anhedonia.*

344

- Eating disorder present.
- Stress (due to losing Ph.D., moving home, recent police interview, childhood – seems severe).
- Personality difficulties of borderline type? (Responsible for patient management problems)?

Patient's comments:

- "I did not phone ward to ask for help."
- "Clear intent of suicide."
- "I will do it again."
- "I absolutely do NOT give you permission to speak to my family."

Actions to be taken, patient fully aware of:

- Patient strictly ward-based, on 10-minute observations.
(Room has already been searched).
- Add risperidone [an antipsychotic] *for impulsivity up to 3mg nocte.*
- Urgent referral to Dr. Pearce, patient informed of this.
- If Katy attempts to leave she is to be restrained and put onto a section 5 until a section 3 can be arranged.

That time in my life is still a blur for me. I am amazed I was not described as psychotic, but perhaps my impassivity explains why not. All I remember clearly was that I was *intensely* furious. I didn't actually connect with anybody – even if they think I did. I don't think my anger was picked up on by patients, staff, friends or family. Caroline kept her distance, for which I did not (and do not) blame her. When we later discussed that time we agreed that I had completely "lost it." There was nothing of me, nothing of Katy Sara, *nothing*, in the shell that was my body.

Katy Sara's mind floated around, up on the ceiling or in the sky, skitting in and out of her body, sometimes nervously, sometimes in a dance-like motion, *always angry*. Her mind was not always present, at times she was numb and unaware, and remained so for considerable periods of time. She had no grip on reality, and no desire to get one: for doing that would mean accepting facts she did not wish to face. It meant being depressed and agitated; it meant brain-noise: not an attractive proposition. She kept going over and over the feeling of peace from when she injected the heroin, to try and calm the fire she was hiding inside herself. She thought about heroin a lot. Her body was on autopilot.

Two days after her near lethal OD the nurses recorded her as:

"Playful."

"Not depressed."

"Bright."

"Reactive."

"Flavour of slyness." [Thanks for that one Rich, false].

"Sarcastic." [And for that one Rich, but true].

Three days after the OD I made a half-hearted attempt to leave. I really don't remember it; I was thinking about heroin. Apparently Rich told me to turn around and I did. I was described as:

"Cold."

[Rich wrote]. *"Patient stated that she had proved she was serious about ending her life after the staff had told her she wouldn't kill herself. I asked if that was a verbatim quote. Katy said she was 'too tired to argue the finer points other than to say it was a fairly accurate quote, and more importantly, it was how the staff had made her feel.'"*

"Tearful."

"Playing games."

Four days after my OD I succeeded in escaping the ward by climbing out of the smoking room window (like Declan always did). If you ever see that window you'd be amazed. It is very high and very small, and I am nearly six foot, which meant big bones however thin I was. I did that to test if "they" would keep me safe, partly because I was angry, going stir-crazy, and also because I thought lividly: *"Fuck 'em."* I don't know if I was psychotic, but I do know that I came back to the ward quickly (unnoticed) because I felt so unsafe. I had proved my point – they had not kept me safe. I'm not quite sure to whom I was proving this.

Six days after my OD it was time for ward round again. Katy Sara was not really present in heart or mind, only body. I remember very little, just a vague calmness instilled by Dr. Ogilvie, which made me want to tell him the truth. The notes show I was honest and my thinking decidedly unbalanced – I say that because, what I admitted, was pretty stupid if you remember that my aim was to be allowed off the ward a.s.a.p. However, if you suppose that I was a person who wanted to be helped; then what I said wasn't stupid at all: it may have been an unconscious manoeuvre by myself. The notes say:

> - *Katy said she "now feels in control" because she has found "the <u>perfect</u>" way to kill herself and she "<u>knows</u>" she has the "strength to go through with it again."* [Dr. Ogilvie looked at me unblinkingly].

> - *Admitted that she only said she was "grateful" and "lucky to be alive" to make other people happy.* [Dr. Ogilvie: unblinking].

> - *Admits to strong suicidal ideation.* [Dr. Ogilvie: unblinking].

> - *Admits she has ripped all the stitches out of her leg because "they itched," and then admitted she was also "pissed off and angry."* [Dr. Ogilvie: unblinking].

[I said I was **ANGRY** – was anyone listening?]

- *Does not appear objectively low.* [Anger was the dominant emotion: which was not an improvement, it was just a change].

- *Reactive.* [Well not really: I was angry and very practiced at responding to people, no matter how shitty I felt. I have a very good autopilot].

Actions to be taken:

- *Remain ward-based (section 5 if attempts to or does leave).*
- *Increase risperidone to 6mg.*
- *Remain on 10-minute checks.*
- *Regular meetings for discussion of future with Dr. Steve Pearce.*
- *Staff to be made aware that Katy is more likely to abscond following ward round.*

Exactly as Dr. Ogilvie predicted I *did* try to leave. I wasn't deceitful but I was subversive: I tried to walk out of the ward's main door. I obviously didn't give much thought to it because I can vaguely recollect that I was not dressed properly. I think I had a T-shirt, my Derby County team shorts and a dressing gown on – with my Derby County team socks to keep my feet warm.

This bit I do remember. George was holding the door closed: using his strength to stop me from opening it.

But I wouldn't stop; I wouldn't go away. I nearly climbed up the door to use my entire weight to pull back on: to no purpose. I remember saying to George that he couldn't section me if I told him I wasn't going to hurt or kill myself. He corrected me, so I went away quietly.

By this point, I didn't believe they would ever section me because it had been threatened so many times with nothing happening. Even if they did section me, *I wasn't me*. Whoever I was, I didn't give a flying fuck if Katy Sara's body was sectioned, restrained, drugged, harmed or killed, whilst the real me was floating way above all of this, seemingly unable to affect anything, *screaming* and *shouting* so loud in *agony* and *anger:* without making a sound that anyone could hear.

One week after my death, I spoke to Rich telling him I was desperate to self-harm. There was insubordinate method in this, as I intended to *appear* cooperative. Sure enough, in my notes it says, *"more rational."* Oh what a manipulative management nightmare I was: how was I to be helped if I would not accept the help on offer? On the eighth day following my death I started to refuse my lithium claiming I felt sick. And on the tenth day after my death, I tried and succeeded to leave the ward.

Whilst I was in hospital, I took virtually every chance I had to abscond, so I was going to succeed sometimes. I wasn't trying to be difficult or manipulative, like I said, I wasn't in my own body at the time. I walked to the door on the ward that opened into the garden, said I was going shopping; I was advised strongly to stay by a nurse assistant whom I really liked, but I left anyway. No one stopped me. By brain was floating on the ceiling, laughing, in and out of consciousness – but I do remember a distinct feeling of guilt for putting her in that situation. Had it been a male nurse who knew me, I would never have "escaped." I didn't (and don't) *ever* really confront men.

I was immediately AWOL'd to the police, who no doubt went looking for me at my flat. But I didn't go to my flat. I went, of all places, to Tescos, and bought some cup-a-soups. After that, I went cycling to appease my eating-disordered conscience, and then back to the ward before the police found me. I was searched, the AWOL was cancelled, and I apologised to the nurse who I had walked out past. I didn't mean to get her into any sort of trouble – I think I did. (They let me keep the cup-a-soups).

What is odd from that time is how numb and inaccessible most memories are to me, even now. I don't remember if I slept, if I saw the-Dark-Dark-Man-over-my-shoulder, if I drank, if I ate (and this is a person who can list almost everything she has eaten since she was 2½). I don't remember if I smoked, watched TV, spoke to people – it's all one big blur. Perhaps that detachment was and is for the best. I can guarantee one thing: If you thought you spoke to me back then, you didn't. I was a ghost. I had more than lost hope; I had forgotten what it was.

> "The sudden disappointment of a hope
> leaves a scar which the ultimate fulfilment
> of that hope never entirely removes."
>
> ❧ Thomas Hardy (1840-1928)

I stuck a quote from Kay Redfield Jamison's *Night Falls Fast* (p.24) on my wall for the duration of my hospitalisation. I read it over and over. It reads like somebody is replacing your spinal fluid with ice-cold water. I read it now, differently to how I read it then. When I stuck it on my wall in the Summer, I was trying to feel "normal" and *communicate* (without self-harming) how dreadful I felt, *and how serious was my intent*. However, when I read it now, first I see the part about the devastation left behind. In 2002 my family didn't know anything; I refused Dr. Ogilvie permission to tell them. They still don't know much of what happened because they tell me it is "too painful." My dad doesn't believe I have attempted suicide. (Denial is powerful and comforting). Back in November 2002 I stared at that passage for hours. I had died by suicide, with every bit of suffering as Kay Redfield Jamison described; but I had also been brought back, which meant the only person in mourning was myself.

I thought they were all laughing at me. Was that a delusion? I became more and more livid. I was already furious enough for a small country where everyone was on make-me-angry pills. My anger was so intense that it physically hurt. I wanted that pain to stop. *I wanted everything to stop.*

Twelve days after my death, Ray was back on the ward and in charge. My only feeling was being angry because I *knew* he would stop me from leaving if I tried. I did not want him (or anyone) to keep me safe. I did try to leave, and was (according to my notes) "*accosted by staff*" and thereby detained on the ward, still a voluntary patient. Did I feel safer for it? Honestly - I don't know. My memory and diary from these days are blank.

I recall one very rebellious piece of behaviour, not intended to annoy, but which was probably very irritating! I still *needed* the staff to prove to me that I was safe. It was one of those days where I was hyperactive but trying to hide it. Late in the afternoon there were 5 nurses on the ward (including a female student nurse). From the smoking room, wearing pyjamas and a dressing gown as I had all day, I sauntered towards the main corridor where the nurses' office was, trying to look calm – just to see if there were any possibilities for escape. The female corridor, and my room, was opposite the nurses' station. Without stopping, I walked passed the office and into my room, having noted that only the female nursing student was blocking my way. I didn't think anyone had noticed my surreptitious investigation.

In my room, I quickly changed into my cycling gear, and walked to the end of the female corridor. This took about 60 seconds. I hesitantly peeked around the corner towards the ward entrance, expecting to see the student nurse alone. Three male nurses stood across the doorway (which was not ever locked – always guarded); the student nurse was not far away, standing in front of the locked garden door. John was sitting nonchalantly on a chair, reading a magazine, not that far from the female corridor; obviously not wanting to get drawn into any of my "games." So, they *had* noticed. I walked towards the ward's main entrance, and was promptly told to turn around and not come within 5 metres of the door. *"Stupid idiots,"* I thought pompously.

What they had not realised, was that whilst all the staff were busy in the corridor, the nurses' station was left unmanned – and unlocked. Quick as a flash, I dived into the office, and straight out of the back door into the hospital grounds. I had no idea where I was going, that didn't matter. I remember thinking how intensely funny that all of this was. Until, despite running as fast as I could, three male nurses landed on top of me, and forcefully dragged me back to the ward, my arm pinned behind up behind my back. It was just like a scene from (the wonderful) *One flew over the Cuckoo's Nest*, akin to every stereotypical image you have about mad people being restrained in mental institutions. I just laughed and laughed like it was a great joke. Not that it was really funny.

At the next ward round, I was told by an unsmiling Dr. Ogilvie that I remained ward-based on 15-minute observations, and if I so much as attempted to leave, I was to be held on a Section 5 until a Section 2 could be arranged. (A Section 2 is 28 days of involuntary admission for *assessment* – which seemed odd since I had been an inpatient for 6 months at this point. I didn't argue: 28 days sounded better than a Section 3 – i.e. 6 months). My meds were unchanged, the antipsychotic risperidone remained at 6mg. Not that I always took what I was supposed to.

That evening, following (without any realisation) the pattern of absconding/leaving following a meeting with Dr. Ogilvie, I tried to leave the ward three times by the main door and garden door. I was prevented but not sectioned. I spoke to the ever-trustworthy John to ask him what would happen if I left because I was "confused." John went to read my notes and told me it was "comprehensively documented" that if I "left or tried to leave" I "should be sectioned." I said, "Thanks" and went for a smoke.

I then proceeded to climb out of the tiny smoking room window. Another patient gave me a leg-up so that I could reach it, as long as I promised him that I wasn't going to kill myself. I met up with Tony outside, as we had become a couple. I hope he wont be offended when I say I remember nothing about how we got together – other than being repeatedly told off by staff for "inappropriate snogging." (Come on, get real). My low self-esteem meant that at the age of 27, Tony was my first real boyfriend, and sadly, I had to be psychotic and absent from my body for that to happen. Again, that is no reflection on Tony, it is just the truth about the person I was at that time.

An hour after I'd left, I phoned the ward from my flat to tell them I was fine and not to send the police. I only did it because I liked John and felt bad for running off. They hadn't even noticed I was gone, despite the fact I was on 15-minute checks. That *would not have looked good*. I was immediately AWOL'd and shouted at to get straight back.

I said I would be back soon, and I was. When I stepped back onto the ward, (literally as I stepped back through the door) I was immediately sectioned. I was put on a Section 5(4): a nurse's holding power for 6 hours. I didn't understand the logic of sectioning me once I came back to the ward. *"Who were the mad ones again?"* The duty psychiatrist was then called to see me. He asked me questions I don't remember, other than him asking if I would agree to stay. I thought: *"You twerp, you haven't read my notes? OK, tell him yes."* "Yes, I'll stay," I replied calmly. Despite the self-harm implements I had secreted into my pockets whilst at my flat, I lied saying, "I have no plans to harm myself in any way." So he took me off the Section 5(4); I think the nurses expected him to impose a Section 5(2) hold for 72 hours at least.

Of course, they wanted to know how I had gotten away and I didn't want to say. They knew I hadn't walked out of the main or garden door, and they knew I'd been seen last in the smoking room. I tried to ignore them. I sat in the smoking room trying to concentrate really hard on smoking my cigarettes, when the "interrogation" took place; they frightened and intimidated me, so I pointed at the tiny window. They looked very surprised. The window was soon covered with bars to stop anyone using it again.

Oops.

The notes say:

> *"Acting   recklessly."*
> (Understatement of the century).

On the 27th of November, 6 months after my referral, I saw Dr. Steve Pearce for assessment. Call me a cynic, but it's funny how killing your self can "oil the NHS clogs" and suddenly make available a top consultant psychiatrist *and* consultant psychotherapist, based at the Warneford Hospital, Oxford. He was there (so I was told) to give a second opinion regarding my diagnosis, being an expert in difficult cases and personality disorders. Rich sat with me because I was very nervous about meeting this new man.

I remember telling Dr. Pearce that I didn't think I would have much to say because I felt disconnected and ashamed, but as the meeting progressed I had a great deal to say. To some extent this meeting partly restored Katy Sara to her body: although she was still very, very ill; alternating between being numb, angry and then depressed. I also remember feeling very tired. So *tired* that there aren't adequate words to depict how it felt. I don't just mean tired because of lack of sleep (although that was a factor). I mean tired of _everything_: bored with my _life_, numbed by my _death_, tired of _games_, bored with _depression_, and tired of appearing to _conform_. I was utterly ashamed by the presence of my feelings of rage, and my whole body exhausted by this _furious anger_. I was resigned to the _anorexia;_ my arms, legs, and bones hurt to the point of collapse, and I was _absolutely_ exhausted at keeping a "brave" or "happy" face together. Despite this exhaustion, I was unable to rest even for a moment, or stop myself trying so hard to appear chipper. In many ways, I had nothing to loose. So with Rich's help and Steve Pearce's expert manner, I told the truth about all this.

Already trusting Rich and instinctively liking Dr. Pearce was helpful. We discussed many things. To elaborate would be a whole new book or repetition. The final outcome was a decision that I definitely did _not_ have a personality disorder, but that I had a severe depression[26] that was complicated by my anorexia, creating some borderline-type features (i.e. self-harm,

---

[26] Manic depression with dysphoric (angry/irritable) presentation, or more correctly "mixed bipolar I affective disorder with psychosis." Often a mixed state was prolonged (I mean months), in my case it lasted for a period of years, followed by long periods of major depression with and without psychosis. At the time I was being treated for treatment-resistant, (?psychotic) major depressive disorder, which _was_ usually dominant, at least outwardly and I hid most signs of mania when the doctors were around – I do not know why. I was not easy to understand due to my blatant lack of honesty and insistence that I not show anyone the intensity of my anger/distress because I thought it made me a bad person. My own dishonesty along with anorexic symptoms further complicating issues did not help my doctors make what was a difficult diagnosis. I'm bipolar.

attempting suicide). To further clarify this Dr. Pearce wrote:

> *"A 'personality disorder' is not the correct diagnosis. Katy's psychological problems might best be described in terms of an attachment disorder. My use of the phrase 'attachment disorder' does not indicate a diagnosis: the term refers to a set of problems stemming from childhood relationships, in particular relationships with major caregivers. It indicates the root of psychological problems rather than a diagnosis.*
>
> *Katy responded well to a direct approach. From the notes and her account, she does not appear to display impulsive traits: her self-harm is planned meticulously."*

I was in agreement with this opinion, and grateful for the open nature with which Dr. Pearce explained everything. This fitted with what Dr. Ogilvie had told me he thought to be wrong with me: a diagnosis of severe, long-term, treatment-resistant depression (with deliberately hidden/confused mania, or more usually mixed episodes, and psychosis). But I did have one very BIG doubt: I always believed that my brain chemistry had played an important role too. I based this on the fact that I had first been depressed/anxious/busy/emotional/overwhelmed/suicidal when I was 5 years old, (really kicking in at age 10).

I had always been restless, agitated, unable to sleep, unable to relax; long before childhood/adolescent events took place, which no doubt made things worse and left me scarred. Almost all I had known was an existence with depression and had a brain that was *never quiet, never peaceful.* Although I could not verbalise this to anyone in Oxford at the time, I do not believe either nature or nurture were solely to blame for my illnesses: I think *both* played parts.

Dr. Pearce then described to me, his understanding of my internal angst. He said it was like I was sitting on bubbling pots to keep them shut; that they kept opening under pressure of the steam within, and I had to quickly move from pot to pot to stop the force of the heat and steam opening them. But that all the time I did that, the pots, (i.e. the problems), were still bubbling away under the surface, always ready to explode, never dealt with. Not a safe situation. *"YES!"* I shouted (silently in my head). I was so grateful that someone could put my feelings into words: who saw that I was angry, edgy, resentful, always busy, sad, afraid, damaged, emotional, negative, forever terrified of failing, and that as a result, everything would overpower me, tearing me apart like we all unthinkingly, angrily, tear up junk mail. He saw that to protect myself, I swallowed my (many) intense emotions, and had been doing so for *years*, and that my mind was forever unquiet.

Dr. Pearce and Dr. Ogilvie then decided that what I needed was to be made to feel safe. That was something I had been trying to explain to staff for a long time. My notes reveal that no connection had been made between my absconding, and my motive being to test the staff in that way, to help myself feel safe. A behavioural plan was drawn up by Rich and myself whereby I was allowed out gradually, half an hour more at a time, but whereby if I self-harmed I would be ward-based for various lengths of time depending on the severity of the self-harm. If I cut myself, I would be ward-based for a day. If I attempted suicide, I would be ward-based for the foreseeable future. If my haemoglobin fell below 6.2 (which was it's value on the day we made the plan, although it is an unbelievably low threshold to have set, safety-wise, normally requiring a blood transfusion) I would be ward-based for the foreseeable future. And so on.

If, however, I said to the staff, "I feel unsafe today." I would be ward-based for the day, but rewarded for not self-harming. I never actually got rewarded, even if it was deserved – terrible examples of them not holding up their side of the bargain. (I know the NHS is busy, but don't promise things you can't do). The two suggestions given were being taken to the cinema or going for coffee. I wanted to be "good." I vehemently wanted to get well. But I still wanted to self-harm and die, and the less I felt people cared, the more I hurt myself. John thought the behavioural plan was condescending to me, and said it would either work wonderfully or "teach me to lie." Ultimately the latter proved to be the case.

At first I was reduced to self-harming on the ward, as I still wasn't allowed out. Each time (if caught) it resulted in a room search, and each room search left me laughing smugly at how crap they were at searching rooms. Sixteen days after the heroin OD, I tried to leave the ward and made it into the garden to where my bike was locked. Rich commanded me back, and I did as I was told. He took my keys off me; I felt like a child. I was ill, not a child. I hated feeling like a child. I asked Dr. Ogilvie for permission to go to a football match, I was told no. (By the way, I don't disagree with any of those decisions, however unpleasant it was having them made for me at the age of 27).

Eighteen days after the heroin OD I managed to get off the ward again. Two bank staff (i.e. temporary) were on duty and so when one of them was guarding the door, I put my cycling gear on, and walked past, I even smiled and said, "Hi, wont be long." (Yes, I had a spare key for my bike). I went straight to buy needles and a blood giving set. Then I went back to the ward, sneaked back into my room, got changed, and I hid the needles.

Later I chatted to John, and told him I'd left the ward because the bank staff hadn't recognised me as a patient who should be confined to the ward. I said it made me feel unsafe. He said, "Mmm." I later read an entry to my nose from John that day:

> *"Katy states she left the ward to go cycling whilst the bank staff were by the door (and didn't recognise her)."*

> *"There is no proof that the Pt. has left the ward."*

[Oh dear John: that sounds like you **didn't** believe me].

Later that night the duty psychiatrist was fast-bleeped to Vaughan Thomas because there was an emergency. Katy, who "obviously" had not been able to leave the ward, but who had been searched innumerable times so could not have owned anything harmful, had collapsed unconscious, and could not be brought around. Closer inspection of her room found three litre jugs and a blood-giving set, purchased that very afternoon. Two of the jugs were full, the other part-full of warm blood. Her pulse was fast at 130 beats/min *minimum*; her blood pressure (BP) was low at only 71/31. An hour later it had gone up to only 75/37. (I have little faith in the accuracy of these recorded observations – my heart rate was nearer 200 beats/min according to my measurements. I don't believe they got a decent BP reading).

If you are wondering: was that a suicide attempt? The answer is: absolutely *yes* – not her ideal method, but the best she could come up with at the time. It was not an unpleasant way to go. It also took place because bloodletting would quiet and calm her anger, for a time at least – but it was mainly a suicide attempt of 100% lethal intent. For months she had been losing blood and she was anaemic. On top of this, even without that fact, she knew that venesecting past the 2 litre point put her in the most serious grade of hypovolaemic shock, and that even with treatment for fluid depletion, she ought to die.

Was she sent to the Emergency Department? No. Did she get a blood transfusion when the importance of one was explained to her? No, she refused one, and told them she *already* understood the importance of one. Did she die? No, she defied all the odds and clinical expectations: and lived, although she felt very ill for a long time. Yet again she felt angry at her apparent immortality. Did she get ward-based for safety or as "punishment?" Yes. Rightly so.

Following this bloodletting, her anger stepped backwards to allow depression to take centre stage once again. But anger stood in the wings, waiting for its comeback.

Three weeks and one day after death-by-heroin-OD, ward-round with Dr. Ogilvie:

[Before patient entered room].

Fellow patient (Declan) states Katy has asked him to get her some more heroin so that she can OD again. He reports that he has refused.

[Patient entered room].

- Patient subjectively and objectively low in mood.
- Permission to go to football refused again.
- Pattern of absconding, commonly after ward-round, has been noticed by Dr. Ogilvie, and this had been explained to other staff and patient.
- Patient's (haemoglobin) Hb has fallen below 6.2, which means she is strictly ward-based.

Anger returned with the refusal to let me out. I only remember, with my medical notes here to prompt me, that I had asked Declan to get me some heroin. He bragged of connections, but refused to help me because he didn't want me to die. Sometimes he would bring it with him, or be high when he arrived; but he adamantly refused to help me kill myself or have any heroin from him. (Although providing any other drug was fine).

I proved Dr. Ogilvie right yet again. Immediately after ward-round, I attempted to leave the ward – again.

At first I was stopped, but according to my diary, on my next attempt I made it out. I did some cycling (not much because I was so physically weak) and bought a bottle of wine and some soup. I had been immediately AWOL'd; the wine was confiscated upon my return. I had to see my favourite SHO, Dr. D. M***** who told me unequivocally that if I ever did anything like that again he would section me. *"Yeah, yeah,"* I thought. *"That's what you people keep on saying. And anyway, I don't give a fuck if I am sectioned anymore. What does it matter if I am dead soon? I'm dead already."*

Perhaps I should have known Dean meant what he said about sectioning me. Actually, I think I did know: I just didn't care. My favourite SHO (Dean) was still the duty psychiatrist that night (though I didn't know that). At 8.30pm my room was searched, and this upset me, so I walked out. The room search was stopped, since the patient is supposed to be present during a search. I walked towards the main Vaughan Thomas doors, where the nurses very strongly advised me to stay. They surrounded me, four or five nurses, some female, but they did not actually restrain or even touch me. I ignored them, and they parted as if I repelled them, and I went straight into the main part of the hospital, and started walking down towards the front door.

As "luck" would have it, my favourite SHO was walking in the opposite direction, carrying a pizza that I am sure he would like to have eaten hot. (Sorry). I smiled at him, and said calmly, "I'm going Dean. If you want to keep me in this place you are going to have to section me." I made it all the way to the main front doors of the Warneford, just reaching out to push the door. At this point I had four nurses and my favourite SHO surrounding me, asking (well, telling) me not to leave. I remember George telling me, "Whatever you do, don't touch that door, if you do, we'll section you and take you back." My arm outstretched, I paused. In a not entirely logical sense (considering what I had just said to Dean), at this point I decided to be "good" and avoid the section.

I went to my room, the nurses dispersed, and then I set off again. I cannot explain why: my rational brain knew it was a fruitless action, but my ill brain was in the driving seat, and still wanted out of the hospital. Logic had very little to do with my actions. I didn't get beyond the ward doors that time; I slumped back to my bedroom. I think that by this point, I was the subject of discussion in the nurses' station. My favourite SHO requested that I come to "have a discussion" with him. I refused. So, he came to my room to assess me there. I said, "I really don't feel like talking Dean." To which he replied that it was inappropriate that I called him by his first name.

I took this as a personal insult – rightly or wrongly it felt rude, and I refused to speak to him at all. No doubt he thought me rude; I still don't care! He called me by my first name, so I would call him by his, as I had been doing up to that point: doing otherwise would have suggested that he was a better person than me. Dr. Ogilvie allowed me to introduce myself to him – I could have called myself Ms Culling had I wanted. I called him Dr. Ogilvie out of respect that was earned, not demanded. Generally I don't believe in titles, not for anyone. Sometimes I use them for an easier life, for categorisation purposes, or just to be polite, but I don't use them in my head. If using a title is important to someone, I am even more sceptical about it.

I said (under my breath) that I would call him Dr. whatever-he-liked, *if* he called me Professor Princess Banana Creamboat Culling – fitting into my philosophy that neither person should have an unfair proportion of the power in any relationship. He called me Katy; I called him Dean. That is my own personal view on things; I stand by it. Somehow it was different with Dr. Ogilvie – I felt he was more distant, and he scared me quite a lot (because of my neuroses, not because he is particularly scary).

Responsible for such a strong reaction were many things: my own dashed dreams of becoming a physician; the subjugated child *and* adult within me; a damaged young woman; a recently and terribly abandoned academic; lots of anger; excessive head-noise; and the depressive (existential) nihilist[27] that has

---

[27] Nihilism is the belief that all values are baseless and that nothing can be known for certain or communicated; though nihilism has other complex interpretations. I strongly believe that the only values/morals I have are those I have formed, not those imposed by society. I have no problem with people using drugs because I don't care what the law says; it is a personal – serious – decision. I refuse to believe, I refuse to obey. I'm not an active anarchist; I'm too passive. I reject authority and disagree with law – so I am more accurately a non-conformist. I am pragmatic, which means I don't waste my time worrying about what I cannot change. I do not *ever* reject personal morality. I do not reject faith, I *do* reject religion - though do not impose this belief on others. Nihilism refutes the existence of god(s): as do I, utterly.

Existential nihilism is the notion that life has no intrinsic meaning or value, which is the most commonly used and understood sense of the word at present day. This I do believe, *especially universally*. This clashes with my humanitarian values, which I hold dear to my heart, but cannot *connect* with if I am of low mood – making me a depressive nihilist. I don't believe that *nothing* can be communicated – or why write this book? Resigned to eventual defeat? Yes, that is I. If I exist, I do so without reason.

always been in me, that becomes more rebellious and negative the more ill I become. Of course I was overly sensitive about the whole "doctor" issue. Dean was (is) my age. I had studied medicine at Oxford just like him; had I not become ill, I might have been the SHO looking after a patient. I had once gone to him to talk about losing my D.Phil. position and he had expressed regret. It felt like he was slapping my failure in my face. He knew I wanted to be a doctor. Were roles reversed, I would not demand to be called Dr. Culling if calling me by my name made him more comfortable. Some people like saying Dr. Ms. or Professor; it can put people at ease… For me, it was a *delicate* issue.

After being "told off" for calling Dean Dean, I curled up insolently on my bed, and covered my head with the sheets, and refused to talk with him. I don't think I ever spoke to him again. He had a one-way conversation for a while, then left. Nurses reappeared to sedate me, and I was put onto a Section 5(2): a 72-hour hold, with one-to-one nursing observations. *"Oh great; being followed to the toilet,"* I thought. *"Must have really pissed him off. Good."* My room was searched very thoroughly: all the Christmas presents I had brought were unwrapped, and the alcohol within them confiscated (and never returned). Nobody opened up Rammie though, nor checked inside books or behind posters. They found empty pill packets, but no full ones. They missed the

---

In psychiatry, nihilism may be classed as delusional: such as when I truly believed that I did not exist. Usually depressive and existentialist nihilism are distinct, but in my case, they were conflated in 2002: meaning that I rejected the authority of the hospital, laws of the country, thought that *my* life had no purpose or value, and I felt invisible, unimportant and unreal, as did my surroundings. *In my recovery, I've learnt not to think on a universal scale too often.*

bottle of wine hanging out my window too. Dean's summary of me in the notes was:

> *Patient room searched: alcohol, razors, various other sharps including venflons and needles, suture kits, lignocaine, sterile wound dressings found.*

> *Pale, no eye-contact, difficult rapport, lying on bed, baggy clothing.*
> *Speech: no spontaneous conversation, refused to answer questions.*
> *Mood:*
> *Subjectively angry*
> *Objectively* angry.*
> *Insight: FULL.*

> *Plan: Section 5(2), 1:1 observations, sedation – see meds card. If attempts to leave, to be restrained. To be searched for alcohol and self-harm implements at nurses discretion. Bags of visitors and anything given by friends* [Clare bought me "edible" food most days] *to be searched by staff. No visitors allowed in her room.*

*I (of course) would argue that an "objective" opinion (truth) is an impossibility. Yes I was angry. But nobody could "objectively" state this, all opinions were subjective: with my opinion being the nearest one to "truth." I after all lived in my head.

There is little difference to being sectioned and ward-based – in principle. One is involuntary, one meant to be voluntary: although we all know by now that people are often not true "volunteers." The biggest difference (in my case) was legal: meaning people worried *less* about legal ramifications if they interfered with my personal freedom. Many (not all) nurses hesitate to restrain or chase you if you are voluntary, but if you are sectioned it is their job. You will *not* be asked "politely" to think again about leaving; instead you *will* be stopped from doing so. That means you *will* be restrained, you *will* be chased, you *will* be medicated, and you *will* be AWOL'd to the police if you escape. So, all in all, not much changed for me.

Four weeks and a day after my death-by-heroin, it was time for ward-round again. That meant seeing Dr. Ogilvie, which I liked because he seemed to be one of the few people within any insight who listened to me: although it scared me because I knew that he saw through some or all of my bullshit! I think he frightened me because I knew I was pushing him hard to take control, yet at the same time desperately not wanting him to take it. I knew he was in charge, and I knew he could take more control. It also frightened me that he wouldn't like me. And it frightened me that he would not deem me worth saving. Unfortunately due to a crazy workload, I didn't get to see him as much as I would have liked.

According to the ward-round notes I *"flatly denied any suicidal intent with respect to all my attempts to leave hospital, or times I actually left hospital."* I doubt that anybody believed that: I didn't believe that. However, my 72-hour section had passed and I was not placed onto a longer section. The strict but common sense boundaries that Dean had implemented were kept in place by Dr. Ogilvie in order to try and make me feel safe. The only changes were that I was placed on 15-minute observations, a reduction from constant 24-hour observations, and due to my insatiable eating-disordered anxiety, it was agreed I would be allowed to leave the ward for a very strict, timed 15 minutes a day to cycle – in theory not enough time to get to my flat or town and back. (At least, that's what people thought).

My room, my friends, and I would continue to be searched on my return from cycling, or at the nurses' discretion. Were I to be found in possession of drugs, drink, needles, blades, or anything dangerous, I would immediately be placed onto constant 24-hour observations. If I self-harmed or attempted suicide, I would be back on 24-hour observations indefinitely – a threat that Dr. Ogilvie had astutely gathered would often dissuade me from misbehaving. I remember thinking (somewhat dismissively) that I wouldn't ever be on constant observations for long because it took up a lot of staff time. Only a day later my notes say:

> *"Katy has not left her room since early morning: following her 15-minute cycle she has remained in her room asleep all day."*

[Yeah, that'll be because of attempted suicide with a large overdose of sleeping medication].

The same is recorded the next day, the next, and the next. By this time we are talking about absolutely fucking-ridiculous quantities of zolpidem, zopiclone, and various other sedatives I tried. I used to hide them in my socks and trouser pockets – none of which were ever searched. I always mixed them with alcohol to heighten the chance of death: given to me by Ash, Declan, or both. None of these suicide attempts were particularly well thought through: I merely took everything I could get my hands on and hoped for death. The suicidal intent was 100% serious.

I mostly stayed in my room and I didn't get dressed properly much. I tended to wear my Derby County shorts & knee socks, and a tight designer T-shirt, covered with my flowing, purple dressing gown or a fleece if I nipped for a cigarette. I swapped my football shorts for cycling shorts when I cycled and only got dressed when it was ward round – so that I looked "normal" for the doctors. It's true that the whole time I was on Vaughan Thomas, I got a lot of male attention – but only because the men had a limited choice. I now swung between a stuporous state in my room due to overdoses, and running here, there and everywhere on the ward, manic: very different to the low profile I had previously kept.

At this time I was engaged to Tony, and completely faithful: although some male patients stated (lied) otherwise. So I wore my happy face for the 30 minutes a day that Tony visited me on the ward – he hated the ward, and Rich was very territorial and/or protective. I did hug and cuddle Ash regularly, but in an understood, asexual, between-friends way when he was upset or just needed a patient comrade. My notes say:

> *"Fears for Katy's naïveté with respect to men on the ward were discussed. She said she simply was not aware of ever appearing provocative as she had always believed she was rotten-filth."*

*"Katy showed us her engagement ring –
she's engaged to Anthony Carrick."*

Of course, being engaged was of questionable timing, and produced an interesting dichotomy. I was, on one hand, planning (not very seriously) to get married; on the other I was planning (seriously) my suicide. The suicidal side of me won most of the time. Since I would be dead shortly, it was easy to say to myself: *"Fuck it. Get engaged, have a boyfriend, consider marriage – because this is the only chance you are going to have. Go out with a bang as they say."* (That should not be read as a poor reflection of Tony who is a wonderful man). Personally, because of many fears, I could only maintain a relationship whilst I was kept "safe" and distanced on the ward – <u>not</u> that Tony would *ever* have hurt me. If I felt low, I could hide on the ward. Tony had been released from hospital by this time, and had moved into my Iffley road flat.

Everything I felt seemed so *intense* and *powerful*. It is probably of notable importance that this occurred when I had been refusing my lithium for some time, on the basis that I felt "sick," or I pretended to take it (and saved it for a future overdose). Often I didn't take my risperidone either. Nobody really suspected me of not taking my meds, so it was easy to get away with.

I was supposed to be in love… but my head felt like it was going to explode. Most of the time I felt like I was being pelted with rocks and jeered at by people who I knew weren't really there, but I saw and heard them all the same. Sometimes I thought everything in life was an illusion, or that I was ethereal. Reality was distorted: people moved and spoke in slow motion, but my brain buzzed. I was overwhelmed with thoughts, and thoughts about my thoughts, and thoughts about having thoughts about thoughts. I looked calm, but nothing could have been more inaccurate. At times when things slowed down, I had the sensation/belief that I was melting or disappearing, like the water-doused Wicked Witch of the West in *The Wonderful Wizard of Oz* (by L. Frank Baum). I watched myself, and my life force flickered like a weak flame in the wind.

> "O, hark! what mean those yells and cries?
> His chain some furious madman breaks;
> He comes--I see his glaring eyes: Now,
> now, my dungeon grate he shakes. Help!
> Help! He's gone!--O fearful woe, Such
> screams to hear, such sights to see! My
> brain, my brain,--I know, I know I am not
> mad but soon shall be."
> ❧ Matthew Gregory Lewis (1775 –1818)
> *The Maniac.*

Pain was exquisite, my *fears* all-consuming, my fiery *anger* volatile, and the *irritability* was "…aarrgghh" indescribable. My mind was racing so much I wanted to pull my brain out through my ears and have a good scratch around inside my scull. This was *exhausting*; yet mostly contained from everyone. I was incapable of explaining any of this: too frightened, too lost for words, too puzzled, too ashamed and far too uncooperative. If I walked about anxiously on the ward, people assumed it was anorexic behaviour, and I encouraged that thinking. Actually I didn't care about my weight, I just couldn't keep still. I didn't know quite where to put myself, what to do, how to cope, or how to stop myself falling to pieces in front of anyone.

Warnings of being sectioned again meant little by this point – and my notes show I was on a Section 5(2) a few times without my knowledge (or at least, not that I can remember). Dr. Ogilvie and Dr. Pearce explained to me that they did not think the ward environment was helping me, but I did not want to hear that because I could not contemplate any other way of surviving. It was true that I was in a far worse mental and physical state by December, than I had been upon my admission in June. They explained they wanted to send me to a specialist unit (the Bethlem Unit) in London: I flatly refused. I was too scared of a large city and not being able to cycle. I am a country girl, and although Oxford is a city, it is small – and at that time, it was my *home*. They told me I had to improve (i.e. self-harm less, eat, not attempt suicide and bloody well cheer up), or I would be put onto a Section 3 (*initially 6-months, but extendible for treatment*) and sent to London against my will.

So, I decided I would have to lie in a believable, gradual fashion that I was recovering. However, I was *far* too ill to be convincing; Dr. Ogilvie and Dr. Pearce were *far* too perceptive for that plan to work. I remember once Dr. Pearce came to visit me on the ward, but I had overdosed and couldn't speak properly. He recognised the symptoms immediately, and cut our session short, but sent the nurses en masse to search my room – that scared me. By that point I really liked Steve Pearce, and I was scared that I had made him angry and hateful – projecting my thoughts about myself on to him. I handed over some booze and risperidone that I didn't mind losing: keeping the "good stuff" in my hot water bottle Rammie. They picked him up, squeezed him, and went "Ah how sweet." I thought, *"Only half the story sister. Oh I am evil."*

One gorgeous nurse, whom I really liked, Margaret – got me some signed Derby Country gear. Her notes say:

> *"Katy is of low mood, having suicidal thoughts saying. 'I've nothing to live for.' Gave 1-1 time and reassured her that we are aware of her situation and we are there to help."*

> [Not one word of that reassurance sank into my consciousness – my brain was impervious].

My diary at this point became a rant about having biological depression:

> *It's biological! Psychological aspects played a "vital role," but BIOLOGY is where it all began. It's the fucking chemicals in my fucking brain you imbeciles. Buzz buzz. Please shut up in my head, in my room – peace, rest, just a moment's peace. I beg you. The noise. The people.*

> *I'm confused.*

> *The strain... I think I am going to shatter into a thousand pieces. Maybe that will bring peace? Ahhhhhhh... Go away. Fuck*

*off. Who are you? Just go the fuck away. I
don't want you here. GO.*

I felt that nobody was listening to me. Up, down,
buzzing, angry, irritated, suicidal, round and round and
round: it would drive *anyone* insane with misery. I was
doing my best to keep still. All my movement and
energy was concentrated in my brain, my head ached,
my eyes were sore from flickering underneath my
eyelids and the long sleepless nights. Outwardly I was
compliant, still, and non-complaining. At this time my
grandmother, "Nanny" Betty was dying up in Derby; I
wondered if it was easier for the staff cope with
bereaved-Katy instead of all my usual shite. My notes
say:

"Quiet."

"Withdrawn."

"Flat-effect."

"Preoccupied."

"Bored."

"Cooperative"

*"Isolated – spending all her
time in her room."*

"In bed."

"Subdued."

"Spends all her time alone."

Under strict parental supervision and aided by temazepam, Dr. Ogilvie allowed me to go and see my dying grandmother. I whispered into her ears that we were all there and that we all loved her. She could not respond but I believe she heard me; hearing is the last sense to go. I sung into her ear for a bit, told her what a wonderful life she had had, and that I was proud of her. I told her I was still working in Oxford – something I knew made her so very proud. To me, seeing someone die, being there, holding their hand, leading them through their fears at their death, is all about them, and was all I wanted to do that day. Once she was gone, she was gone… and so I whispered in her ear until dad said we had to go.

She died in the night, peacefully. At my Nan's house I was told I could take something to remember her by. I didn't need possessions because I was about to die myself. I had memories: that was enough. So instead, I reprehensibly stole all of her diazepam (valium) because, well, she didn't need it anymore. I downed it all in one go, and headed back to Oxford.

Leading up to Christmas there are a number of false allegations made against me in my notes – including claims I was dealing marijuana on the ward and was in three new suicide pacts with unnamed patients. I had learned my lesson with my pact with Caroline – the allegations were completely unfounded. I was not even being sociable at this time. I was never given an opportunity to clear my name, indeed I did not even know about these lies. One day, Jean asked me to teach her how to insert a needle into her arm so that she could get blood or inject air into a vein to commit suicide. I flatly refused, however, in my notes, Simon recorded:

> *"Katy was overheard teaching Jean how to inject air into her veins in order to kill herself."*

What I *actually* said was that I would *never* teach her that, and I suggested she not bother injecting air into her veins because it wouldn't kill her. The notes up to Christmas continue:

> *"Patient slept soundly for long periods."*

I wonder why? Surely those overdoses were obvious? At the time I was grateful for the lack of interruption, but looking back at what went on, I am surprised. I continued to be allowed out some days for just fifteen minutes. Sometimes I had sedatives to overdose on, sometimes I didn't. So I was either comatose or overactive. Often my body would be motionless, my mind a busy ticking bomb. On Christmas Eve I was noted to be *"up all night writing."* I only wrote a few words:

> *MERRY CHRISTMAS*
> *AND*
> *A*
> *HAPPY FUCKING NEW YEAR*
> *(IN HOSPTIAL).*

On Christmas day I attempted suicide by venesecting with a blood-giving set but was caught. I denied it was a suicide attempt despite having planning it for…ooh, a week or two. Bloodletting as a form of self-harm had the added advantage of calming my anger – by causing exhaustion or unconsciousness. I managed to hide the collecting jugs behind a huge box that Tony had put my Christmas presents in; and, lying on my bed under my dressing gown, I could raise my head every 15 minutes to keep shouting at the staff doing checks that I was trying to sleep (hoping they'd leave me in peace and not notice when I died).

It worked for a bit, until Simon came to give me 1:1 time (talk to me) and he spotted the blood immediately. My room was searched briefly. I was put onto constant observations until 8pm. Thankfully John was allocated that task, and we talked for hours. I did fully intend to die, it was not for anyone's attention, but making the best of talking to John was the sensible option. I refused to be physically checked and was noted to be:

"Non-remorseful about bloodletting."

"Of very low mood."

"Sleeping from approx. 8pm onwards." [I overdosed on sedatives as soon as I was removed from constant observations].

On the 26th I saw Dr. Ogilvie who added Mirtazapine to my drug regime in order to help me sleep – not only as an antidepressant but to help with my marked early wakening at around 2am. It worked very well to sedate me, but had no noticeable effect on my mood. On the 27th I took another sedative OD. On the 28th I was escorted to see Derby County play; and privately I said goodbye to all my fellow supporters – though, of course, they didn't know that. I came home singing, "I am Derby till I die, Derby till I die." I looked a few people in the face whilst I sang, willing them to understand I was *meant* to die. That's one (the only) Derby song I don't sing anymore.

On the 29th I took a massive overdose, over 1,000 zolpidem and several hundred Zolpiclone. The intent was death; the result was:

"Katy spent lengthy periods sleeping."

"Seems a bit vague."

The following day:

"Katy is still in bed."

"Sleepy."

"Refused blood test to check lithium levels." [Scared they'd pick up on the overdose or that I had only sporadically taken my lithium].

"Katy told me [George] *that she has to die before her 28th Birthday so that she is forever 27."* [Oops didn't mean to let that slip].

The following day I overdosed again, sleeping until 10am where I was described as:

"Oversedated?"

"Groggy."

"Unsteady"

"Pt. claimed she would be fine to cycle; returned within allotted 15 minutes, but then has spent all her time asleep in her room. [Yes, I'd taken more sedatives with the intent of dying].

You might question the severity of my intent to die with these sedative overdoses; surely I should have learnt that they were not "working?" My intent was clear and absolute. Each time I overdosed, I *honestly* thought it would be my last time, or if not, the cumulative effect would kill me reasonably quickly. I also, rather snootily, believed absolutely that most of the hospital staff were incompetent enough to miss the difference between me sleeping…and me dead.

At the beginning of January 2003, Tony (whom I had broken up with) phoned the ward to inform them I had "smack" (heroin) at home, with which to overdose. That, in fact, was incorrect. Since Achilles had disappeared, I had no idea how to get hold of heroin, and it is not as simple as you might think. You can't just walk up to someone in the street and have him or her sell it to you. Supplying drugs carries a life-sentence; you need to be known, or "introduced" to a dealer in order for them to trust you. As a result of this (false) allegation I was ward-based by Dr. Dean (who I did not see) and Simon, and placed back onto 15 minute observations. I was compliant because of the threat of 24-hour constant-observations. My room was searched unsuccessfully.

A day later I had (honestly and convincingly) persuaded them that Tony was misinformed, and was told I could go out and cycle. Before I left, I opened my mail, and received my mobile phone bill, redirected from Derby. On it was the mobile phone number of Achilles' heroin dealer. So I called him. Just like that, I picked up the phone and plunged straight in: "Hi, I, erm, need to buy some heroin." I said I was Achilles' girlfriend and needed some heroin. We arranged to meet in town – and I slipped out of the ward unnoticed. I met two men, one took the money, then the other put the heroin on the floor after taking it out from under his tongue in little balls. They could have raped, stabbed, mugged or killed me: I didn't care. I bought £60 worth in three £20 baggies, put £40 worth in my flat, and kept £20 worth on me, in my sock. I felt *terrific*. I finally had more heroin, such a delightful way to die that would:

    a.) Work

    b.) Not hurt.

    c.) Be neat and tidy.

    d.) Not endanger anyone else.

I had to get back to the ward quickly so as not to rouse suspicion. I must have walked with a bounce in my step and a grin on my face because Rich was immediately on to me. He said in quick succession: "What is it? What have you done? Something has happened. You've got more heroin haven't you?" I tried not to smile, but did. He told me to hand it over and I laughed nervously, lying, "If I really had bought heroin, which I haven't, do you honestly think I would be so stupid as to bring in with me to the ward again after last time." Images of strip-searches went through my mind, but my cold smile did not waver.

That night, a Friday, I "tested" the heroin. Just to make sure it was the real deal. I knew £10 would be lethal, and used approximately £3 worth. (2002 prices). Because Clare had thrown away my citric acid, I used a small amount of an effervescent vitamin C tablet to help the heroin dissolve. I felt calm, soothed, warm and sleepy: such a relief from my vitriolic anger. I did the same thing on the Saturday and Sunday night, actually feeling better because *I felt I had my life back in control*. In other words, it was now *mine* to end whenever *I* liked. Rich allowed me to leave the ward to cycle if I promised not to go home – a promise I kept. Then Monday arrived and at 6am I went out cycling; after which it was ward-round.

When I saw Dr. Ogilvie it was afternoon. I was *immediately* ward-based on the basis I admitted (or more accurately did not plausibly deny) having heroin at home. I don't remember admitting anything, but I am capable of being enough of an arrogant twit to do exactly that. Maybe that was an unconscious cry for help. The police were informed, and I was told they would search my flat. (Actually they refused to do so). The threats about sectioning, increased observations and AWOL'ing me were reaffirmed. Before I was even allowed to leave the meeting room where ward round was held, Dr. Ogilvie insisted that all the ward staff be told that I was a flight risk, and that I was not to be allowed to leave. Not much got passed Dr. Ogilvie.

Obviously I left the meeting practically shitting myself that the police would go around to my flat and I would get charged with possession of heroin again, (remember that at this stage, I still didn't know I'd been let off the first charge). There was absolutely no way of getting out the front door, so I looked in the bathrooms, kitchen, meeting rooms and bedrooms – to no avail. I went into the smoking room, and looked sadly at the new bars on the high windows: impossible to get through. Then I noticed that one of the lower windows was broken, and with a bit of a squeeze, I climbed through, scraping my arms and legs red-raw, my low weight an advantage. I cycled home initially intending to dispose of the heroin, but when it came to it, I couldn't bring myself to throw it away: instead it mesmerised me, and I hid it in my socks.

I cycled back "home" to the ward, the AWOL was cancelled, and I told John that I had been forced to leave in order to destroy the heroin to avoid a conviction. My story made sense, and I confirmed several times (with puppy-dog eyes) that I had destroyed the heroin, and challenged them to search my room or my pockets. As a result I was not sectioned; and only 15-minute observations remained in place. With my door locked (giving me enough warning time to say that I was fine, just getting changed) I cooked up £20 worth of heroin. I waited until a nurse went by doing the 15-minute checks, then I swiftly injected the entire syringe of heroin into a vein. I heard the beautiful, galloping horses once again, and quickly settled/fell into my bed, certain that I would appear to be sleeping – at least, until it was too late. Eternal sleep.

My next memory just a flash of John and some other people lifting me on to the floor of my bedroom, and someone saying, "Get another dose." Then darkness. Apparently the first dose (I don't know how much) of narcan (naloxone) had done very little to help, and I still wasn't breathing. The notes say they used a guedal airway to help me breathe, and also gave me oxygen. Next I remember a female doctor shouting in my ear, yet she seemed to be shouting from far away – me in Oxford, her on top of Mount Everest kind of distance. She shouted that she was sectioning me under the Mental Health Act, then darkness again.

When the paramedics arrived they gave me more narcan. John would later comment that he was impressed at how well narcan worked, having never seen it in action before. He said I had been completely lifeless but the three intravenous doses meant that in matter of minutes I was actually able to walk (with help) to the ambulance. I was then taken to the John Radcliffe Hospital Emergency Department. I remember very little other than being pissed off at the rude interruption, *again*.

In my room were a large number of suicide notes – none that were ever intended for reading, just ones that I wrote because I was that way inclined. Unfortunately, the nurses took them away and opened them all to read. In the John Radcliffe I was allowed the sign myself out AMA (against medical advice) but that meant I was sent straight back to the Warneford Hospital, as I was under a Section 5(2).

I remember Jean was working that night, and she was very welcoming. I was informed that I was not allowed to go back into my usual bedroom (number 9), as it had to be thoroughly searched: a fact I found most distressing. All change was difficult, but especially difficult as I knew there was heroin in my teddy bear Rammie. Instead, I was to be back on the acute ward, but I asked Jean if I could just get some nightclothes and a book – some things to keep me comfortable that she could check. Harry (the nurse in charge) agreed, and I picked out my Rams shirt and shorts, my black combat trousers, a book ...and Rammie.

My brain was buzzing, my body the opposite, and I wasn't allowed my usual night meds (a decision I cannot argue with) and so I found myself very much awake on the intensive care ward being watched. Whilst given a few minutes of privacy to get into my nightclothes, I swallowed a few packets of zolpidem and risperidone.

I was on constant, strict, 24-hour observations; not unsurprisingly since I had nearly succeeded in killing myself whilst in a psychiatric hospital. I clung to Rammie all night, and wondered what to do about the heroin in him. The next morning, whilst a male member of staff was doing my observations, I asked for permission to partially close the door whilst I got dressed. My wish was granted: as I dressed, I removed the heroin and a large number of zopiclone from inside my trusty teddy and secreted them in my socks and combat trouser pockets. I then went to the toilet, and was allowed to close – but not lock the door – customary for female patients being watched by a male member of staff. I removed the heroin, wrapped it in tissue, and flushed it away. Had I known at that point in time, that the heroin dealer would *never* trust me again, I would have kept it. Instead, fortunately, I felt no qualms about my decision, and watched the heroin disappear.

Only 2 minutes later, Dr. Ogilvie arrived to see me, even though he was not on duty that day. On that day I was terrified of him: he seemed huge. He looked angry through my eyes. He seemed, and was, omnipotent. He reminded me that I was under a Section 5 and told me that before it ran out, I was to be placed on a Section 3 (i.e. *6 months* involuntary detention, renewably, for treatment). He also told me I had very nearly died. In my diary I wrote:

> " Dr. Ogilvie said I 'nearly died.' So I nearly died... apparently."

I told Dr. Ogilvie that it had not been a suicide attempt, that I had been "testing" the heroin for recreational purposes, but that it must have been purer than I thought. (Plausible?) When I said that, I did believe it, but looking back it was a form of denial. *I knew* damn well I had taken over 6 x a lethal dose for me, and had avoided discovery as best as I could. Whilst I cursed myself for not putting my teddy under the bed, Dr. Ogilvie saw and immediately removed him from my possession. The ward manager opened him, finding sleeping pills, a spoon, needles, a couple of 5ml syringes, but no heroin. It was handed over to the police for testing. The notes by Dr. Ogilvie say:

> *"Tearful, unsettled, not to be allowed any personal property in her room, not even a teddy bear. No access to nurses' office. Patient was ward-based as soon as I learned that she had purchased heroin; but she escaped, returning to the ward saying she had destroyed it. Katy has been lying to staff. Danger to other patients? To remain on constant observations, detained on a Section 5(2) to then be held on Section 3."*

I told Dr. Ogilvie I wanted my suicide notes back, explaining that they had not been intended for reading –

which *was* the truth. He agreed; though many had already been read. I felt emotionally violated. None of those words were intended for reading. I continued to press my case that the heroin overdose had just been a terrible accident, and that I was fine and grateful to be alive. Dr. Ogilvie's unequivocal response was that it didn't really matter if I intended to die or not: my self-harm had reached such drastic proportions that I was going to end up dead if they did not take over all responsibility for me. I *hated* Dr. Ogilvie that day; but I also felt intense gratitude that he felt me worth keeping alive. So *finally* I had forced him to take *all* the responsibility for my life from me; I was sat in a room with nothing but a bed and someone watching my every move, and I immediately wanted responsibility (control) back. But that was not going to prove so easy to get.

The next thing I remember, (bearing in mind I was feeling quite poorly), was seeing Neil, Dr. MacLennan, walk into my room. I was curled up in my horrible hospital duvet staring at four walls and a nurse, thinking I was going to die with the boredom of having nothing do; frustrated, angry, and I *hated* Dr. Ogilvie for making me seem transparent, and for making decisions about *my* life. Then I saw Neil's friendly face, and, after an initial fear that I was seeing things, I welcomed the sight of a trusted person whom I had not seen for a few months: although he looked sad. A social worker followed him. We talked about the recent heroin overdose, and I swore it had been an accident: again, convincing myself of that lie. Dr. MacLennan told me he had been asked to sign me onto a Section 3, but having seen me he wanted to speak to Dr. Ogilvie first. Dr. Ogilvie quickly persuaded him, and all the papers were signed.

As it happened, that week I decided to let my family back into my life. I saw it like this: I was going to die, so why not? Theoretically, my next-of-kin (my father) was supposed to sign his consent for the Section 3. My dad refused to do so until he had spoken to Dr. Ogilvie; who told him that his consent was only a formality, and that I would be sectioned with or without his sanction. All of this took place on a Friday before a bank holiday weekend, meaning it was 4 days after my 2nd heroin overdose before I was able to sit in a room with just Dr. Ogilvie.

I asked him not to section me. I said I would behave, comply, and not try to run away again. I meant it. He believed me: agreeing not to make the Section 3 papers official, but reminding me that they were completed and would be handed in immediately if I stepped out of line. As far as other staff were aware, I had been placed on a Section 3. (The papers were completed and entered into my record – with no amendment that I was, in fact, voluntary again).

I genuinely meant it when I told Dr. Ogilvie I would comply. What I don't know is why on Earth he believed me. When I asked him years later, he simply said, "You persuaded me." That was how, just 4 days after attempting suicide, I started to be allowed a timed 30 minutes a day out to cycle, (any bags I brought back with me searched), and was reduced to 15-minute observations. I was soon recorded as *"compliant"* and being of *"low risk of absconding,"* because that was the truth.

Behind that truth was a decision by myself to comply in order to get released, so that *then* I could kill myself in private. Dr. Ogilvie met my parents for the first time (I had previously exercised my right to confidentiality). They were rather shocked, though of course, the picture that was painted was not actually as dark as the reality: even so, it was pretty bleak. Dr. Ogilvie told them I had died, twice, and *just* been resuscitated: it's hard to get much more blatantly sinister than that.

Dr. Ogilvie told me that there was still a high possibility of my being sent to London, and that if that time came around and I didn't agree, the Section 3 would be enforced. What actually happened in my head at this point was that I (in the words of my diary) became:

> *"Shit-bored with this place. I am NOT going to London. I'm going to "behave" and do everything I can to get out of here as soon as possible, and then take care of "business." Time to stop fighting the system...Hide the busy-busy feelings, try to look calm, hide self-harm, look happy."*

My notes show I was not so good at hiding this as I thought at the time:

> *"Katy is compliant due to perceived threat of London, not because she wants to be safe or in psychological control."*

> *"The transfer to Bethlem Hospital has been cleared."*

For the next week, questions were constantly being asked about how drowsy I appeared. I had used the small amount of time I was allowed to cycle to get equipment and medication with which to hurt myself. I was able to honestly deny using heroin, and deceitfully lie about using anything else. In fact I attempted to kill myself (or at least shut up my noisy mind) with whatever mixture of sedatives I had, in ludicrously high doses and with no real interest about getting caught. There was no logic: it directly opposed my plan of conforming, but I could not help myself.

> *"Katy denies being sedated during the day."*

> *"Unsteady, withdrawn, lethargic and flat. No attempts to leave the ward."*

> *"Patient very drowsy; though denies this. Slow, slurred speech, low mood, subjectively and objectively."*

On morning, Ash and I sat slowly smoking cigarettes in the smoking room, drinking the "lovely" decaf coffee you get in psychiatric hospital, and he suddenly said, "I'm going home tomorrow." Ash was as textbook-mad as he had ever been, and had never mentioned anything about going home before that morning. He was madder around staff than patients. When alone with me he was fairly normal. It took a moment for this information to register in my brain, before I asked, "You mean you are being let out of hospital for a bit – on leave?" Ash replied, "Yeah, kinda. I'm being discharged properly, but I don't like where I am going: some druggie half-way house." "Oh." I said. "That's good for you though, getting out of hospital… They must think you are ready." We returned to our cigarettes in silence. I thought *fucking hell! They are letting Ash out before me. Shit, that is not good, I must be ill; I must get out.*

Ten days after the near-lethal heroin overdose, my room was searched again, and I was immediately ward-based because of what was found. They found about 10% of what I was hiding. They mainly found the stuff I put in places to be found:

> *2 strips of zopiclone (one empty, one full 20-blister pack)*
> *Anadin (4 used out of 6)*
> *Paracetamol (2 used out of 6)*
> *6 packs of risperidone, 3mg tablets, 10 used.*
> *1 full packet of dihydrocodeine*
> *5 diazepam used, 5 left in packet*
> *4 chlorpromazine (6 used)*
> *Smally bottle of brandy (full).*
> *4 cans of lager, 3 empty cans in bin.*

The next day I was allowed a nurse-escorted walk in the grounds. The following day, despite being *"pale, tired and avoidant,"* I was allowed out for a short cycle. That was 10-days after the 2nd heroin overdose; and the first day I requested that I be discharged from hospital. On the 11th day after the 2nd heroin overdose I requested discharge more firmly, able to say with honesty that I had not purchased any illicit substances. (Defining illicit as "illegal," not as the word was misused by the staff – according to them alcohol, paracetamol and laxatives were illicit. No: they are substances I should not have had and could have abused, but they are not illegal). Even the sedatives I imported were legal at that time. (No longer). I agreed with no hesitation that I would continue to see Steve Pearce to discuss my long-term care.

The following day, and every day after, I requested discharge from hospital stating that I felt trapped, disrespected (by some nurses), distrusted (which I deserved), and because they could not keep me safe. I was described as:

"Isolated."

"Slowed-up."

"Pleasant."

"Warm."

"Sleepy/sedated."

The next time I saw Dr. Ogilvie I repeated my request for discharge. "We" planned to hold a discharge meeting in four weeks; which seemed an eternity. But by then I had been in hospital for ¾ of a year, and so discharge is taken most carefully. Especially as most suicides are people who have just been discharged: and hey, let's face it, I must have been a near sure-bet for that eventuality. The day after, I began requesting that my discharge be speeded up.

On the 25th of January, 19 days after the 2nd heroin overdose, I turned 28 years of age. I was somewhat furious because I still believed I should have died whilst forever 27. If anyone knew of or remembered my delusion about this, they did not say so. But I was not allowed leave before my birthday. I did not share my disappointment at being 28. I was the only patient not to receive a cake from the hospital on her/his birthday, making me feel undeserving and reinforcing feelings about not-deserving food. But my medical notes show that people were starting to believe I had "turned a corner" and that I was improving. They record:

> *"Pleasant and tired."*

> *"Interacting with staff minimally."*

> *"Uneventful day."*

> *"Any of recent changes could have produced the current positive change in picture."*

> *"No management problems."*

> *"No deliberate self-harm."*

> *"Patient has ripped up and binned all of her suicide notes."* [Yeah, and she did it in front of you deliberately, to make you think she was better].

All of this was my playing at being "good." Nothing had actually changed; I intended to kill myself. Not everyone was fooled. I know John wasn't fooled: he told me so, and I didn't deny it because I respected him far too much. I doubt that Dr. Ogilvie was fooled either; but thankfully he did take in and digest my points that I hated being on the ward, and that *they could not keep me safe, or make me feel safe.*

In early February, Dr. Ogilvie granted me permission to go on leave from the ward. That did *not* mean that I was discharged, but it meant that I was allowed home (to Derby in my parents' care) on a trial basis for varying lengths of time. I remember quite clearly the meeting with Dr. Ogilvie – I went in, and immediately asked, with some desperation, to be allowed home because "I could not bear being in hospital any longer." Dr. Ogilvie spoke unflinchingly, saying a firm, "No." Then we discussed it, and, after some time, I remember him saying, "It's important to recognise you are a voluntary patient, and if you feel you would do better at home, and the risk of being at home is not that much different to that of you being here – where you have proved we cannot reasonably keep you safe – then I am inclined to agree, and let you go home for a few days to see how things go."

A few days turned into a couple of weeks with regular reviews with ward staff and Dr. Ogilvie or his SHO.

I continued saving up my lithium with which to overdose on. I would be back.

Chapter 12. Will all this end?

> Razors pain you;
> Rivers are damp;
> Acids stain you;
> And drugs cause cramp.
> Guns aren't lawful;
> Nooses give;
> Gas smells awful;
> You might as well live.

∾ *Resume* by Dorothy Parker, (1926).

I was so tired of life. I realised that time does not heal all like they promised. Some things go on, and on, and on... Back in early 2003 in the Warneford, I still hated everyone for saving me and wanted nothing but my death. I thought I understood my circumstances completely and that I was an utterly lost cause. Nothing was any better, and I was still haunted by a long and painful past. I had no faith that anything could improve my situation and I gave up (even more). My end would be a relief for all: so I believed with unreserved sincerity.

I wanted death to take me more desperately than I had when I had been admitted to hospital in the first place. All day, every day, and most of every night, I dreamed of finding a way to pacify my distempered spirit permanently. Nothing appeased my despair, nothing calmed my anger, nothing brought me any enjoyment, nothing caught my interest, nothing seemed worthwhile, nothing lowered my anxiety; and when, at the end of an endless, tortured day, I lay down and closed my eyes, the noise in my head just got louder. I yearned for death. I didn't care about anything, especially myself. I didn't want protecting, and I didn't want to be loved, because that made what I had to do more difficult. I was of the opinion that I had the right to extinguish my own existence, and nobody had the right to stop me or save me.

So in early February, in this extremely mixed/depressive state, I was (frankly) amazed to find myself allowed home for 3 days. Not alone at first, but into the care of my parents, living in the family home near Derby, a hundred miles away from Oxford. My bed on the ward was saved for my return from leave. The "agreed" long-term plan was that I would spend time in Derby, some time on the ward, and gradually more and more time at my home in Oxford – alone. I understand why I was allowed out. I had said all the "right" things, and even if I wasn't believed, (which I probably wasn't), the risks of me being out, were not that different to those of me being in hospital. True, hospitals are meant to keep you safe, but I had demonstrated repeatedly that I would attempt to take my life wherever I was "living." The ward offered no real shelter to me anymore.

My plan was to live in Derby, be "good," and kill myself as soon as I was allowed a night home alone in Oxford. I had been saving lithium for that exact purpose – hence I was not properly medicated. Not the wisest decision, but my choice at that time. It meant I was fairly strung-out on my own brain-chemicals: tense, angry, un-sleeping, irritable and on edge. After my initial 3-days at home, and a consummate performance of being "calm," I saw Dr. Ogilvie again and was allowed leave for 1½ weeks, back in Derby, and that time my bed was no longer kept open on the ward. I was due to see Dr. Ogilvie again at the end of my agreed leave, and, to test how I was alone in my Oxford flat; I was to spend the night before alone in Oxford

So, my patience paid off, and on a Thursday I drove from Derby to my flat on Iffley Road, where I ate three sandwiches, threw up, and stuck on the TV. A reality TV show set in a hair salon was on. I sat on my floor, and counted up my pills. I remembered that I had saved enough lofepramine to theoretically kill me many times over, (based on a dosage a playwright had used to kill herself). I'd also got lots of venlafaxine XR, chlorpromazine, diazepam, lorazepam and nearly two thousand zopiclone (sleeping) tablets. I also had Metoclopramide to stop myself vomiting; and, of course, the lithium which I expected to be lethal. I'd have liked something more dangerous like barbiturates, but I could not get hold of them.

For over an hour, I popped all the pills out of their blister-packets: designed thus to slow people down when they are overdosing and suicidal. Losing consciousness before I could pop out a lethal dose to swallow would not catch me out. I poured them neatly into medical containers, "ready to go."

Then Clare phoned.

If you remember, she lived in the same house as me, along with a number of other twenty-something year olds, students and post-docs from Oxford. I told her I was going to bed and didn't want company. With no prompt from me, she simply said, "Please don't do it." I denied any knowledge of what she was talking about. (Warning: explicit details of self-harm).

I took a few pills, fifty or sixty plus: a mixture of zopiclone, chlorpromazine and diazepam. I did it to make me sleepy, and to make the act of taking the prepared massive overdose easier to go through with. It was easier if I couldn't think too much about those I loved. But I couldn't forget Clare's words. She sounded desperate and sincere; she knew perfectly well what I was doing, but no one ever listened to her. All through my hospitalisation, she was my confident (not about everything, but about a lot – nearly as much as Dr. Ogilvie). She was my closest friend; she came to see me almost daily, and knew more about me, and my situation, than my own family. I was still very ill, very uncooperative, and hell-bent on self-destruction. I did not ask for help when I needed it, nor take it when offered. Usually.

I loved (still love) Clare deeply, and her literal begging had faced me with the reality that my death would cause others pain. Not wanting to hurt her, made me do something unusual. I voluntarily telephoned Vaughan Thomas ward at about 7pm, and told them I was in great distress and needed their help. The female nurse who answered (and knew me) told me that the ward was full, there was no bed for me, they couldn't help, and I should come in to the ward in the morning to see a doctor.

This ignited my fury at the total and utter stupid inconsistency of "care." I was not happy with this state of affairs, and nearly threw myself out of my window in anger. (It was a four-story, old, Victorian house, and would have killed me). I cried, cried and cried. Then I drank a bottle of wine, and sat staring at my hoard of pills. I realised it would be pointless to take them now, because I would be missed in the morning were I not at Vaughan Thomas ward and needed longer to be certain I was dead. So I hid them all, around the room, in my bag, the many pockets of my combat trousers, and some in a bottle hidden down my socks.

Then I phoned "my" heroin dealer, hoping to get some heroin, because I knew that would kill me too quickly for them to be able to save me in the morning. He told me to meet him in the usual place. I waited and he didn't come. I phoned again and he said he would be there, but he didn't show up. I phoned again and he cancelled my call. I phoned again and his phone was turned off. I nearly threatened to tell the police on him if he didn't deal to me, but then thought I'd end up with a knife through the ribs. And then I started to wonder if *that* would be a so bad, after all I wanted to die. I considered asking around in town, but did not dare. Instead I went home to my flat, fuming with rage. I couldn't think; I didn't know what to do. I felt like the whole world was conspiring against me. Obviously I was not rational in any sense of the word. I took a handful of pills without looking what they were, just wanting to sleep.

I called Clare and asked her to come and stay the night with me. When I woke up the next day, Clare was still half asleep beside me, and my parents were sitting on my sofa. I didn't understand how my parents could be there; shouldn't they have been in Derby? They frogmarched me to the Warneford hospital. Apparently there had been a lot of communication between Clare, Vaughan Thomas, and my parents during the night – none of which I could remember. Clare had phoned them all. The ward had told Clare to take me to Accident and Emergency during the night, but Clare hadn't done it because I had refused to go, and I said I would refuse to go in an ambulance. I'd obviously taken something, but admitted to twenty zopiclone tablets thinking no one would care about so few tablets, but everyone seemed terribly alarmed. (I took approximately 100 tablets in total, plus the bottle of wine). It was a small dose by my recent proportions. However, at that time nobody knew of the previous year's constant and large overdosing. There is also no such thing as a "safe" overdose.

I was immediately readmitted to Vaughan Thomas, and ward-based (restricted to the ward without any leave), although I was not sectioned. I was once again "voluntary" in name only. A chat and a bed the night before might have prevented the need for readmission – meaning I had to face being back on the ward for an indefinite period. I was very angry. But unfortunately, the NHS never has enough beds for the people who need them.

By this point I was obviously well past the point of being trusted, which felt absolutely horrible, but I cannot argue that it was not deserved! My bag was thoroughly searched by the ward manager, and of course there were bottles and strips of medication in it, including all the saved up lithium. I had to watch as she poured at least five hundred zopiclone tablets in the bin, thinking that they were my property: surely I should get them back? What gives anyone the right to throw away over five hundred pounds worth of *my* property? I was fuming. She also removed the alcohol, but that didn't bother me at all; apparently I would get that back. (I never did).

Then, when I thought things could get no worse, the ward manager told my parents to take me home to my flat, and remove any pills, or medical equipment with which I could do myself harm. The medical staff could not do that, or ask the police to do it as long as I had nothing illegal, and I didn't. I have no idea if this imposed search was legal; I argued but was bullied into compliance, in fact given no option other than to comply. My dad scared me far too much, and my mum appeared to have completely lost the plot, she was so stressed and angry with me. Again, I cannot argue that the search was the morally right thing to have happen, even if it pissed me off royally.

My parents had stayed in my flat on a couple of occasions whilst visiting me in hospital, and I soon discovered they had searched it before, but had not moved anything for whatever their reasons were. Now they had "permission" from the professionals, my room was ripped open to expose my most precious (and harmful) belongings, my parents heading straight for my hiding places without any hesitation. All my lignocaine, scalpels, blood-giving sets, needles, first aid equipment, chlorpromazine, diazepam, lorazepam, zopiclone, zolpidem, lofepramine, venlafaxine, metoclopramide, and even flipping cod liver oil tablets and vitamins were collected from their hidden and obvious places respectively. Nothing was missed, and all was handed over to Vaughan Thomas.

The principle of that search really upset and annoyed me. Yes, fine, I had dangerous items *in my own home*, and yes I was suicidal. That doesn't, or at least shouldn't mean I do not have basic legal rights. Nothing that was taken from me was illegal to possess or use, (this has since changed with regards to benzodiazepines being illegal to possess without a prescription, although I did have a prescription). Not one thing was ever returned to me; dangerous item or not. These things were *my* property. I felt as if I had been burgled, and my most important and treasured items (even if my "treasured" items were strange ones to be cherished), were taken or destroyed. Would I do *exactly* the same thing to my own child, friend or a patient, were the situation reversed? *Yes, of course I would: absolutely, thoroughly, and in a heartbeat.*

And so, my parents left me in Oxford. Once again I found myself trapped and angry, back on the (fucking) ward, back on the acute corridor, which I loathed. Clare stayed with me for a while, scared I would hate her for helping me, but I could never hate her. A year later, my Mum told me, that on that day, she said to my father that she could never live with me again, as it was too upsetting, and more than she could handle. I was crying as they left, feeling abandoned; watching them leave through the glass windows in the doors, and then the window. Apparently my head bowed, and I was dressed in my customary black. Stripped bare of all the items I had for years collected, saved, and spent money I didn't have on. My carefully planned exits from the world all gone and I reached a new low. I had nothing. Except the pills in my pockets and socks that no one had searched.

On 15th February I wrote:

> *"I'm back in the fucking hospital. Just had last two weeks out, mostly at home (Derby) with my parents. They know I smoke. Had a wobbly night at home (Oxford) alone: Clare ended up staying over. Now I am forced back into hospital where I do not want to be. I don't want to be anywhere. I don't want to be alive. They've taken MY stuff. I still have pills, but not enough to kill me. I am trying to*

think of another way to die. I am afraid to attempt suicide in case I am caught and have to stay here even longer, or I am sectioned, or I am sent to London.

It occurs to me that Ray was right all those months ago. He predicted that this would happen.

The only good thing is that Declan is back in here – so as least I have someone who cares."

So I spent some more time in hospital: on the acute ward where there is a window in your door and things are never private. After a few days, the getting-out plan Richard and I had previously created, (at the suggestion of Dr. Steve Pearce), was reinstated. I was to start from the beginning and start to work my way up from being ward-based again. I argued that the plan had been conceived at a time when I was afraid to leave the ward, and that as such, I had made it a very slow plan. I didn't want it to be so slow. Dr. Ogilvie took this plea on-board, believed me; and I was being truthful. He cut the time I was to spend at each level (of greater freedom) in half, thus halving the time to reach potential release from hospital. But it was still going to take many weeks, and I just didn't think I could bear it in there for another day, let alone weeks.

Everybody wanted to enable me to leave the hospital, but I had proved myself completely dishonest and disinterested cooperating for a meaningful recovery. I was failing more and more, which just meant I was going nowhere (except maybe London for treatment).

The fact that I had not been taking my lithium and risperidone had been noted and people (almost always) made certain I took what I was prescribed, when I was supposed to.

I discovered something unpleasant. Once upon a time I had wondered what on Earth I had to do in order to get noticed, and how to get help by being hospitalised. I thought hospital would help me. Now I had reached the stage where it was hard to get out of hospital even when appearing relatively OK. Thoughts of death and suicide that were at one time just noted, but not acted upon, were now holding me back. And since I had had suicidal ideation of varying intensities for my *entire life*, it was unlikely those feelings would go away. They didn't go away, but I realised I was going to have to be creative about that fact.

A small incident of self-harm, and I was back to square one again. I knew the consequences of my actions but was unable to choose to keep myself safe. The threat of being sent to a specialised unit in London for the foreseeable future hung over me again. I was no longer scared of being forced to leave the safety of ward: I couldn't stand being there anymore, largely because I was not trusted and was subsequently searched often. Nor did I feel particularly comforted by the place, or safe. I had to prove myself willing, work my way towards freedom. Or rather I had to *appear* willing, and lie.

Dr Ogilvie told me that I had to realise that if I was to persist in admitting to feelings like that I wanted to kill myself, even if I had no definite plans now: I would have to stay in hospital. Like him, *I listen* to people, and I took his words on-board. I decided to lie about some of my feelings from then on. I find it difficult to tell a straightforward lie – if I can twist someone's words, or my response, it is easy; but telling a direct lie is hard. But, I decided it was the lesser of two evils: how could I be honest when it faced me with a penalty too terrible to contemplate? A single day in hospital seemed like a year. I had lived for twenty-plus years with serious suicidal thoughts and if I had to stay in hospital until they went, I would be there a VERY long time. So I kept quiet, hid my self-harm, and lied.

I began with half an hour outside one Saturday to cycle. I actually went and bought a lethal dose of paracetamol and some booze. My thinking went along the lines of *OK you bastards, you've taken away all my easy suicide methods, so I'll have to die horribly and in pain, once my liver is failing you wont be able to help me, and then you will know that it was you who forced me to die so horribly.* This was extremely irrational and a direct response to my intense anger. There is no mention of my anger in my medical notes: I can't believe nobody could tell. I popped out all the paracetamol, had just swallowed three, when George popped his head around my door. I slid the pills under a book.

George asked me to remove the poster from the inside of my door because the staff needed to see into my room, because (apparently) I was on fifteen-minute checks. I told him he must be mistaken because I wasn't on any checks, and wanted more privacy. I truthfully pointed out that I was surrounded by men on the acute corridor: they were always looking in, sometimes just standing there, looking at me, sometimes trying to come in. I was sincere in both respects. I didn't know and had not been informed that I was on any observation checks.

Dark Clouds Gather

George was, and I assume is, a very thorough nurse, and was not afraid to do things necessary for my safety even if I hated him for it at the time. I remember one time he muttered to me, "Not you, I'll do anything it takes" by which I he meant he was not going to let me "succeed" at committing suicide. We had come a long time from the pleasant summer chats in the hospital garden about his football team Newcastle United; and my team, the best team in the world, Derby County. (Best team, delusional…? Ahem). I liked George and got on well with him, but he began to meticulously upset me by *forcing* me to be safe. Of course, I've gained perspective with time, and am now thoroughly grateful.

The power had shifted, nurses didn't treat me as friends, rather a menace that needed managing. (I cannot argue that I was not a management nightmare; manipulative, clever, deceitful and unwilling). I was voluntary in name only. At the time I quite cruelly wondered how much George was enjoying having power over me. It is entirely possible that he hated it. He went to read my notes. I was going to regret challenging him about my checks because it said in my notes that I was to be searched when returning to the ward from cycling. As I hadn't been searched at the time, my whole room was searched instead, and the drink and paracetamol was found. I did not actually ever intend to mix these together. I was going to drink instead of overdosing if I couldn't muster the emotional energy to overdose. George counted the number of paracetamol tablets, and compared to the packaging he realised three were missing, which he challenged me about.

I said I had a headache.

"Taken from Katy's bag:

35cl bottle of Scotch whisky
1 IV blood giving set.
Ex-lax tablets, 1 full box of.
Paracetamol tablets: ***. (Missing 3
according to package?).
1 razor [For my legs, but never
mind].
1 pair of scissors."

George would make a point of talking to patients
before he wrote up his notes. When he asked me if I
wanted a chat, and I decided I would talk to him: as a
damage limitation measure. I knew that he wanted to
get out of me all the juicy details of any plans so that he
could write them up. At the time I thought it was his
ego, wanting to be the nurse the "difficult patient"
confided in; but now I see he was doing his job and I do
believed he chose to do it because he is a caring man.

He asked me if I had planned to attempt suicide, and I
had to say, "Yes," because it was blatantly obvious
what I had intended. I added that it was just a thought, a
moment of weakness, and that *I had changed my own*
mind about going through with it, before the pills were
found. Obviously this was not going to look good when
I next saw Dr Ogilvie and asked to be allowed to go
home! George advised me to be on my "perfect
behaviour" if I was to have any chance of leaving the
ward soon. As it happened I didn't see Dr Ogilvie until
Wednesday, I think it was the very next week, but it is
entirely possible that an additional week, or two weeks
passed that I do not recall.

Dark Clouds Gather

Declan and I spent a lot of time together; we were close. He was making a lot of illicit money, but despite our relationship, (or perhaps because of it), he refused to sell me anything. We were always getting in trouble for being "inappropriate," but as far as I am concerned that was a stupid rule that nobody had the right to impose. We were adults after all. There was nothing rebellious, dangerous or inappropriate about our close relationship. I actually loved Declan – as much as you can when mania makes you, how shall I put it, more available to men and women than usual. The notes say:

> *"10.30pm. Katy found in Declan's room with him in it. Reiterated boundaries re: not going into another patient's room. Katy left. She was then observed to be sitting in front of the TV with Declan's head in her lap.*
>
> [The following day]. *Declan was found visiting Katy in her room. Boundaries were reiterated."*

After that event, my diary reads:

> *"Control freaks. Go on all you want bitch, you don't make the rules in my life. No one rules me. You can try, but I'll ignore you because I don't recognise your so-called authority. I might just blow up in your face, so watch out."*

OK, so there was a touch of rebellion in there, but only once my private business had been nosed into.

My mother had an idea that I write day-poems, one word per line, to describe each day, and to see how days were gradually improving. I wrote three of these day-poems waiting to see Dr. Ogilvie (which is what makes me think I saw him the next week). By the way, "fag" is an English slang term for two things: when I write fag here, I mean a cigarette.

Monday
Clock
Fag
Soup
Clock
Clock
Fag
Clock.
Fucking clock
Clock

That was a whole day on the ward for me. Not fun, and exceedingly boring. The next day, my parents arrived and I was allowed out with them during the day.

Tuesday
Fag
Decaf
Fag
Cycle
Fag
Phone
Fag
Parents
Soup
Fag

Car
Town
Benefit office
Fag
Coffee
Walk
Beer
Fag
Clare
Cinema
Fag
Beer
Football
Baileys
Car
Hospital
Goodbye
Cry
Meds
Bed
Sleep.

Much as I would love to have been more poetic, I couldn't be. But such candid expression is quite true to the direct-natured person that I am. Poetry is something I very much appreciate, but have absolutely no talent in producing. Time passed at a snail's pace. My notes say:

"Moping around."

"Compliant   but   increasingly isolated."

"Heard discussing suicide with a number of other patients." [Come on; be realistic! It's an adult, general psychiatry ward; suicide gets talked about a lot by *everyone*].

"Quiet, no interaction with staff."

Despite my mum saying she could not live with me, my parents were in Oxford to see Dr. Ogilvie and hopefully take me home with them again. I was desperate to leave, and was determined to leave or die that week. Nobody knew that of course, and telling anyone that would not have done my case for release much good. Wednesday arrived; Judgement Day. I packed up all my stuff, took my posters down, unable to comprehend the possibility of being forced to remain as a patient any longer. Apparently the ward my parents were told I would not be allowed home before the meeting began. Instead, I was staring in the face of a Section 3 (a six month involuntary detention for treatment) and transfer to London.

I sat in the chair in the middle of the main corridor, waiting my turn. I was called in. I lay down my copy of the book "An Unquiet Mind" by Kay Redfield Jamison, and the first words out of my mouth were that I wanted to go home. Dr. Ogilvie replied in his Scottish tones, a gentle, but firm, "No." And… the world as I perceived it started to crumble around me into intolerable agony. I crumbled too, the faces of the people talking at me crumbled, the walls of the hospital crumbled, and I knew that I must and would die, if only to escape the hole in this hospital/prison that I had built for myself.

George was there, and he described the paracetamol incident. The crumbling continued as they began to talk about me continuing on my behavioural program, being allowed out a little more each day. At which point my mind left my body and paid no attention, the words in the room were too painful to hear. Then at some point, I re-focussed and turned and addressed Dr. Ogilvie as if he was the only person in the room. I spoke directly and honestly, saying I could *not* remain on the ward because it would break me: he had to let me go. I wanted to go home. Wherever I was, life was horrible, but things were slightly less horrible at home. That was all truthful. I then added a lie that he needed to hear, which was that I had no plans to kill myself. I doubt he believed me because Dr. Ogilvie understood me very well by then. Still I had to say it because he could not release me if I told him I had suicidal thoughts or plans. He asked if I wanted my parents to come in and join the discussion, and so they did.

My mum was quite strident about her fears of having me home, obviously not wanting me released. I was shocked and angry with her at the time, not understanding why she wasn't helping me to become free. Now I know she was afraid, couldn't cope well, and certainly couldn't protect me. My dad, who has never liked psychiatrists or therapists "interfering," seemed keen to help me get home. Both my parents have always wanted to keep family problems in the family and not bring outsiders in (to judge). I have a good idea why. I used to think it was because I was bad, disgusting, wrong and shameful.

Dr. Ogilvie changed his mind, and said I could go home. I think that is the sign of a secure clinician, to be able to listen and change an opinion that is quite literally life or death. Dr. Ogilvie's answer to my mum's fear was that I was at high risk both on the ward, with the availability of illicit drugs, and off the ward, at home.

My packing was already done and so I practically legged it out of that ward. I sat in the back of my parent's car: Oxford passed me by, then the motorway, and then fields, and then I was home. I was happier for a day or two, because I was free. I did little, and had no energy. After a few days the novelty wore off, but at least I was able to drive to the shops everyday, and could buy alcohol that wasn't allowed on the ward. I got through each day by telling myself I could go to sleep at the end of it. I had sleeping pills to help.

Sunday

Home

Bed

Fag

Stroke Bob [dog]

Decaf

Cycle

Fag

Decaf

Drive

Supermarket

Drive

Home

Fag

Peas

Fag

Walk Bob

Papers

Fag

Write
Sick
Bath
Fag
Write
Bailey's
Fag
T.V.
Read?
Paint?
Diary
Pills
Fag
Dinner
Bed
(Hospital tomorrow).

I don't remember much from this time of my life. It's probably for the best, because I was so incredibly low. Gone was any energy, except mental, and even that was slow. I hit a low, major depression and got stuck in the murky mud down at the bottom. Beth said I didn't wash, eat much, and I wore the same baggy black clothes all the time, even with food stains on them. Apparently I was "zombie like," totally oblivious to life passing me by. Memories are hazy. This blurry life was only punctuated by visits to see Dr. Steve Pearce or Dr. Ogilvie. I was living in Castle Donington, Derby: and being cared for by the Oxfordshire mental health services.

When I woke up, (always early) I felt appalling, and I dreaded the long day ahead. I had nothing to do that I enjoyed so would sit around doing nothing, and play with my dog for ages. My main memories are of staying hidden under my duvet until nearly midday, because in bed I didn't have to face the world. I'd stick on my TV, but there was nothing worth watching on it. Periodically I would sit and stair out of my window at the trees in the garden, looking how they intertwined, or lean out of my window to smoke, whilst staring at the patio. Sometimes I'd paint, without much talent. One day I poured my medication on the floor and painted a picture of them all, there were so many different pills, most of which I thought were useless. I thought the venlafaxine XR made me worse, but I kept taking it. Some hypnotics helped me sleep a bit, and this time I stuck with lithium because of the strenuous recommendation for it in the book I had just finished reading by Prof. Kay Redfield Jamison. I felt that, at any moment, I might implode with the enormous boredom and uselessness of it all.

This went on for weeks, as I waited for drugs to arrive over the Internet (to my Oxford address of course), and planned various suicide methods. I was far lower in mood than I had ever been, so low in fact, that I barely managed to put together a cohesive plan. I managed to spend a few nights in my flat in Oxford, which pleased Dr. Ogilvie, but he didn't know of my ulterior, (in fact only) motive: waiting for the arrival of pills from over the Internet. They took ages to arrive so I went home to Derby. Then they arrived and I picked them up on a trip to Oxford to see Dr. Pearce. I told him about them, for some reason I am not aware of, but I didn't tell him that I had them with me in my bag at that actual moment. Whilst driving myself home I took three 100mg chlorpromazine tablets. I knew this was dangerous, (remember one 100m tablet had paralyzed me once) and I did want to crash, but I *didn't* want to hurt anyone else so I did not attempt to crash. (I have not counted this as a suicide attempt, even if it was stupidly reckless).

All I have in my diaries from this time are odd words or those strange poems. I know I came to see Dr. Ogilvie many times, but I can remember nothing: not the journey, not being seen on the ward (technically I was still an in-patient), or seeing Dr. Ogilvie himself. I do know I came down to see him a few times. My medication was not changed, because I had to get used to living in a new environment again, after years living independently and then in hospital. Moving back in with my parents after years of (ill) autonomy) is a hard thing to do, and would ideally have been avoided.

[My last ever diary entry]. "*It's Monday sometime in early March 2003. I went to see "The Hours" today. It's about Virginia Woolf's suicide, life, enduring life, enduring hours, thinking about death and suicide, and the trivialities of life. I had to go secretly as it was billed as having a "strong suicide theme." It was very good. She and I have a lot in common. It has made me think about drowning myself though. What if I attach myself to our big old barbeque and jump in the pool when no one is around? That should hold me down once I lose consciousness, and prevent me from changing my mind once I'm down under the water.*

I wish I could take a leaf out of Robbie's book and say, 'Wherever it may take me, I

know that life wont break me,' but I can't
because I am already broken."

I saw Dr. Steve Pearce every month, to discuss my future, and if I wanted to get further treatment. The suggested option was that I join a therapeutic community. I liked talking to Steve Pearce, even though we talked about difficult topics. He was very good at putting me at ease. On one visit I told him goodbye, because I was going to overdose on paracetamol. If had he not talked so well and so convincingly about it being a shame if I died, I would have decided he didn't care, and would have walked away feeling I had his permission. He was rightly concerned, and for just a moment I worried he might not let me leave and insist I came into hospital. But he didn't, so I left, and a few days later, at the end of March, I took the overdose exactly as I said I would. In my medical notes he wrote that by warning him, I must have felt ambivalent and wanted help – but no action was taken to stop me. Never expect anyone to miraculously save you – you will die. (Warning: explicit details of attempted suicide).

After many weeks of trying to think of a way to kill myself I tried putting a plastic bag over my head on a couple of occasions, but never managed to lose consciousness before I panicked. (I haven't counted these as suicide attempts or even self-harm, as I was more "testing-the-method for tolerability" than actually attempting anything definitive). After this, with nothing to hand with which to end my life the way I would like, desperation lead me to consider a method I never wanted to use. Mum had just searched my room and removed £400 worth of sleeping pills I had waited so long for, which made me angry. I didn't want to die from a paracetamol (acetaminophen) overdose because I know using just paracetamol alone is a slow and painful way to die, taking a minimum of five days, but up to two or three weeks. I know of another substance that I had better not name, that I could mix with the paracetamol that would lead to death in less than an hour, but I had no way of getting hold of this medication; nor did I expect a doctor prescribe it for me, and anyway, my GP was still Dr. MacLennan, a hundred miles away in Oxford.

With a paracetamol (acetaminophen) overdose, almost universally, death is the result of liver failure; the patient usually dies in a long drawn-out hospitalisation, which I did not want to do. I wanted to die outdoors in the Derbyshire countryside. I did not want to have days or weeks where I would be ill, but conscious, and have to face my family and friends, knowing I could not be saved. I didn't want to do that to myself or to them.

But I was desperate, angry, needed immediate gratification, and was too low in mood to plan anything more elaborate. Maybe simplicity would finally bring success? Paracetamol certainly kills. I found myself staring at a half-used single packet of paracetamol that I still had hidden. I knew that to be reasonably certain of death, I needed more than twelve grams of paracetamol, and I only had eight. I also knew that paracetamol is one of the only drugs that when overdosing, you don't mix it with alcohol. People tend to mix overdoses with alcohol to improve the chances of dying, usually a "good" idea; but alcohol actually competes for the same receptor in the liver as alcohol, so taking alcohol at the same time is actually protective of the liver. Anyway, it was early in the morning, and I realised I would have to get my hands on more paracetamol. I wasn't allowed to drive to the shops by myself, and certainly couldn't return home with boxes of pills that would be checked for. So I took Bob for a walk.

In the United Kingdom, paracetamol can only be bought in little boxes of sixteen 500mg tablets. This is to try and reduce its use by the general population for overdosing, as it is the most common cause of "intentional" self-harm[28] in the UK accounting for approximately 70,000 cases per year, a small proportion of which, die. Paracetamol is the commonest cause of acute liver failure, which means certain death unless a liver transplant is performed. Once again, my knowledge made me more lethal, I knew I needed more paracetamol, and I knew the antidote (administered intravenously) needed to be used quickly ideally within four hours. I believed that if I was not discovered within the first ten to twelve hours, nothing could be done; except maybe a liver transplant that is unlikely to be approved and which I could refuse. The dose I eventually took was lethal several times over.

Bob and I walked down into the centre of Castle Donington, where there are a few little shops. I managed to buy *** more boxes with sixteen tablets in each. Now I had ***g of paracetamol. (Enough to kill 5 men). I bought a bottle of diet coke, deciding caffeine

---

[28] This figure comprises paracetamol overdoses presenting for medical treatment: overdosing for self-harm's sake *and* for attempting suicide with serious suicidal intent. From many internet forums, it has been my experience that many people take "small" overdoses of paracetamol to self-harm, possibly daily and for long periods of time – These are not reported, hence cannot be part of the 70,000 recorded annually: their long-term affect is unknown.

would best aid my task, and stood in the middle of the street, swallowing all *** tablets, in plain view, and with my little dog at my feet. I didn't care if anyone saw me, as long as I didn't see anyone I knew (who could tell my parents and thus stop my plan). People did look at me; I didn't care, believing myself unbeatable. I threw all the boxes away in the village centre, and we walked home. On arrival I asked dad for a couple of paracetamol for a headache, which I promptly swallowed. In retrospect I think that was rather cruel of me, but meant I totalled *** + 1g of paracetamol. I was convinced that if I could keep quiet until eight that evening, I would certainly be dead, still alive, but beyond treatment that could keep me alive.

I can't remember what I did with myself during that day, but I was calm, content and resolute. I do remember dad offering me a sleeping pill around lunchtime: something he never did before or again, so that I could get some sleep. Of course, I was so used to large numbers of sleeping pills that it did nothing. I tried to sleep though. Then dad knocked on my door at about three in the afternoon, and asked me to come downstairs. They had called out an emergency doctor. I didn't speak, waiting to see what the doctor and my parents knew first, and I soon realised that they didn't know about the paracetamol, they just wanted me to go back into a psychiatric hospital. Now since I could no longer cope with hospitalisation in Oxford, on a ward with staff I trusted and patients I knew: I certainly could *not* cope with a hospitalisation in Derby, on a new, strange ward.

The emergency doctor referred me to the hospital, and I had little choice other than to go, because had I been unwilling to be assessed, it would have been suggestive that I was hiding something. I didn't foresee any chance that they might hospitalise me, as I would give them no reason to do it. I saw a young female doctor, who asked me all the usual psychiatric history questions. Of course, I couldn't deny I had got depression, as it would have been blatantly lying. I needed to be considerably more devious than that. I denied *any* current thoughts or plans of suicide and self-harm, I acknowledged the past but said I was much better, was enjoying some things, had no harmful intentions, and was at absolutely no risk. During all of this time, the paracetamol overdose was swimming in my bloodstream, but I uttered not a word, nor did a single give-away expression cross my face.

They told me they would still like me to come into hospital; that they recommended I come in voluntarily. I didn't show any emotion, no fear, I reiterated that I had no desire to hurt myself and was happiest at home. Then they used that time-old scare tactic of threatening to section me if I didn't agree. Now there are times like this when you don't push back in case you are sectioned; but I was more than prepared to risk it. If I ended up in hospital it no longer mattered to me if I was sectioned or not. I decided to call their bluff. I was reasonably certain that they couldn't really section me based on what I had said.

I could feel the exasperation with me permeating the entire room. My parents, the doctor, and the two nurses who were there. (Two nurses, did they think I'd run? Where the hell to?) The only tenuous reason they had, was that I had purchased a large number of sleeping pills, but as I pointed out, I only wanted them to sleep, it was cheaper to buy in bulk, and I knew it would be impossible to overdose lethally on the amount of zopiclone ordered, which was all I had been able to afford. I reiterated again and again that I had no suicide plans. So I had given them no reason to involuntarily admit me, yet the young doctor still wanted to hold me. (She will make an excellent psychiatrist). My parents were desperate to get me admitted, but since I didn't tell them how I felt, they couldn't honestly answer that I had indicated to them, any risk to myself.

Bored by now, I demanded to see the consultant psychiatrist, so the young doctor phoned him, and (without seeing me) he agreed with me that if I said I was not in any form of risk, or was not doing anything that suggested I was intending to put myself at risk of harm, they could not force me stay. I am not writing this as a criticism of anyone; I took the law and used it to my purpose: not disclosing anything to anyone, not even my parents, meant I was able to make it impossible to section me even when it was plainly obvious I needed help. It was my doing, my choice.

Had I been seen in Oxford I would have been whipped into hospital faster than something very, very fast. If I'd seen Dr. Ogilvie, I would have been unable to lie. Or if I had tried to lie, he would have known, and would have been able to force me to stay based on him knowing my history and suspecting my lies. Derby did not know of my lies. All my medical records were in Oxford.

When I was told I could go, I had to force myself not to skip out of there with glee! I think that despite their lack of knowledge of me as a patient; lack of proof I was suicidal; together with my outright denial of all suicidal intent; they still been very close to forcing me to stay. My tired (and I suspect frustrated) parents decided to pick up a Chinese meal on the way home. I looked at my watch, nine o'clock. *That is it I'm dead: finally!* I thought. By half past ten, I was lying in my bed, after picking at my prawns in garlic sauce. I'd taken my night meds, and was preparing to attempt sleep.

I didn't even think of the paracetamol by now hammering at my liver, I had decided instead, to enjoy the last day or so of my life before I was hospitalised to die. My mood was certainly improved at the prospect of death. I wonder if my parents had spotted that improvement in mood earlier and called the doctor – I doubt it. I still don't know why they did call him that particular day. As it happens, if I *had* been admitted to that psychiatric hospital, I would probably be dead now. Once again I was exceptionally lucky. My extreme efforts to kill myself and not get caught or hospitalised, actually lead to me being caught.

Clare phoned me on my mobile. If I had been forcibly hospitalised earlier, I would not have had my phone with me, and therefore would not have spoken to her. There was a mistake in my knowledge. Although a paracetamol overdose is *best* treated within ten to twelve hours, (preferably less), the antidote, usually *N*-acetylcysteine, can be effective up to twenty-four hours, and occasionally even forty-eight hours after the overdose. I don't remember what time Clare called, but it was sometime before midnight. I was dopey because of all my meds, and combined with me thinking it was far too late to save me, I decided to say goodbye. I can't imagine what that must have been like for her, especially when she was not well herself. I told her that I loved her, what I had done and that it was too late to save me now.

Clare would later tell me that she actually felt relieved. Then she felt guilty for feeling that. She thought that after supporting me through the previous year's hell, my lifelong pain would finally be over soon. She had lived battling her own illnesses whilst being a damn good friend to me with my depression and constant suicide attempts. (Sometimes even helping me when advised to distance herself for her own sanity). I will also support her to the end, hers or mine, and I think I would have been similarly relieved were our roles reversed. But none of that stopped her from phoning my parents, who immediately burst into my room, and took me to the hospital I had been turned away from a few hours before. I was sleepy, I don't remember it that well, but I have wondered since if that young doctor was still there. The Psychiatric Hospital sent me to the Derby Royal Infirmary, to the only Accident and Emergency department in Derby.

It was eerie. I had been to the same A&E department many times. Once as a kid when I broke my wrist, and had to wait hours to be seen. I also worked there as a student, when the A&E Consultant made me his pet student to take and see all the interesting cases. It's where I first saw the results of a car crash close up, and nearly passed out when I saw a boy, approximately six, with holes where lots of his face was meant to be, and he lived. I held his face and calmed him whilst he was being anaesthetised. I've hardened since then. I still prefer to be the health carer than the patient.

This time, I was definitely a patient and there was no wait at all. I was rushed in since it was approaching fifteen hours after my large overdose, and too late to pump my stomach, (paracetamol is adsorbed very quickly anyway). I vaguely remember being asked a lot of questions, mostly things like what medications are you on, do you smoke, nothing about the intent of my overdose, or my past attempted suicides. I was told I'd be admitted and on a drip for quite a while. I asked if I could have a cigarette before they put the drip in, so I left and went outside. I was followed, and so I returned. Then I don't remember much until a few hours later, I was having trouble breathing and was given oxygen. Then I woke up properly at four in the morning, turned off and took out the saline drip in my right arm. Then I turned to my left arm and just started to take out the *N*-acetylcysteine drip, changed my mind and pushed it back in. I decided that if I were discovered to have pulled my drip out in the morning, I'd be put in restraints and probably involuntarily admitted to a psychiatric ward once the danger from the paracetamol had passed.

The staff were not friendly, but nor did they treat me badly. A few nurses and two doctors were actually very good during my three-day stay in hospital. Of course I had to be psychiatrically assessed; performed by a senior nurse who specialised in people who had just been admitted for emergency treatment following attempted suicide. There was no doubt in anybody's mind that I had intended to die, because of the size of my overdose. (I'll repeat that I don't think the possible lethality of a chosen method of attempted suicide should be the only indicator used for future risk). Anyway, it wasn't the only parameter they used, because they also wanted to talk to me. And I, as was by then customary: lied, smiled, and expressed regret.

I said it had been impulsive and that I had intended to kill myself; I'd just been upset. I said I had not ever attempted suicide, and they had no medical history to check. I'd met a girl with liver disease in the smoking room, and described her, saying how scared I was at the thought of ending up ill like her. I said I didn't realise how dangerous paracetamol was, or what sort of dose was dangerous. I said I definitely wouldn't do it again, and I wouldn't try to leave the medical ward I was on until I was told it would be safe for me. I noticed this experienced nurse was nodding and smiling at me; he said I would be able to go home soon as he didn't think I needed admitting as a psychiatric patient. I explained (lied) that I was depressed and wanted more help, and that that was why I did it: to get help, not die. He promised to put me in touch with a Derby psychiatric team to help me, promising they would call me in less than a week. I never heard from them.

The specialist nurse said that if this had been our second meeting, or if I had committed another separate suicide attempt, things would be different, but since this was my first time and swore I hadn't really intended to die, he was inclined to believe me. First time? Try at least 443rd time. Obviously I was lying to this man, the reason being I didn't want any help. I felt that I was *beyond* help, and that death was just the next suicide attempt away. I'd had help, good therapy, good nurses, good doctors, good friends, my family, and medication after medication: the result? Living hell. I had diagnosed myself as untreatable. I felt it was a clear decision, not clouded, not filled with blame or poor self-esteem, but factual. I knew the depression would be biasing my decision, but I felt that if I had to go on living with the depression, the decision deserved to be biased. But for now, I had to play at being sane so that I could get out and try again, maybe in a new way. I could be patient for a while, as long as I could plan an ending to it all.

Despite my Oscar worthy performance, the nurse specialist must have had some reservations. He told me he'd get a psychiatrist to see me, just to back up his recommendation that I didn't need follow-up, psychiatric, inpatient care. He said the dose I had taken didn't fit in with his idea of a first time, impulsive or non-serious attempt. I can't argue with those facts. However, I am a very persuasive (manipulative) person. If he'd thought about it a little longer, he might have questioned why someone who had studied medicine didn't know what dose of paracetamol was dangerous, and why, acting on impulse, she calmly went to several shops to buy several packets of paracetamol, and then told no one for hours, even sitting through a psychiatric assessment, until she thought she was beyond saving. Stupid man.

My parents arrived a bit later in the morning to see me, and brought a packet of cigarettes. I didn't know it at the time, but when my parents left the hospital the previous night, they had been told to prepare for the worst. My bed was at the window end of a female ward, and the window overlooked the guest car park. I saw them arrive, though they didn't see me watching. My mum stepped out of the car, and I have never seen someone look so tired, pale and terrified. Later I would learn that mum had repeated that she couldn't live with me any more, but dad told her that she would have to. I suppose dad felt obliged to do this? I expect living with me, and loving me, would have broken most people. I do not blame my mum for reaching breaking point; I blame myself for pushing her to reach it.

I was on the *N*-acetylcysteine drip for a night and a long day, until ten in the evening. I was pushing to go home, but was told once the drip was finished they'd need to repeat liver enzyme tests on me to make sure I was recovering as opposed to going into liver failure. By this time, I was suitably pissed off with being hospitalised to wish that my liver was OK and I could go home. There was no fun during this brief hospitalisation, no wonderful "mad" people to talk to, no comfy smoking room, and no understanding psychiatric nurses. I was on a women's ward, everyone at least fifty years older than me, and mostly asleep or comatose. I was so bored!

My sister Beth, and her friend Matt (who is now a friend of mine) came to visit me at my request. I was bored stupid, and feeling very low. They came quite late in the evening, and Matt gave me what I suppose was meant to be an anti-suicide pep talk. It can be very hard to understand why someone does not just act differently, think differently, and "get a grip." But it is *never* that easy, and expecting it to be easy can make things worse for the sufferer because they feel they are failing.

Whilst Beth and Matt were visiting, my drip finally stopped. I was so pleased and went to take it out, as I have done countless times. My sister said, "Don't! If you take that out I'll kill you!" There was a silent pause, with me thinking, *yes please, that's fine with me, I seem to keep fucking it up.* When we realised what she had said, threatening to kill her sister who was in hospital for attempted suicide, we laughed; it was the only thing to do. Beth cried and told me she was so angry with me that she almost hadn't come to see me. I felt bad. Then Beth and Matt left, and as soon as they did, I removed the drip from my left hand, and went for a cigarette in the dingy smoking room.

A set of bloods was sent off that night, but the registrar, who was very decent and treated me as a totally worthwhile human being, said I would need to stay the night, whatever the results, it was after all, going on for eleven at night. He wanted to press and squeeze my abdomen, obviously hard for someone who hates her body, and at one time would have been impossible for me. But I seemed to be somewhat better able to cope with such things, and didn't care that much. I expect he was checking for a tender abdomen, and/or an enlarged liver, which would obviously be a worrying sign. I still felt absolutely fine.

The ward sister came over to tell me off quite loudly for taking out my own drip. I was annoyed. I said, "Look, I asked for one of you to take it out, and nobody showed for over an hour; since I've put in and removed thousands of these things I was fairly certain I knew what I was doing, I wanted a cigarette, the drip had finished, you told me so yourself." She scurried back to her desk, but rather than treat me as someone she was pissed of with, she seemed to have more respect for me.

Then a psychiatrist also came to assess me and I lied again. It was easier to lie to strangers. I went into some detail about the girl I had met with liver failure, all her drips into veins all over the place, her arms, her hands, her stomach, and her unhealthy yellow skin colour. I claimed that meeting someone with real liver failure in the smoking room meant I would never do it again. He was easier to persuade than the nurse specialist. From that point on, theoretically I was declared sane (enough).

Dark Clouds Gather

I was stuck there for another day, and spent most of it smoking in the smoking room. There was a lovely bunch of Derbyshire people there. The was a guy of about twenty-two who had taken a slightly smaller overdose (about 2/3rds of what I took – he had been very serious in his intent also), and who had passed out and been discovered within two hours. He had been in hospital for nine days because his liver enzymes were not returning to normal. I remember a thought that I'd never last that long in this place. I was going to leave that day even if it meant walking home.

Despite being such a popular choice for self-harm and attempted suicide, deaths from paracetamol overdose are fortunately rare: around two hundred a year in Britain according to the British Medical Journal. My liver enzymes kept coming back too bad to enable me to be discharged, until eight in the evening, and the ward sister (the same one I had had the altercation about removing my drip with earlier) said I could go, they were still bad, but getting no worse. I was told to get them checked again by my GP for a while, and letters were sent to various people.

The next day I drove down to Oxford to see Dr MacLennan. I gave him the letter from the Derby Royal Infirmary, and he read it, and then looked at me. I suppose he didn't know what to say as I was proving difficult to be help. I wish I could have read his mind, what on earth would he be thinking? Probably, "Oh no, not again." (Re: the bowl of petunias in *The Hitchhiker's Guide to the Galaxy* by Douglas Adams). I was very low, I don't remember anything much of that appointment. I think he checked my arm, and it had no new cuts on it, but an experienced eye would know I had either been injecting something, or bloodletting. I think I'd been bloodletting, though I may well have crushed some sedatives to inject, I don't remember. The times I have self-harmed or intended to take my life are blurred from this time. I hated life, and wanted out, but I was exhausted from the effort. I know Dr MacLennan would have been very kind, considerate and warm to me, he always was.

What I do remember thinking, was that it was ironic that I was far, far, FAR more depressed and suicidal that day, than I was on the day about a year earlier when I had first been "voluntarily" admitted to hospital for my own safety, at his advice. It didn't make sense. But there was no way I could go back into hospital, nor was the subject even broached. I had exhausted the benefits of hospitalisation, and now could no longer cope on the inside. I would have to survive on the outside, or not at all. I intended it to be *not at all.*

"If you don't know where you are going, any road will get you there."

– Lewis Carroll (1832-1898)

And so I returned to Derbyshire, and was invited to a barbeque by Matt at his friends' house. I went and it was a good day. It was the day I decided that I was going to eat anything I wanted, no more eating disorder bullshit. I had a hotdog and ice cream. I haven't looked back since. Unfortunately, starting that week, I also spent time driving around to find a spot where I could jump in front of a high-speed train. Such a method broke many of *my* suicide rules. It meant risking hurting other people, totally freaking out the train driver, and quite definitely would *not* have left a reasonably looking, or even intact body to be found, which I assume would need to be identified by my family. I expected it would hurt a lot too, but only for a second. Then I wondered if that last second would seem long to me?

But I was desperate with a minimum 443 failed attempts surely I couldn't fail if I jumped before a train. (Knowing my luck, I'd probably survive, but without any legs). According to a suicide website, it was one of the most highly lethal choices. So I looked for a spot, and mentioned none of this to anyone. I stood close by trains, pulsing past me, centimetres from death. And every day I wanted to jump, and everyday I could not manage it. I just did not have the energy or confidence it would work.

It was on one of these days, less than a week after attempt 443, whilst driving around I saw a nineteen/twenty-year old girl plummet to her death off a bridge and on to the side of the road I was driving. I'd like to say that it opened my eyes and made me stop feeling suicidal, but it didn't. I don't like driving under bridges anymore, especially if I can see somebody on top. A girl who was between eighteen and twenty died in a horrific and violent way, right before my eyes. I empathised, I knew how she must have felt, and as I was still quite ill myself, I was actually jealous that around ten years my junior, she had succeeded at something I had repeatedly failed at. I was the most depressed of anytime in my life.

I was in Derbyshire driving on a road that goes under a high bridge, thinking my usual dark thoughts, heading for home. I have no idea why I particularly noticed her, but in the distance I saw this dark-haired girl walk on to the bridge. There is something about a person similarly afflicted that a similar soul can pick up on – I saw her and I just knew what was happening, even at a distance. She walked straight towards the edge, and without a moment of hesitation, she just almost jumped over the rails, and … stepped off. She did it as if it was nothing, almost if she expected to fly. She hit the ground sideways but mainly feet first, smack, and crumpled like a compressing concertina. I almost felt her head crack as it impacted the road. I pulled over the car, and stopped to "help," call an ambulance and if needed, perform CPR.[29]

For a moment, I thought her heart was still beating, her chest moved as if she was breathing, but I'm not sure if I imagined that. Some of her head and brain was missing, and the lower half of her body was totally crushed. Fortunately she was unconscious. Moments later she had definitely stopped breathing.

I chose not to perform CPR. I have tortured myself about this decision, with thoughts that someone who was less sympathetic to her suicidal aim would have tried to keep her alive. I am, after all, trained to resuscitate, and people chose to resuscitate me when there was almost no hope. On that terrible day I did think, and I still think, that the girl dying before my eyes wouldn't want to live so severely disabled. But in honesty this is all moot. I knew at a glance that her injuries were lethal. She was so broken that there was nothing to save. I didn't see a point in pointlessly prolonging her death, and at least someone was with her when she died. I closed her eyes, leaving my hand over her eyes for what felt like an age, and hoped she was at peace. I don't even know her name.

---

[29] Cardiopulmonary resuscitation.

I continued to look for suitable spots for myself, and I also bought six more packets of paracetamol. Every morning, I would open a little plastic bag that I had popped all the pills in to, and sat with them in my hand, ready to take. But I never did. I just didn't have the energy to go around that loop, or any other suicide loop yet again. I guess I had reached that low-point of depression where you are so low you cannot find the energy to kill yourself. I was run down.

I continued to regularly visit Dr. Steve Pearce down in Oxford at the psychotherapy department. He was supposed to be helping me consider where to go from "here," how to cope with certain issues, and to stay out of hospital, in order to one day get back a more normal life. He's tall and thin, and would fold himself into one of the chairs in his office, arms behind his head or folded, his legs disappearing off into infinity on the weird red rug on his office floor. I told him about the paracetamol not working, but as I am not a mind reader I don't know what he actually thought about this, especially since I had told him I was going to do it before I did. He did say he was pleased it hadn't worked because it meant I had a chance to be helped and recover instead of having no chance.

Steve Pearce fascinated me in the respect that I could not work him out, something I am normally quite good at with people. I liked him, but in a way feared him too, because I was meant to talk to him about the worst things in my life. He is clearly intelligent and experienced, but I did not fully understand him as a person, coping with doing the job he does; and in that respect I felt awe. Part of me was scared to be under his care because the people he helps seem to me to be those people who are most damaged, possibly with the poorest prognosis, unresponsive to medication or not suitable for medication. I certainly was (am) very damaged, and my prognosis was terrible, and is still lower than what I am really capable of, though it does seem to be improving.

Steve Pearce and I spent several weeks discussing the possibility of me going to a therapeutic community, to live, and heal, for a year of my life. This idea did not appeal to me at all, especially when you can't be on medication. I've also lost far too much time to illness already. Steve Pearce said he would find out if Dr. Ogilvie thought it was possible for me to come off my medications. The answer was a resounding "No!" So Steve found a therapeutic community in Leicestershire where you can take medication. But I didn't want to go. I gave it consideration because I felt I should consider all the advice offered to me, but I did not want to go. I have had so much group therapy, sitting around, discussing life, art therapy, life-skills, illnesses, so on and so forth. I felt with some assurance that another year of doing just that, when I would be bored and unable to open up about myself, would be The Wrong Choice.

And so I returned to Derby, then Oxford, and then Derby: back and forth. I had an appointment with Dr. Ogilvie, and dutifully attended. I told him about the paracetamol incident, since I assumed he would have heard from Steve Pearce or Neil MacLennan. I did not mention about my current searching for a train spot, or the girl who died dying before my eyes. Dr. Ogilvie told me that he wanted to make sure that *I* knew that *he* knew I was more depressed than ever. It was a relief to hear those words, to be understood. There was no mention of re-hospitalisation by either party.

At some point, I cannot recall exactly when, I had an official discharge meeting from Vaughan Thomas ward. Present were four nurses, two social workers, Dr. MacLennan, my parents and myself. I think I recall Steve Pearce being there briefly, and Dr. Ogilvie was off work poorly. I was touched that so many people actually turned up. Chris (a social worker) ran the meeting, and I was officially discharged from the Warneford Hospital. I continued to see Dr. Ogilvie and Dr. Steve Pearce as an outpatient, as I had been doing whilst technically an in-patient.

On one visit, Dr Ogilvie suggested I could try amitriptyline with lithium, instead of the venlafaxine XR (and lithium). Then he seemed to reconsider. I realised why he hesitated and told him that I knew it to be dangerous drug in overdose; but pointed out that if I want to kill myself I could overdose on heroin or paracetamol. Providing me with amitriptyline would not *cause* me to attempt suicide, if I was going to do it, I would do it irrespective of the drugs at my disposal. (Although, I did think to myself that death via amitriptyline would be preferable to death via paracetamol). And so, amitriptyline was prescribed on that understanding and I was to work up the doses until I reached 150mg to begin with.

In 2004 Dr. Ogilvie would explain that based on his experience and the medications I had tried, he had though amitriptyline might help my depression, with the added benefits of sedating me and helping me gain weight. Of course, the first thing I did when I got the amitriptyline was to start to save it up to overdose. I said goodbye to Beth, Clare, and other friends, and told them I would be gone within two weeks. They all had opinions on this, naturally, but none of them managed to scrounge the smallest detail of my plan out of me. However, what I never considered was that my father would be counting my pills to make sure I was using them up. So I arrived home one day, to find all traces of amitriptyline gone, and my parents sitting on the sofa, waiting to speak to me.

He phoned Dr Ogilvie, and then following his directions, gave me the right amount each night, increasing it, and watching me swallow it. About two weeks later, I don't remember this, but apparently I walked downstairs and said to my parents, "Do you know what, I think it's working!" Within a month I was feeling considerably better. I saw Dr. Ogilvie and he increased my dose to 225mg, and I remain on that to this day, and will remain on amitriptyline, lithium, (and some other medication) for life. Dr. Ogilvie was obviously really pleased that I had made such a sudden but apparent recovery. I still had a way to go, but the difference was marked. His delight was visible. If he is a doctor for the same reasons I wanted to become a doctor, then I think it will have been most rewarding to see such a complete turnaround. I remember it was a hot day, and Dr. Ogilvie suggested I visit Vaughan Thomas to see old friends, but also to show the staff what a recovery I had made.

I was nervous to go back on to the ward, mainly because I had gained weight and felt people would be critical of this. That was "good" old anorexic thinking at work. Nobody commented or appeared to notice my weight gain. I sat in the smoking room and talked to Jean for a while. At that time she was hoping to be moved to a group home environment in the next few months. Everything is still so slow, I thought to myself. I also saw Rene, still sitting in broad view with a can of special brew; we talked about football for a while. Most of the other patients were new to me by then. Caroline had left the ward not long after me, and was living in London: we are in touch. I saw some staff too. Rich had left the hospital by then, and Ray was on the Runis Unit (a locked ward), George had vanished, but I saw my other two favourites, John the hippy and Margaret the fellow Derby County fan. I chatted for a while, but John had to get back to work. Dad was with me, and asked Margaret "What happened to that little chap?" We both looked at him questioningly, and he said, "The Crystal Palace fan that Katy took to see a match at Derby?"

"Declan!" I said. Suddenly thinking that it was a long time since we had spoken on the phone. Directly, as there was no easy way, Margaret told us he was dead. I shivered and had trouble registering her words. (Warning: explicit details of suicide). She explained he had recently jumped in front of a high-speed train. I felt cold. "NO!" I screamed in my head. Not another person, another loved friend gone, dead, a suicide victim. That Declan was able to go through with such a violent, grisly act did and did not surprise me. He had a precipitous nature, and had been consistently, at first surprisingly, violent towards himself. I was still ill enough to feel jealous that he had "succeeded" at suicide: I wondered if he was at peace, whilst I struggled through the early tentative stages of recovery. I have spent many hours mulling over Declan's brutal death, and it still hurts so much that I end feeling numb. There simply is not the human capacity to feel sufficient pain for his loss: resulting in a sensation of being stunned. Yes I am sad when people die naturally, but there is something about losing someone, someone you love or just someone, to suicide that is inexplicably awful. Knowing someone is going to commit suicide does not prepare you for it when it happens. Nothing prepares you for suicide.

> "He would say, 'How funny it will all seem, all you've gone through, when I'm not here anymore, when you no longer feel my arms around your shoulders, nor my heart beneath you, nor this mouth on your eyes, because I will have to go away someday, far away...' And in that instant I could feel myself with him gone, dizzy with fear, sinking down into the most horrible blackness: into death."

> ∾ Arthur Rimbaud (French poet and writer, 1854-1891)

I understood Declan well, and I knew of his disappointment about not feeling worthy of help, and his frustration (very similar to mine) with the seeming inconsistency of mental health care provided. Declan was more that just a friend, we had had fun; or at least as much fun as was possible for two people hurtling towards death by any manner possible. Yes, I even took him to see his team Crystal Palace play Derby County one Saturday when he couldn't afford a football ticket or transport. He told me he hallucinated all through the match, but you couldn't tell. He has met my football friends. He has been to my home, both in Oxford and Derby. I didn't ever stop him smoking dope. If he had no money, I'd give him some, though he always paid me back eventually. He used to take the piss out of me for smoking menthol cigarettes, saying he didn't like them because his "last girlfriend had smoked them." But he'd soon pinch my menthols when he ran short.

One thing Declan did for me was save my life. He knew I'd overdosed on heroin and always refused to help me get more – although he could have done. He said he cared too much about me to help me kill myself. I'd attempt to argue that if he cared about me, he'd help me go in a pleasant way, so I didn't suffer. He didn't fall for that one. I even asked for smaller amounts as if I was going to take it for fun, but he (rightly) didn't believe me. He said that he couldn't live with himself if he helped me die: I was "too good" to kill myself.

Then he killed himself.

A few weeks later, feeling significantly better, but still far from normal, I decided I would have to make plans for my career. I was still adamant that I did not want to spend another year sitting around in therapy: I wanted to move on. I talked things over with Dr. Ogilvie, and he said he'd back me fully if I applied to medical school again. I was somewhat shocked at this level of confidence he had in me and couldn't understand why I deserved it. Maybe he saw the potential I would have as a fellow psychiatrist. It was a very different power balance from (not that long ago) when he was dictating if I could go out cycling, or even have a teddy bear in my room. Suddenly I felt I had regained trust and respect as a human being. I had rejoined the human race.

Although it was ultimately decided that manic depression (mixed bipolar I affective disorder), complicated by anorexia, was the best explanation for my illness, Dr. Ogilvie likened me to Susanna Kaysen, the famous recovered borderline personality disorder survivor. After returning my DVD of that film to me at our last session, he said I should look at my life in the sense that I too had been a girl, interrupted.

I remember thinking that 25 years of my life was a little more than "an interruption." However his suggestion was a positive one, and perhaps a useful way to look at things: so I adopted it. My other thoughts were that I could try and get my D.Phil. place back, or I could apply for a social work masters degree, I also wondered about doing a Ph.D. in Psychology. More than anything, I wanted to write. In actual fact, I did all of these things.

To condense many months of gradual improvement and changes: I finally wrote up my D.Phil., I applied to medical school, I applied to study for an MA in social work, and to study psychology. I got offers from several Universities but decided to write this book instead. Whilst doing all this I joined a drama group, "Blue Balloon," and started having a social life. I sing and act for the exhilaration and the exhibitionist in me. Dressing up as a huge purple fairy for the pantomime, or a French resistance member/prostitute/nun in a play, or the nose-picking comedy character "Sniff," in this year's pantomime. Singing in shows and at parties. If anyone had suggested I would *ever* sing solo on stage prior to this last year, I would have suggested they undergo a Mental Health Act assessment.

Gradually I was getting well. I made the decision that I would not continue to live in Oxford, but would live near Derby. I began moving my health care providers up north, first my GP. I loved Neil MacLennan: he was utterly fabulous throughout our time together. He was my confident, concerning himself with such a difficult, messed up patient; even turning up to hospital meetings for me, which made me feel I had value. However, returning to my GP in Castle Donington meant I was back with Carol McGrath, who is an outstanding doctor and phenomenal person. Is it possible that I have had the two best GPs in the world? It feels like that.

My sessions with Steve Pearce were tapered off, which was very hard, and not what I wanted, but I understood why it had to happen. I was put on a ridiculously long waiting list for therapy in Derby, and then chose to turn down further therapy. Then, hardest of all, was changing psychiatrist. I did not want to lose Dr. Ogilvie because as well as respecting and liking him, I trusted him and no one else with my life. But eventually, I was transferred into the care of a Derbyshire psychiatrist, who, alarmingly for me, was an ex-pupil of Loughborough High School just like myself.

During this time, two people I knew committed suicide, one strangled her self just after being released from hospital, and one man jumped to his death. So that totals four people I cared for, lost to suicide, forever, just that year. But I coped. My family and friends rallied around me with support, and after the initial sudden improvement, I went on to continuously yet gradually improve over the months. Emma (Bell) and I resumed our close friendship, and her two boys are as dear to me as the children I wish I could have, but never will.

It has been a very difficult time and I've worked very hard. My eating went through stages of improvement. Time, death, suicide and reasonably controlled manic depression have all remained constant in my thoughts: they are, perhaps, still obsessions of mine. I do not feel safe: I still expect to die by my own hand. I am reluctant to say that at this time I finally saw the light at the end of the very long, dark tunnel that had been my life. But I still do not feel whole.

Someone, I don't know who, once said, "Beware of the light at the end of the tunnel, it is the light of an oncoming train."

No matter how much time passes, I cannot shake that thought.

Chapter 13. Equilibrium, sort of.

"O Me! O life!... of the questions of these
recurring;
Of the endless trains of the faithless--of
cities fill'd with the foolish;
Of myself forever reproaching myself,
(for who more foolish than I and who
more faithless?)
Of the empty and useless years of the rest
-- with the rest me intertwined;
The question, O me! so sad, recurring --
What good amid these,
O me, O life?
Answer.
That you are here -- that life exists, and
identity;
That the powerful play goes on, and you
will contribute a verse."

ॐ Walt Whitman (1819-1892), *O Me! O Life!*
(Extract).

However bad things become, it is possible to claw your way back. The light that is my life has gone out many more times than most, but that shows how many other human beings have rekindled it, and thought me worth saving. I suppose *I* fought for my life too, it just didn't feel like it at the time. A few times, my light went out and should have stayed that way, only for people to *battle* to relight it. My light has also flickered and dimmed, but ultimately been sheltered by other people. There are so many people who have helped, *none* of whom I have forgotten; from those showing me the smallest kindness, to sharing friendship, to loving me, to hearing me, to counselling me, even to the terrible experience of physical restraining in hospital, to the more subtle and clever mental restraining, to the restarting of my lungs, to… to… I owe a large debt of gratitude to many wonderful human beings.

And so I found myself alive. Which was a shock: unexpected, and unplanned for. You cannot go through what I did without it marking you profoundly, both physically and mentally. I found myself wanting to end the nightmare, but not by giving up: *by fighting on.* It was a peculiar existence: unpleasant, frightening, overwhelming, reminding me of being a helpless, vulnerable child again. I was faced with impossible choices that had to be made blindly. Nothing was certain and I didn't know which way I was heading, or how to get there. I needed to create a life for myself, but had no dreams, no hopes I thought I could achieve, and much I knew would be forever unfulfilled. I had no point of reference for "normality." I finally had a diagnosis of manic depression/bipolar disorder, after a long discussion with Alan Ogilvie where I was honest about ALL my symptoms. Four doctors, and an expert clinical psychologist who "scored" the level of my bipolarity from 1-100 have confirmed this diagnosis. Apparently I am an 80-90, yeah, serious.

> "What we have done for ourselves alone
> dies with us; what we have done for others
> and the world remains and is immortal."

> ❧ Albert Pike (1809-1891)

So I started to write. I wrote this book for you. Yes, YOU. Helping people is, after all, of paramount importance to me. It is who I am, what I do and how I measure my self-worth. Although, before now, I was always expendable. In actuality I needed to be well in order to be able to help others. So unfortunately and ironically, my illnesses have prevented me doing what I desired. But now I have my writing, other research I have done and published, research I intend to do, time I devote to help people who are still struggling, all of which let me help others enough for me to feel a success. I now work for Alan, for Equilibrium - The Bipolar Foundation.[30] I hope that wonderful things will come from this work, and I am committed to making a difference for all sufferers of mental illness. I have many roles, but my main one is running the Bipolar Testimony Project, building a collection of stories from every country in the world (slowly, one by one), about life in that country, living with the disease. I also spend some time working in medical research, and helping fellow survivors of bipolar disorder and eating disorders online. I have a particular interest in improving diagnosis and treatment for mixed bipolar disorder states as they are hard to diagnose, and that nearly cost me my life. I am not a practicing physician, the dream that I endeavoured for and dreamed of all my life, but what I am doing is starting to be *enough*.

Without really knowing what I would create, several people said that writing this book might help me: it

---

[30] http://www.bipolar-foundation.org/
See me on page: http://www.bipolar-foundation.org/index.aspx?o=1030
See the Testimony Project at: http://www.bipolar-foundation.org/index.aspx?o=1085

might be salutary, and I think that is true. It took me on a journey of remembrance that was most illuminating and calming. Perhaps I have laid some ghosts to rest, and by doing so, if I have helped you, then I have succeeded. (Be you ill, a friend, family or a professional). By making open to the public my private, personal, theoretically embarrassing, very definitely painful experiences, I hope that fewer people will make the same mistakes that I did. I hope that people out there will feel less or no shame. I hope people will feel less alone. You are not alone. And above all else, I wish to have given you back some *hope*.

Do any of you still fancy a bit of anorexia, just for a few months? I know some of you will, I know others will already be tired of it. Or are you questioning whether you may have depression or bipolar disorder, and realising that you could seek help *with hope* and *without shame*? Do you think some time in a psychiatric hospital will lessen the burden? It might possibly help save your life short-term, but long-term: no way.

If I've learned one thing it is not to wait to be saved by anyone. I am responsible for my own life, my own salvation and any solace that I seek. People can help me, certainly, but only if I try to find their help and then accept it. *Do not wait to be saved*. Nobody can read your mind. Nobody will come – unless you ask. Much can be done – much. There are many ways to ask: a simple phone call, letter or meeting will get you further than grand gestures of self-harm or lunacy (if possible for you).

On an intellectual level, I have enjoyed writing. I rise to challenges, and enjoy being busy. In fact, I *have* to keep busy. I knew some parts would be emotionally difficult, but I underestimated this. Opening my diaries was particularly hard, as I will explain momentarily. Whilst I was fairly certain that I would be well enough to think about my past, I am suffering from the sores left by opening old wounds. That is, however, an overly dramatic description of my existing distress, because, to an extent, "the sores" are always open. The memories do not fade or disappear, the fears remain, the rage still bubbles under the surface. Writing this book did not make those things significantly worse; it just necessitated me to focus on them more than I might have liked.

Be still my pulsing brain.

The sheer volume of thoughts in my brain can be overwhelming and is beyond my control. I often wonder, my mind drifts and settles on unpleasant issues, or horrific factors in my history and possible future. I am easily distracted into thinking dark thoughts, and get excited by gruesome details of suicide and death. I always have to be mindful about how unwise it is to dwell on such topics.

Opening my diaries from school, I decided, was impossible. My diaries from Nottingham University are upsetting, although I love the University and the few friends I made there. I had a tendency to keep things, tickets, photos… crammed full with normal student mementos, split with my ill self's purged feelings: all my thoughts, all the things I had no other way of expressing. Drawings, paintings, and pages crammed with words, always angry and dark.

With my years-of-having-therapy trained mind, I can see in the words I wrote, how all-or-nothing, black, depressed, excitable, angry, eating disordered and filled with self-hatred my thinking was. I am grateful to have learned, with a lot of hard work, how to challenge those thoughts, even though they persist. In most instances, as soon as they pop into my head they are shot down by thoughts of self-preservation and rationality – yes me, rational! I mainly have my wonderful Oxford psychotherapist to thank for showing me how to do that. And... I have myself to thank for that, because I didn't get where I am today by waiting for someone else to cure me. I put a lot of effort into my therapy, I did my "homework," I took everything in, all the time, even when it seemed like I was getting nowhere or worse. The messages taught in Oxford are ones I have learned and still practice.

Some people have said how unlucky I have been: that is true. I also know that I have been lucky; these words to you are almost from beyond the grave. *I should be dead.* Looking at my diaries from my time in hospital in Oxford is like torture. Again I kept everything, sticking things in with glue. There is a page of dictated instructions for cooking heroin, heart monitor pads, and a while later, more pads from the second heroin overdose, then hospital tags from the paracetamol "incident." There is a page with taped-in razor blades that no room-search ever found. There are pages of words I do not remember writing; there are also pages written in blood.

I collected signatures, quotes, even drawings from patients, some of whom are now dead, some are still ill, and some have left hospital only to return. Some are fine, at least I assume so. Many people disappeared, I imagine them getting on with their lives. Then I see the little notes that Declan wrote to me and which I saved.

Oh they rip at my heart now that he is dead and gone forever. I cry as I write this.

There is no return from suicide. No changing your mind, regret or second chance; at least not usually. In 2004 I lost four friends and one stranger to suicide. In 2005 I lost one anorectic friend to the effects of starvation and in November, one dear, oh so brilliant and dearly loved one to suicide (Lisa had bipolar II disorder). Her suicide hit me harder than anything in my life ever. It's one thing that stops me from inflicting the same pain on those who love me. The guilt I feel for not saving her is tremendous. The pain of her loss lasts forever, and tears well up in my eyes as I write.

I suppose knowing so many people who are ill means I am going to encounter suicides. I have known many fantastic people who have butchered themselves. I have witnessed and personally felt the devastation those deaths leave behind. I think it will be hard for me to forget that.

And I owe it to them not to forget them.

For those that have died, there are many more who have survived and moved on: we ought not forget them either.

Someone suggested I should get some "normal" friends... But the truth remains: I am drawn to damaged people. I connect with them, lose some, and feel proud of those who prevail. Many friends I made along my route are well now: Ayeesha is now a London Barrister, Harriet will soon be a doctor, Becky is well, and settled happily in Oxford. Ash writes to me often, sometimes three letters a day, and his writing is getting much clearer; that pleases me after the hours I spent helping him read and write. He couldn't do either when we met. He tells me about the latest book he is reading, creating alternative endings, and I take him out for lunch whenever he is allowed – not often. He's been in hospital constantly since the brief period he was released in 2003. I guess I *did* get to leave hospital before him after all.

Clare (Baker) is doing so well. Alcoholics Anonymous (AA) or "The Fellowship," has really helped her turn her life around. She has not touched alcohol since she gave it up. Her depression is mostly controlled, she does not self-harm, and she gone a record time without bingeing and purging. Like me she has accepted antidepressants and mood stabilisers are a very necessary part of the solution. Nothing makes me happier than to see another person seize back their life, even if I can't understand her spirituality. She has qualified as an Archivist and Records Manager with an MA, and works in the House of Lords! She has a partner and is planning to buy a home. Bloody good for her! I know what a battle it has been to reach this stage in her life, and seeing her success makes me feel all warm and shiny, delighted for her, aware of the effort and bravery that make it so much greater a battle to have won. Listen folks… You must take inspiration from Clare's story also. Three years from rock bottom booze, bulimia and depression, to heath, love, stability, and working in our great capital's Parliament. You see anything is possible *if you don't give up*.

I am in a similar group, the Manic Depressive Fellowship, MDF; now renamed the MDF Bipolar Organisation. (Which doesn't require a spiritual/god part). I find them a supportive, vibrant, caring, funny. Some MDF bipolar friends had comments:

"You are someone with incredible determination, an amazing mind and empathy that is unmatched. You are a person who is making things better for all of us; you are standing up and speaking out. For all the strength you give to others – may just some be transferred back to you when you feel the need."

"KS. I have come to the conclusion that you are nuts. Hahahahaha!"

(Affectionately!) *"What's not to love about you? You are impossible, self-obsessed, aloof, foul-mouthed, brainy, neurotic…"*

"Do you know my first port of call if I need information? YOU! Yes YOU! Anyway - you are my true heroine this year [2005] - you have been a support and inspiration to us all - we all love you to bits - I love you to bits - and if I could give you a big hug I would."

"Reading your book: I want to say that my heart went out to you. Magnify what I have been through by a million and even then you would be only just approaching. That someone can go through so much and survived, let alone be brave enough to

*revisit those places in order to reach out
to others, just blows me away."*

Julius (Julie Potter-Tate, from my Leicester hospital days) is still in my life. She is happily settled and planning to marry. Her anorexia is now mostly past, though she still struggles with food, living mainly on baked beans on toast (the British delicacy). She has now has two sons; they are the cutest. I make the most of my friends' children. Other friends from the Leicester days have settled, have children, and some are married.

Caroline and I are still close, though not as close as I would like – the distance does not help. Her illness, almost certainly mixed bipolar disorder like myself, still plagues her. We shared so much of our raw selves without judgement that it would be hard not to feel connected to her, and her to me. I suppose we lived in each other's pockets during the darkest time of our lives. She is now back studying law and thinking of teaching law. If either of us have the need for an ear we can trust, we know the other can provide it.

*SO MANY PEOPLE WHO WERE HOPELESS ARE NOW
SUCCEEDING IN LIVING THEIR LIVES.*

❧

Some things never change. My family are there for me, as are many dear, dear friends. I still follow Derby County and always will. The singing today was full blast, as you might expect when the opposition is being slaughtered in a crucial match: Derby won 3-1 against Preston, reaching the Championship play offs. (To then be knocked out, go up via the play offs in 2007, and have the worst Premiership season on record). I took Emma's boys, Liam and Aaron with me, and pretended to be a mum for a few hours. I sat silently as fans sung that they are "Derby till I die." I looked up as that chant started, saw the infinite sky, some clouds, noticed myself breathing in, and then slowly out. I thought *if only*, and paused in fear. Then I returned to the fun.

I hit thirty. I went out of my twenties with a bang! Surrounded by people I love at a big party. Caroline metaphorically held my hand, Clare never left my side, Mia was there, Julius too, Emma, Liam, Aaron, all my family, and all our close family friends including the Gatleys, Sumners and all of Blue Balloon. I would have liked Ash there, but it was not possible. My dad gave a moving speech... all about *me,* in which the most important factors in my life were not even mentioned. I retorted so as not to embarrass (i.e. I unwillingly avoided mentioning illness), and then I kicked off the karaoke singing Green Day (who else?)

Throughout the evening I was distracted with incredulity at the fact that I was actually *still alive*, and I wondered how many of the people there were quietly thinking the same thing. (Or is it only me that thinks like that). I wondered what all those people would think if they knew what was still going on in my head – I was wondering if I would ever have another birthday...

Am I glad to be alive today? Am I glad for being saved and glad for saving myself?
Yes.

Do I always feel like that?
No.

Now that it is over, am I *grateful* for my life experiences – am I a better person? Was Nietzsche right when he wrote, "That which does not kill me, makes me stronger"?

No.

Firstly, it is never "over." I will never become complacent because my disease is at best controlled. I still have bad times, bad days, and bad weeks. I do not lack insight into my illnesses, but I lack reassurance that they will *not* come back. I know I have over a 90% risk of returning episodes of mania, depression or mixed bipolar disorder. I am not sure if I would survive it – I say that even though I know it is possible to recover - a belief vanishes when ill, when hope is lost. I feel about the return of illness exactly as I imagine did Virginia Woolf when she wrote in her suicide note that she knew she was becoming ill and that she couldn't go through it again, nor believe she could recover.

I will still try to fight it, if or when it happens; but I fear I have very little fight left in me. The statistical probability of me ending my own life is frighteningly high. Everyone breaks eventually. I have always had a suicide plan; even now I have a new plan, the "ingredients" all ready to take my life. I wonder if one day I will feel strong enough to dispose of the parts of that plan or the plan itself. I simply do not know. For now I need the security of a back-out clause. Maybe one day I wont. Or maybe you are reading this when I am dead.

Grateful? NO! No: I am not, and will not, *ever* be grateful for the horrors I have experienced, however much insight I have gained. I am not stronger for having survived, my body and mind are weak and my (mostly internalised) emotions are still intense and out-of-control. Life is exhausting, I still have nightmares, and I still see things that I know aren't there, which I could argue *are* there... My past has been consumed with illness and my present continues to be dominated by it. I'm heavily medicated. My thoughts rest upon death too often. I am, perhaps, more empathic, I am certainly more knowledgeable, but those things may well have been true about me had I not suffered so long, or at all.

Would I want to swap lives with another human being? Would I take away my bipolarity? *No.* I'm me. People have less luck. It might have been, and daily continue to be, hard work being myself, but I'm me. Is it a no-win situation? *No.* I can focus on the positives and help as many people as I can with whatever time I have left. I am the sum of all those difficult, painful and dangerous experiences; a fact I cannot change, so I may as well use what I have learned.

So what am I left with? I'm a *recovered* anorectic and bulimic; one time over-drinker; ex-drug abuser; a person who no longer self-harms or attempts suicide; and someone who no longer has any borderline personality traits. I still have PTSD (post traumatic stress disorder). I believe I am "recovered," as opposed to "recovering" from the anorexia and bulimia. The manic depression, or being technical, the 'mixed bipolar I affective disorder last episode psychotic,' is a tougher problem for me: it's something to live with day by day. I sleep very little. I am reliant on medication, but I do not care if it keeps the mixed manic depression at bay.

Living with weight gain is *hard*: caused by medication; years of abusing my metabolism; a period of eating all the things I had denied myself; and a fear of exercise lest it entrap me like before. I eat in response to hunger and no other reason. I hate being fat with all the passion I have always hated *my* fatness with. *But I hate depression more.* I positively rattle from all the antidepressants, mood stabilisers, the antipsychotic, the sedatives, hypnotics, etc. that I must swallow daily. I would love to have Angelina Jolie's body, or Liv Tyler's soft curves: and I could... The price would be my sanity, any happiness I have, and most probably my life. As my dear school friend Antonia put it:

> *"The fact that you have focused on staying well rather than clinging to a certain body image at all costs, is a victory over the impulse to self-destruction that I respect. I suspect it has been very hard-won."*

I am so much more than just illness: I'm an existentialist, a great ambivalent (always torn), a humanitarian, a depressive nihilist, a pragmatist, a humorist, always a non-conformist, suicidologist, survivor, and writer. I am erratic, volatile, labile, demonstrative, unstable, open to suggestion and indomitably stubborn about some things – I live on the edge. Which is all a posh way of saying I am mad, sad, emotional, lonely, empty, unpredictable, arsy, angry, and cynical; I don't like being told what to do by anyone, I placate and ignore people wasting my time, think life has no intrinsic meaning or value, but at the same time, (thus contradicting myself), I want to help, and I do value people. I believe strongly in personal freedom and responsibility, I think too much, I don't believe in god(s), I am realistic at the hopelessness of it all, I cope with life by laughing at it, enjoy laughing, and I like to tell everyone what I think – despite being totally unable to explain or understand the meaning of life, the universe, and everything.

"Our greatest glory is not in never falling,
but in rising every time we fall."

&. Confucius

I am somehow blessed with the ability to forgive people anything if they do their best or apologise. I have a good understanding of why human nature leads people to do "bad" things. However I am not blessed with denial, and so some things will never be forgotten. But I am not giving up (…today). It is possible to live with pain, possible to distract yourself, and to find a form of peace. Perhaps there are things it is important to remember. Forgiveness does not mean you condone terrible events, but the capability to forgive is liberating. Rising above any perpetrator and forgiving them makes their actions unimportant, thus removing the power they have over you. But time does not heal *all*, nor is it possible to forgive *everything*, nor forget the pain.

So after all we have shared, would you like a happy Hollywood ending or a dismal, angry, and perhaps poetic "life sucks so just get on with it"? I prefer the truth, which is some where in the middle: good days, bad days, or whatever I can make of life. There is no such thing as a perfect ending in *real* life. I think it is a fair conclusion that I am absolutely crap at committing suicide. But if there's something to be bad at, then maybe that isn't such a bad one. At least, I feel that way today, and hope I still feel the same way tomorrow. I am still convinced that next time it will work. I *am* grateful for my stupid, little life, but not for every single moment.

The truth is: I am not particularly happy, but sometimes I am. My outlook on life has improved. I am far more settled than once I was, but more melancholic than most people ever get in their lifetime. I feel empty, yet about to burst: *torn* in two or more directions at all times. I often feel overwhelmed. I could venture down the pathway of insanity again, to some extent it is my choice. Or it could just happen. I will always have manic depression and various idiosyncrasies. People say I laugh more these days. Real laughter.

My mood goes up and down, just not *so* far in either direction. I get angry easily, I get upset easily, I catastrophise: I think I always will. If I have a bad day, I am terrified that it is the start of sinking in to another depression, one I would not survive. I shelter myself from stress and boredom. My favourite time of the day is still climbing under the duvet, hiding from everyone including myself, and snuggling down to sleep. Semi-sweet oblivion: where my life-long adversary Time does not haunt me. He does not exist whilst I am asleep. Sleep is always a busy, tiring sleep, often filled with nightmares of hospital, being chased as I try to run away, being made to feel small, being arrogant, eating food I don't want, and heroin. I dream about heroin a lot: injecting it, cooking it, buying it, dying, calming the fury within, and hearing the galloping horses. I usually wake up and think "Oh no, another day." Then I somehow bounce out of bed at about 3am and start working.

Time to exist. It goes back to the oldest problem I ever had and still have. That problem is time. Too much time means boredom, and boredom is something I simply cannot deal with. My mind is always active: a busy, busy, busy mind. Resultant boredom can be a downside to intelligence, and potentially a massive hitch if you are predisposed to depression and self-damaging behaviour. I need things to do, *all* the time, every single moment. I am either planning things to do or doing them. The anxiety surrounding this is extreme, but getting better. Days need jobs and fun, as much work as I can achieve, as much pleasure as I can fit in: keeping the sadness at bay, and my thoughts more quiet. It is hard work keeping myself satisfactorily busy. It remains an anxious obsession of mine: to fill time, to avoid boredom, to occupy my neurons and glia, lest I go mad once again.

Too long have I merely existed. My life's essence so far is best summarised as that of someone who has been damaged, has been very ill, who knows illness will return, and now tries to survive. But I want to do more with my life than just cope. The truth of the matter is that I have been very ill for a very long time, and I suspect that it will take a lot more time before those feelings go, or diminish. I am thirty, and haven't yet lived a fully healthy year in adulthood.

Stars, bridges, and trains: just three examples of ordinary things that will always look different to me. I shudder at the sight or sound of a train, thinking of Declan, and thinking about standing at the side of the tracks myself, whilst a train sped past two inches away from my nose. Stars always remind me of my dead friend from San Francisco, and the pointlessness of life in this vast universe. I have real trouble driving under bridges, one in particular. I still get very agitated, angry, and sometimes darkness clouds my head and everything comes flooding back. Certain songs remind me of sad times or people lost. I always feel everything so intensely – I've almost forgotten what "normal" is. I have to force myself to take the lithium because I hate it dampening my mind, and drying the voice out of my swollen body. Other times I am grateful for anything that calms my sense of intense fear, anger and anxiety.

> "It is what a man thinks of himself that really determines his fate."

> ❧ Henry David Thoreau (1817-1862)

Sometimes, more and more, I am reminded of what it is like *not* to live on the precipice of various catastrophes. More often I am fortunate enough to be able to process emotions: I may cry to mourn those people and things that are lost forever, I may laugh and joke. Other times I know I appear impenetrable, even fooling myself, and feelings are absorbed into my subconscious for later management. I am not impassive, I am deeply emotional – you just can't see it.

All I can tell you, is that I have come through illnesses I thought impossible to beat and witnessed others do the same. For the first time in my adult life, I am "living." I have career plans, drama, and football matches (however agonising the result). Oh how I love, with my concentration now restored, to lose myself in a book. I always adored reading and found it most distressing when I couldn't do it.

Dr. Alan Ogilvie used to ask me if I found enjoyment in anything I did, and I didn't, not *ever*. But I do now, thankfully. I can take pleasure in things, and I know what it is like to live with a heart of stone and unseeing eyes, I appreciate the difference greatly.

When people meet me, they meet *me*: or at least more of the real Katy Sara than has ever been on show. You do not meet an arrogant, aggressive anorectic: which is all that most people have seen since my early teens. I shudder remembering some of my behaviour towards people. But if people don't like me now, then that is their problem, not mine. That sounds braver that the truth: if I was not accepted, *I* would be the one doing the running away.

I used to be afraid that if I was myself and had self-belief, then "they" wouldn't like me and I would be left all alone. Thankfully I have discovered that I have more friends than ever. My illness cost me one friendship unexpectedly, but made me some amazing friends that are more than worth the exchange, and it made me value those friends who have stood by me all the more. I have been able to reconnect with some friends I once lost due to the self-imposed isolation that an eating disorder, depression, psychosis etc. causes.

I am not so dichotomous as once I was; I'm *less* split into two people, one for show, and one who is ashamed. But I'm still split. What you see is still rarely representative of all that is going on inside my head. I fear that I appear too confident. I hide that I am unstable, easily hurt and break easily. I ought to wear a big "handle with care" badge. Tiny events set me off hurtling down into despair; though usually I pull myself clear of danger in time: for now at least. I don't expect that someone so fragile yet also opinionated and apparently full of convictions to survive for long. I know I will go to my death "early."

In the past I have been exceedingly angry and out of control, but the wrath was always ultimately directed inwards at me. I am less angry now. But consider when you tip a little bit of your cup of tea or coffee down the sink, just so that you don't spill it: most of the tea stays in your cup. Most of my anger has stayed in me. I am angry, but that might pass, or it may be useful (protective, motivating) and I certainly don't harm anyone, including myself, because of the anger. I am not afraid to feel angry anymore. I no longer think it makes me a bad person and I understand where it comes from – and that I have a right to feel as I do.

I am still afraid to feel sad.

All in all, this is pretty dull, basic stuff. No grandiose starvation, ostentatious self-harm or extravagant suicide attempts with last minute saves or inexplicable survival. The most dramatic thing I do now is speed on the motorway. Far more boring than being dangerously ill, but I have had my fill of being ill. Being ill is tedious.

Believe it or not, there are still elements of the naive idealist in me, but you wouldn't think so after we have discussed my beliefs, which are very corporeal. I believe in myself, I believe in other people, …and I don't. I believe in instinct, hope, coincidence and luck …sometimes. I don't believe in God or Fate. There is far too much suffering in the world, now and always, which is proof enough for me that there is no "good" higher power. I do not have the luxury of trusting there is always some better, hidden reason to explain why misery exists and things go wrong.

I don't believe I have survived in order to fill some purpose. Nor do I believe there is a reward to look forward to after death to make up for the pain of living; something making suffering bearable because of some impossible dream of eternal happiness. I take no comfort that I will see lost loved ones again in some green field, or on a fluffy cloud, with the sun shining, telling me how happy they are. But I have no problem accepting that other people have different beliefs – I am happy for them if they are happy. In actuality, Atheism is just a belief too. I carry love for people in my heart.

I wont waste my short life waiting on a promise I don't believe, nor be good out of fear of retribution (from an ethereal or earthly power). I do "good" because it is right to do so: my choice. I don't murder because it is morally wrong, not because it is illegal or will condemn me to hell forever. I do not do good out of fear, I do good because I believe in it. I see no point in breathing in and out waiting to die and *then* start living in the afterlife. What a waste life on Earth would be if everyone did that. Surely, if there were a god, she intended there to be purpose to life, or why bother with it? Better to face the truth and make the best of what you have, always prepared to be stabbed in the back by anyone, even by life itself. There are fewer nasty surprises then.

At the end of the day, you can lie and lie to everyone except yourself: so honesty, insight and self-acceptance are *so* very precious. Are these not good things to aim towards? If I can do it, anyone can. I have always been respectful of others, and find that only now am I in the position of respecting myself too. I cherish that. But of course, depression can snatch all of that away so fast, I try not to think of that. I suppose you will only appreciate just how much I treasure self-belief if you know what it is like to live with out it: to have no respect for yourself, to hate yourself, to loath yourself. But to have finally reached the point where I like the person that is Katy Sara is joyous beyond words. There are still things about me that I hate, but nobody is perfect.

I have to be honest. I cannot promise you a cure, or say that if you've read my book and you do x, y, and z you will recover. I can't tell you how to feel any more than you can tell yourself how to feel. Mood disorders, addictions, eating disorders, suicide and self-harm just don't work like that. My only advice is that you accept you are powerless over your illness, it will run its course, but retain *responsibility,* for getting help and a positive outlook (the best you can do) will usually shorten this course.

Stop blaming yourself. You must help yourself, and in many aspects often *you* are the only person that can help. Try, try, and try again to be as healthy as you can. Gladly receive help from friends, family, fellow-sufferers, and professionals. Be loud! Ask for the help you need, and keep being vocal until you get it. There is a lot of help out there. See your doctor, talk to a friend you trust, join a pro-recovery website, get all the information that you can. Remember to give yourself time, sometimes lots of time, and *do not give up*.

Balancing between mania and depression can feel like being on a knife's edge – a razor sharp one. As can the divide between eating or not. Happiness can be so fluid, and is able to disappear for years, or (it feels) forever, resulting in pain unlike any other. But as far as clinging to happiness, I know I did, even if it was perverse at times. I hung on in there all the way.

Dark Clouds Gather

As yet, I am unable to let anyone touch me, physically or emotionally. No one can touch me for I am too vulnerable, emotionally scarred and troubled. I find my whole life altered: most people take a partner, a family, a home and a career for granted – none of which I have, and most of which I never will. Why? Because I am injured, and because time does not heal this damage. I cannot even cope with love, yet how can I live a meaningful life without it? I see others doing it day after day, making it look easy. I fell in love once, but I cannot let anyone close. I am too afraid. I still feel empty. I still feel damaged. But I intend to fight for my life, and never go as low (or high) again.

If you are desperate and suffering from any of these illnesses that I have shared my darkest secrets about with you; ensure that I didn't share them for nothing. Please *try* to remember the things in your life that are worth keeping, worth living for. It can be very hard I know, but try. Think of people you love, your family and friends, the beauty of the evening sunshine as it falls behind the trees, some quirky love that you have of something – for me it's sheep! Think of the future you might have, with your career, your family. You have but one shot at this life.

There is, for most people, a way through the dark times, when you feel there is no hope: a truly dark and dangerous existence. Starving, manic, depressed, addicted, bingeing, harming, in pain... Torn between a life you don't want because you can see no future, and a death you are afraid of but which represents emancipation: an end to your suffering, dreamless sleep forever and ever. I am lucky, *extremely* lucky to have survived what I did to myself.

If *you* feel there is no way out, no point, no hope; please, *please*, do as a wise, long-haired hippie-nurse John, once said to me, with gritted teeth, and a clenched fist, "Hold on."

HOLD ON, those Dark Clouds that Gather, they will pass.

Never lose hope. The dark times that overwhelm do not last forever. Battles with food, drugs and drink are won. The dark cloud that is depression, the lightening that is mania, or the combination of both; that blusters over your mind or fills it with energy; that devastates; that decimates lives; that lingers; that blinds; *will lift.* Clear days lie ahead. Believe it.

♦ Epilogue.

It's the Summer of 2008, just a couple of months ago I finally plucked up the courage to write to a publisher, and now I find myself published! As a final act, to put this thing to bed, I am letting you all know I have survived the past 5 years free of self-harm, free of any eating disorder, and with my moods mostly controlled – the bipolar disorder is as ever proving to be a despicable component in my life, and that of my family. Since Lisa there have been no more suicides, though I still expect to go that way one day – and if I do, I will go down fighting, and you must still fight – imagine me holding your hand.

One thing I did just this week was open a diary I had previously felt unable to read. I did not expect to find anything. Let me take you back to 2004 when I started to write this book... in dribs and drabs, in early recovery. Before I did anything, I chose a title. And I chose it by holding Professor Kay Redfield Jamison's authoritative book on suicide *Night Falls Fast*, in my hands, thinking to myself, I need something like this, 3 words, something dark... And I chose *Dark Clouds Gather*.

Flicking through one of my diaries this week, looking back to when I was a first year at University, it is filled with photos and keepsakes. And right at the back, there is a letter from my mum. My heart almost stopped when I read the words, long forgotten, but obviously buried in my subconscious somewhere. She ended her note:

Don't be afraid when dark clouds gather,

Katy Sara Culling

Somewhere the sunshine is breaking through!

~ Mum xx   28: 11: 1995

❧ Acknowledgements

Where to start? Alan; Dr. Alan David Ogilvie, based at the Warneford Hospital, University of Oxford, Oxford where he is a senior clinical research fellow in mood disorders, honorary consultant psychiatrist, and more recently CEO and founding member of Equilibrium – The Bipolar Foundation (and thus my boss). Thank you for listening, I mean really *hearing* and being open to adaptation; thank you for your common sense and logic; thank you for your direct approach and precise use of English that meant I could not lie as much as I wanted to; thank you for your insight; thank you for your time; thank you for standing firm; thank you for not being afraid to make me angry in order to make me safe. Sorry for being a patient management nightmare. Frankly, without you, I would be dead. Without your encouragement this book would never have been written – and so my readers thank you also. I am eternally in your debt Alan. Thank you.

I also owe my life to Carol and Neil, the two best GPs in the world: Dr. Carol M P McGrath (Castle Donington) and Dr. Neil MacLennan (Oxford). Both of you have kept me alive. Both of you have fought for my life when I could not. Carol your supporting, genuine, respectful approach, and understanding is unparalleled. The time and friendship you gave (and give) me is appreciated and treasured. Neil, you made me laugh even during the darkest years of my life, you bothered enough to turn up to hospital meetings, and gave me a reliable person I could always trust in a city that wanted to swallow me up whole. You too were exceedingly gracious with your time. I only wish I could persuade you to change your regrettable football allegiance (Man Utd).

To my treasured though unnamed psychotherapist at the Oxford Adult Eating Disorder Service – who taught me how to find my wise mind and challenge the core beliefs that tore my heart to shreds. You gave me the tools with which to choose for myself. You gave me a reason to get from Tuesday to Tuesday (the day of our sessions). You remembered; you listened; you explained; you gave me time; you cared, and so you saved me too.

Thank you to all the staff at the Oxford Adult Eating disorder Service – I didn't hate you or disrespect you. I was ill and didn't have the words to ask for the help I needed, nor the ability to accept that which was offered. Thank you for trying.

Thank you to Steve, Dr. Steve Pearce, consultant psychiatrist *and* consultant psychotherapist. Based at the Warneford Hospital, Oxford. Expert in personality disorders and "difficult cases." Thank you for your gentle, relaxed manner, sharp ears, superb tact, expertise, no-nonsense attitude, concern and ability to see right through me to show me things I didn't even know about myself. Sorry I appeared to take so little notice of your advice – I was listening.

Thanks to John, Ray and Rich, and other nurses on Vaughan Thomas ward whilst I was imprisoned there. John your intelligent chats were the best, and you have my deepest respect for being the only nurse who never let me wind you up in the slightest. I was the princess manipulator, but you never took the bait. Ray you are one smart cookie and a beautiful person. Rich thank you for your time, not giving up, and enabling me to cry. Sorry things got pretty fucked up towards the end. Thanks to Margaret, Harry, Neil T, George and Jean too. Thanks to you all for taking me far more seriously than I thought you did at the time – though I was totally misunderstood (I take part of the blame for that).

Thank you to Andy, Professor Andrew M. Salter at Nottingham University. A great teacher, a great support: with an unfortunate taste in football team (he knows I'm not kidding). Thank you to all the other staff at the University of Nottingham. Thanks especially to Ian, Professor I. A. Macdonald, Director of Research, Faculty of Medicine & Health Sciences, Co-Director, Institute of Clinical Research, School of Biomedical Sciences, for spotting me in the crowd, for feeding my intellect, and giving me hope at a time that I so desperately needed it.

Thanks to Professor Keith N. Frayn for his brilliant teaching, guidance, support and concern during and after my D.Phil. studentship at Oxford. I'm glad we finally published my research after all. Thanks for having me round for tea; I don't think many supervisors do that.

Thanks to my Linacre College tutors, especially Heather O, the head tutor, and other staff members, especially the College Secretary Jane E, who all supported me totally, without question, through all my difficulties, and who fought hard for my studentship rights. Thank you to my College Advisors and the two Bursars that were there during my time. Sorry I burned my room down! Oxford University is a Collegiate University for good reason; your College is your friend, and candles are now banned.

~

My heart, as always, for those who are irretrievably lost.
Lisa… Declan… many others…

~

Friendships are treasured: Mia, Antonia, Claire, Fiona actually all of LVIF at Loughborough High School and those who took three sciences with me for A' levels. Thank you to my favourite Geography teacher and both my Physics teachers.

My warm wishes for the future to all friends I have made over the years because of my illnesses and theirs, and who shared their lives with me for a time. Especially Jean, Summer in New York, *** in San Francisco, *** In Ohio, Claire, Lissa, Heidi, Becky, my secret friend from Crieff in Scotland, Rose, Harriet, Ayeesha, Lizzy T, Ivor, Zee, Rene, and of course, Tony. Thank you to all of you on the Stephen Fry SLOTMD forum who are like family, and similarly those on the MDF Bipolar Organisation forum. I feel privileged to have known all of you.

My darling Katie and Caz from Nottingham University: bet you are surprised by what's in this book! Ben the biker and Ben who lent me his bed. My housemates from Keggy. The same goes for all my friends from Linacre College, Oxford – Dr. Mel, Dr. Bethany, Dr. Colin, Dr. Halyna. And to my undergraduate biochem students Andy and Dr. Abbie.

Matt, Linda and John Wesson, Zoe, Lucy Sumner, Luke Burton, Melody, Michael, Ian Clayton and the rest of the Blue Balloon gang, thank you for assisting me to repeatedly make a total arse out of myself on stage for the sake of comedy.

Dave: thanks for your company, debates, being my smoking buddy until you quit, for picking good movies and being you.

Thanks to the Gatley and Sumner families: not only for being lifelong friends, but also for supporting my parents through my illness when they needed people to lean on. I didn't know about it at the time, but thank you. Special thanks to Josie and Jackie for helping mum, and the recently married Mr. and Mrs. Simon Gatley (Si and Clare) for their treasured friendship with me.

෴

Thank you to Stephen Fry for speaking out about bipolar disorder and making The Secret Life of the Manic Depression. (Known by fellow fans as TSLOTMD).

Paula (Radcliffe): You ran faster that me from the age of three. Then you ran faster than anyone in the world, so I feel less bad about losing. Bless ya honey. Love to your family.

Caroline: May you shine in other peoples' lives like you have done in mine – and continue to do so. I love you dearly.

Ash (Power): you can be my god any day Ash.

Julius (Julie Potter-Tate): you share my evil sense of humour – which I love. You have proved that anything can be overcome, and sons Tomas and Dan are tributes to you. Love and hugs always. (Down with Forrest. Up the Rams).

Clare (Baker): thank you, I love you, anything, anytime, don't you forget. What you have fought through is inspirational and awesome. You are in my heart forever.

Maggie (Findley): I love you; you are often in my thoughts.

Emma (Bell): Love to you and your two gorgeous boys Liam and Aaron Richardson. You are my family. Forever friends: forever singing embarrassingly awful late-1980's songs (along with dance routines).

Jill. Xx

Lisa, you are gone, but I still love you and I wish you hadn't done what you did. But it taught me one thing. The pain of losing someone you love to suicide is unbearable, and that has kept me alive for some years now. I miss you. I still have every letter, every email, every web-chat stored, and every text you ever sent, including the one that you sent in the middle of the night, warning me when I woke up that you would be dead. I'll be at peace with you some day.

Beth: I love you too my sweetest even though now you have to live with a boy! (Your husband and my brother-in-law Tom Richmond). How you have kept a level head with everything my illnesses threw at our family I will never know, but you did. You are sane! You are wonderful. You have understood that mental illnesses are not something people choose to have – most of society is far behind you on that point.

Mum (Sue) and dad (Paul): I love you forever. I know you have always been there for me, but I must give special thanks for your acceptance and understanding since the Oxford years. I am truly honoured that you have taken the time to really, REALLY understand what my illnesses mean, and am grateful for the unconditional support that is always there for me.

REFERENCES

There follows a list of the books I have found the most useful over the years, which will help you to understand in more depth about one or more of the particular topics. After the book list there is a list of the details of useful organisations, including websites, which provide useful facts and information, and who you might wish to contact in some way for advice and help. I highly recommend that you do.

Otherwise I refer you to the following journals, my favourites:

The British Medical Journal (BMJ): http://bmj.com

The British Journal of Psychiatry: http://bjp.rcpsych.org/

BNF 49, British National Formulary 49, March 2005. http://www.bnf.org/bnf/
(BNF 50, British National Formulary 50, September 2005).

The American Journal of Psychiatry (AJP): http://ajp.Psychiatryonline.org/

The International Journal of Eating disorders: http://www3.interscience.wiley.com/cgi-bin/jhome/34698

For information I also recommend the World Health organisation: http://www.who.int/en/

Dark Clouds Gather

To look up diagnostic criteria of Mental disorders, the world standard is the **DSM-IV** *Diagnostic and Statistical Manual of Mental disorders*, Fourth Edition, 1994 (American Psychiatric Association, 1400 K Street NW, Suite 1101, Washington, DC 20005-2403 USA). Type DSM-IV and the illness into the Internet and you will find anything you need.

SUGGESTED BOOKS/READING.

Depression.
Darkness Visible by William Styron.
The Bell Jar by Sylvia Plath.

Manic Depression:
An Unquiet Mind by Kay Redfield Jamison.
A Can of Madness by Jason Pegler
A Brilliant Madness - by Patty Duke and Gloria Hochman.
Finding the Still Point - by Gerald O'Mahony
Electro Boy by Andy Behrman
Inside Out - a guide to self-management of Manic Depression. Published by Manic Depression Fellowship (now the MDF Bipolar Organisation).

Eating disorders.
Wasted by Marya Hornbacher (Honest – my inspiration).
Anorexia nervosa and Bulimia: How to help by Marilyn Duker and Roger Slade.
Anorexia nervosa, a guide for family and friends, by R.L.Palmer. (Might seem elementary to longer-term sufferers).
Coping with Bulimia, by Barbara French.
Anorexics on Anorexia, edited by Rosemary Shelly.
Eating disorders and Obesity, A Comprehensive Handbook editors C.G. Fairburn and K.D. Brownell. (2002). Note that some of my research was taken from the earlier 1995 edition.

Self-Harm
Bloodletting: A True Story of Secrets, Self-Harm and Survival by Victoria Leatham

Suicide
Night Falls Fast by Kay Redfield Jamison.
No Time to Say Goodbye: Surviving the Suicide of a Loved One by Carla Fine
The Savage God: A study of Suicide by A. Alveraz.

Other books
Girl, Interrupted by Susanna Kaysen.

SUGGESTED ORGANISATIONS TO HELP.
(& websites where possible).

My website: http://www.katysaraculling.com

DEPRESSION AND MANIC DEPRESSION:

Depression Alliance is the leading UK charity for people affected by Depression, with a branch in England, Scotland, and Wales.
Depression Alliance (England).
212, Spitfire Studios
63 - 71 Collier Street
London
N1 9BE
Website: http://www.Depressionalliance.org
National number: 0845 123 23 20. All calls will be charged at the local rate.
Information about groups:
groups@Depressionalliance.org

Depression Alliance Cymru (Wales)
11, Plas Melin
Westbourne Road
Whitchurch
Cardiff
CF14 2BT
Email: wales@Depressionalliance.org

Depression Alliance Scotland
3, Grosvenor Gardens
Edinburgh

EH12 5JU
Fax: 0131 467 7701
Email: info@dascot.org
Website: www.Depressionalliancescotland.org

Equilibrium – The Bipolar Foundation.
Website: http://www.bipolar-foundation.org/
The sky is the limit. If you haven't already done so, join our Bipolar In-Touch Network
and receive our comprehensive and up-to-date newsletters:
http://www.bipolar-foundation.org/mod_product/register.aspx?o=1288
Equilibrium works with others to transform the understanding and treatment of bipolar disorder.
Registered office: 1 Rivercourt, 1 Trinity Street, OXFORD, UK, OX1 1TQ, UK
(Phone number coming soon).

Manic Depression Fellowship/Bipolar Organisation
UK based.
(Self-help groups across the country, also with Wales and Scotland bases).
Castle Works, 21 St. George's Road, London SE1 6ES.
Telephone 08456 340 540.
Fax 020 7793 2639.
E-mail: mdf@mdf.org.uk
Website: http://www.mdf.org.uk/index.php

BipolarAware: http://www.bipolaraware.co.uk/
Child and Young Adult Bipolar Foundation: http://www.bpkids.org/

EATING DISORDERS:
Something Fishy website.

Without doubt, the best pro-recovery international (available in 3 languages) eating disorder website is the **Something Fishy website**, started by a recovered Anorexic (Amy Medina) and her husband (Tony). At the time of writing this it has 26,225 members worldwide (of which I am one) plus many more visitors. I first visited the site when it started up in 1995, have been a member since, and I have witnessed a small website become the best. The sight ingeniously offers no-nonsense, honest information and support for all eating disorders, including those often overlooked, and includes help for issues that can be combined (in every conceivable combination) with eating disorders. Covered are mental illnesses, self-harm, alcohol and drug issues, sexuality, spirituality, holiday-time survival, family life, student life, living alone, men with eating disorders and abuse issues. For recovered people there is support to prevent relapse. Precautions are taken to prevent exchange of dangerous information. As well as a wealth of reliable information, there are chat rooms and message boards where you can meet people who share your particular problems, and make friends to help each other towards health and better understanding. Visit it.

Website: http://www.somethingfishy.org/

Eating disorders Association (EDA)
UK based charity.
Website: http://www.edauk.com/
Email: helpmail@edauk.com
Adult phone line (18+) 0845 6341414 (Mon-Fri 8.30am-8.30pm, Sat 1pm-4.30pm).

Under 18's 0845 634 7650 (Mon-Fri 4pm-6pm. Sat 1pm-4.30pm).

National Eating disorder Association   (USA based)
Information and Referral Program
603 Stewart Street, Suite 803
Seattle, WA 98101
1-800-931-2237
(206) 382-3587
(206) 829-8501 (fax)
Web: www.nationaleatingdisorders.org
Email: info@nationaleatingdisorders.org

ANRED Anorexia nervosa and Related Eating disorders Inc.
Website: http://www.anred.com/

SELF-HARM
Bristol Crisis Service for Women (UK based)
National voluntary organisation that supports women in emotional distress, particularly women who self-harm. With a national helpline, information and publications about self-injury, with talks and training courses to professionals and support self-help groups.
Bristol Crisis Service for Women,
PO Box 654,
Bristol BS99 1XH,
Office/Admin 0117 927 9600
Helpline 0117 925 1119
Email: bcsw@btconnect.com
Website:
http://www.users.zetnet.co.uk/BCSW/index.htm

SIARI Self-Injury & Related Issues
A free international Internet service of information, resources, and support
Website: http://www.siari.co.uk/

SUICIDE:

The Samaritans
Head office
10, The Grove
Slough, Berkshire, SL1 1QP
08457 909090 (24 hours a day, UK).
Website: www.samaritans.org (Search for your local Samaritans office).

Befrienders International (now maintained by the Samaritans). Suicide prevention worldwide, with 31,000 volunteers in over 40 countries).
Website: http://www.befrienders.org/index.htm

Oxford University's Centre for Suicide Research
Website: http://cebmh.warne.ox.ac.uk/csr/

American Association for Suicidology
4201 Connecticut Avenue, Suite 408
Washington, D.C. 20008
(202) 237.2280
(202) 237.2282 (Fax)
Email: Info@suicidology.org
Website: www.suicidology.org

SOS: Survivors of Suicide: *for relatives and friends* left behind after a loved one commits suicide.
Website: http://www.survivorsofsuicide.com/

Tony Salvetore's website for suicide prevention and to support those who lose a loved one to suicide; described as "A site for those who have experienced suicide loss and those who want to know more about suicide and its aftermath."
The   Suicide   Paradigm   Website: http://lifegard.tripod.com/

General Mental Health:
(General sites that might include depression, eating disorders, suicide, other mental health problems, details about hospital admission and other links).

Mind (National Association for Mental Health) UK based
0845 7660163
Website: http://www.mind.org.uk/

SANE (UK)
Saneline: 0845 767 8000
(Check website for phone line opening times, currently Mon-Fri 12 noon -11pm, Sat 12 noon-6pm).
Website: http://www.sane.org.uk/

NICE: National Institute of Clinical Excellence, National Health Service, (UK).
Website: http://www.nice.org.uk/

National Institute of Mental Health (USA)
Website: http://www.nimh.nih.gov/

***Hyper*Guide to the Mental Health Act:**

Information on "sectioning" (i.e. committal, involuntary admission, 'civil' admission, leave, discharge etc) to/from psychiatric hospital in the United Kingdom. Set up by Nigel Turner and "the longest running site on mental health law."
There are links to updates.
Website: http://www.hyperguide.co.uk/mha/

Alcoholics Anonymous (Global).
Website: http://www.aa.org/

Narcotics Anonymous (Global).
Website: http://www.na.org/

The IBS Network (UK based).
Website: http://www.ibsnetwork.org.uk/

Action for M.E. (UK based)
Website: http://www.afme.org.uk/

For mental and physical advice – e.g. following self-harm. (UK based only)
NHS Direct.
Phone (24 hours) 0845 4647
Website: www.nhsdirect.nhs.uk

General websites that have mental health sections:

The official Stephen Fry website – all of it's good, but there is a subsection called *The Secret Life of The Manic Depressive* (TSLOTMD) where mental health is discussed, with bipolar disorder the main theme, but everyone is welcomed.
http://www.stephenfry.com/forum/

Write to Anyone: http://writetoanyone.org/ Write about anything, anonymously or not, with replies or not, here mental health can be discussed openly, including suicide discussions, often banned elsewhere.

Printed in the United Kingdom
by Lightning Source UK Ltd.
133648UK00001B/1-9/P